THE COTA EXAMINATION REVIEW GUIDE,
2nd Edition

Caryn R. Johnson, MS, OTR/L, FAOTA
Academic Fieldwork Coordinator
Department of Occupational Therapy
Thomas Jefferson University
Philadelphia, Pennsylvania

Tina DeAngelis, MS, Ed D, OTR/L
Occupational Therapist
Crozer Chester Medical Center
Upland, Pennsylvania

and

Occupational Therapist
Bayada Nurses
Home Care Specialists
Philadelphia, Pennsylvania

Arlene Lorch, MS, OTR/L, CHES
Clinical Instructor
Department of Occupational Therapy
Thomas Jefferson University
Philadelphia, Pennsylvania

 F. A. DAVIS COMPANY • Philadelphia

F. A. Davis Company
1915 Arch Street
Philadelphia, PA 19103
www.fadavis.com

Printed in the United States of America

0-8036-0844-6

Last digit indicates print number: 14 13 12

Acquisitions Editor: Margaret Biblis
Developmental Editor: Colleen Ward
Cover Designer: Louis J. Forgione

As new scientific information becomes available through basic and clinical research, recommended treatments and drug therapies undergo changes. The author(s) and publisher have done everything possible to make this book accurate, up to date, and in accord with accepted standards at the time of publication. The author(s), editors, and publisher are not responsible for errors or omissions or for consequences from application of the book, and make no warranty, expressed or implied, in regard to the contents of the book. Any practice described in this book should be applied by the reader in accordance with professional standards of care used in regard to the unique circumstances that may apply in each situation. The reader is advised always to check product information (package inserts) for changes and new information regarding dose and contraindications before administering any drug. Caution is especially urged when using new or infrequently ordered drugs.

PREFACE

The purpose of this review guide is to give candidates for the National Board for Certification in Occupational Therapy (NBCOT) certification examination a general review of the profession and study tools to use while preparing to take the exam. It will also serve as an excellent review for occupational therapy assistants reentering the field or changing areas of practice.

This book's format encourages users to synthesize and apply knowledge and become comfortable with the format of the NBCOT exam. The questions in the certification exam are designed to require candidates to call upon their knowledge of occupational therapy practice and to *apply* that knowledge to realistic practice situations. The questions in this book are designed to evoke these same thought processes. The reader will find that basic knowledge combined with reasoning will lead to the best answer; the questions in this book do not test basic knowledge alone. While the majority of questions in *The COTA Exam Review Guide* have been written in a style that simulates the NBCOT exam, some have been written to maximize review of important content areas.

The textbooks referenced for most answers are those most commonly required for purchase by students in occupational therapy and occupational therapy assistant programs across the United States. In some cases, the authors cite less well-known references because they provide the best rationales. Candidates can access these books through their school's occupational therapy libraries or libraries of other occupational therapy programs. In addition, many of the books cited are available from the Wilma West Library at AOTA headquarters.

Please keep in mind that this workbook will *not*:

- be a comprehensive guide to practicing as an occupational therapy assistant,
- replicate the examination or any of the questions on the examination, or
- offer the student a guarantee of passing the examination.

This workbook *will*:

- provide a general review of occupational therapy practice,
- help readers identify the strengths and weaknesses in their knowledge of occupational therapy,
- acquaint the reader with the format of questions used on the examination,
- help the reader organize and set priorities for study time, and
- provide the reader with a reference list from which further study may be pursued.

THE AUTHORS

Caryn R. Johnson, MS, OTR/L, FAOTA, serves as Academic Fieldwork Coordinator for the Occupational Therapy Program at Thomas Jefferson University in Philadelphia, Pennsylvania, where she has taught since 1983. Caryn received her Bachelor's Degree in Occupational Therapy from Tufts University in 1978 and an advanced Master's Degree in Occupational Therapy from Thomas Jefferson University in 1991. In addition, she is president of Occupational Therapy Associates, a private practice specializing in aquatic rehabilitation. Caryn's special interests include developing fieldwork opportunities in nontraditional community settings and in the development of professional behaviors in OT and OTA students. In her free time, Caryn works with a wide variety of craft media.

Tina DeAngelis, MS, OTR/L, is a practicing occupational therapist with Bayada Nurses where she currently works in the area of home care. Tina also works as an occupational therapist at Crozer Chester Medical Center where she has been employed full and part time since 1991. She has experience in burn, orthopedic, and neurological conditions. In addition to this, Tina recently worked in the Department of Occupational Therapy at Thomas Jefferson University teaching selected courses and managing federally funded grant projects. Tina received her Associate's degree in Occupational Therapy from Harcum College in 1987, her Bachelor's degree in Occupational Therapy from College Misericordia in 1992, and her advanced Master's degree in Occupational Therapy from Thomas Jefferson University in 1997. She is currently enrolled in the doctoral program of Higher Education Leadership at Widener University in Chester, Pennsylvania, and is the mother of two school-aged girls.

Arlene Lorch, MS, OTR/L, CHES, received a Bachelor of Science degree in Occupational Therapy from the University of Pennsylvania and a Master of Science degree in Health Education from Arcadia University. She has been a practicing occupational therapist in acute care, rehabilitation, and long-term care settings for 25 years. Since 1996, Arlene has been a clinical instructor teaching occupational therapy courses and labs in evaluation, intervention, occupation, group dynamics and environmental adaptation in the Occupational Therapy Program at Thomas Jefferson University in Philadelphia, Pennsylvania. As a Certified Health Education Specialist, Arlene is interested in the development of health promotion, injury prevention and wellness programs, combining knowledge of occupational performance with health education approaches. Other special interests include quality of life issues in the older adult population, falls prevention, and the role of the environment in supporting occupation.

ACKNOWLEDGMENTS

The input and enthusiasm of many individuals has made this book possible. We especially want to thank Colleen Ward, Margaret Biblis, and Lynn Borders Caldwell for their guidance and support. We also want to thank Janice Burke for her support and tolerance over the course of the work. Our deepest thanks to friends and family, for tolerating us, present and absent, while we lost ourselves to this project for the past year.

CONTRIBUTORS

Each of the following individuals has called upon years of experience and a wealth of knowledge to develop well-researched and well-written questions. Their contribution to the COTA Examination Review Guide has been invaluable.

Deborah Dichter-Nightingale, OTR/L
Mental Health Consultants
Furlong, Pennsylvania

Brittany Duling, OTR/L
Pediatric Occupational Therapist
Thomas Jefferson University Hospital
Philadelphia, Pennsylvania

Florence Hannes, MS, OTR/L
Chair, Occupational Therapy Assistant Program
Orange County Community College
Middletown, New York

E. Adel Herge, MS OTR/L
Instructor
Department of Occupational Therapy
Thomas Jefferson University
Philadelphia, Pennsylvania

Diane M. Hill, COTA/L, AP
Longwood at Oakmont
Pittsburgh, Pennsylvania

Catherine Verrier Piersol, MS, OTR/L
Academic Fieldwork Coordinator
Department of Occupational Therapy
Philadelphia University
Philadelphia, Pennsylvania

Kerstin Potter, MA, OTR/L
Associate Professor & Program Director
Occupational Therapy Assistant Program
Harcum College
Bryn Mawr, Pennsylvania

Pamela E. Toto, MS, OTR/L, BCG
Independent Home Health Contractor
Pittsburgh, PA

Debra Tupé, MS, OTR/L
Instructor
Thomas Jefferson University
Philadelphia, Pennsylvania

Jeffrey Weest, COTA
Staff Occupational Therapy Assistant
Thomas Jefferson University Hospital
Philadelphia, Pennsylvania

REVIEWERS

Finally, we would like to recognize the efforts of those educators and practitioners from across the country who painstakingly reviewed, critiqued, and validated every question to ensure accuracy and appropriateness.

Roselyn V. Armstrong, MA, OTR/L
Chair, Department of Occupation
Pitt Community College
Greenville, North Carolina

Deena Baenen, MA, BA, AAS, LSW, COTA/L
Preceptor
Department of Occupational Assistant Technology
Cuyahoga Community College
Cleveland, Ohio

Michelle Ann Barr, COTA/L
Thomas Jefferson University
Philadelphia, Pennsylvania

Kay Blose, MOT, OTR/L
Assistant Professor
Occupational Therapy Health Science Program
Mountain State University
Beckley, West Virginia

Liane Hewitt, MPH and OTR
Assistant Professor and Department Chair
Department of Occupational Therapy
Loma Linda University
Loma Linda, California

December E. Hughes, COTA/L
Thomas Jefferson University
Philadelphia, Pennsylvania

Rebecca G. Robler, MEd, OTR
Instructor
Occupational Assistant Program
Pueblo Community College
Pueblo, Colorado

Melinda Deen Sissel, BIS, COTA/L
Instructor
Department of Occupational Therapy
Shawnee State University
Portsmouth, Ohio

CONTENTS

CONTENTS

PREPARING FOR THE EXAMINATION

WHAT IS THE NBCOT EXAMINATION?

Successful completion of the certification examination is required for anyone who wants to practice as an occupational therapy assistant. Passing the NBCOT examination is the culmination of academic and field-work study. The examination tests your depth of knowledge and ability to apply that knowledge to practice. The questions require you to apply knowledge of occupational therapy or synthesize bits of knowledge to select the correct answer. The purpose of the examination is to identify those candidates who demonstrate entry-level competence for practicing as an occupational therapy assistant. Once candidates have successfully completed the examination, they are certified as occupational therapy assistants. The examination is offered at designated times throughout the year. The computerized examinations are given for both certified occupational therapy assistant (COTA) and registered occupational therapist (OTR) candidates. Both the NBCOT exams and practice exams are offered at hundreds of centers around the country. Only those registered for the NBCOT exam are eligible to take practice exams. More information on the exams and practice exams is available at www.nbcot.org.

WHO CAN TAKE THE NBCOT EXAMINATION?

The NBCOT oversees the certification examination and eligibility of candidates. Candidates must be graduates of an accredited occupational therapy assistant education program, and have successfully completed the required fieldwork. Candidates are required to submit either an official transcript or the NBCOT Academic Credential Verification Form from their occupational therapy programs. Many states require students to sit for the first examination offered once they have become eligible; however, this is no longer an NBCOT requirement.

In cases where graduation is not scheduled until after the examination date, students must be cleared for graduation (both academically and financially) by the institution's registrar. If complete official transcripts cannot be submitted, the student must have the "NBCOT Academic Credential Verification Form" completed by the registrar and submitted to the NBCOT. Deadlines are strictly enforced. An official transcript must be submitted *no later* than 90 days after the date of the examination. Failure to do so may result in loss of certification.

Individuals who are not recent graduates (within one year) of an accredited U.S. program, and international candidates seeking to take the examination, must contact the NBCOT for additional information.

ABOUT THE NBCOT CANDIDATE HANDBOOK

The NBCOT Candidate Handbook contains the application for the examination. Detailed and critical information is included in the NBCOT Candidate Handbook, which the candidate should read from cover to cover before completing the application form. The handbook is available online at www.nbcot.org. Students may also request a hard copy of the Candidate Handbook by writing to the NBCOT at: NBCOT Candidate Handbook, PO Box 70, Waldorf, MD 20604-0070. You must include a self-addressed, pressure-sensitive label with your request. Candidates may also contact the NBCOT by phone at (301) 990-7979.

The handbook includes an application for the examination, eligibility requirements, deadlines, and information about test administration and scoring. Read this handbook thoroughly and save it until after you have received your test scores.

HOW TO APPLY FOR THE EXAMINATION

Applications to take the examination are actually submitted to the Professional Examination Service (PES), not the NBCOT, and may be submitted online or by mail. Applying online significantly reduces the possibility of submitting an incomplete application and is strongly encouraged. Candidates should contact PES for questions concerning the online application. The most current address and phone information for PES is available in the current Candidate Handbook. The fee for taking the examination (at the time of this writing) is approximately $395. There is an additional charge to have reports of scores sent to state regulatory agencies and for each notice of Confirmation of Eligibility requested. These items are frequently required in order to obtain a license to practice.

The Candidate Handbook and application forms are usually available online about 3 to 4 months prior to the examination date. The application deadline is usually about two months before the examination date. There is not a late registration deadline and deadlines are strictly enforced. Candidates can check the status of their applications online. Candidates who mail their applications to PES may include a self-addressed postcard, which PES will return to the candidate as confirmation that the application was received. The postcard confirms receipt of the student's application, but does not provide information regarding the status, such as whether the application is complete. Candidates may wish to send the application by certified mail and to receive a "return receipt" from the United States Post Office. Candidates requiring special accommodations are required to submit a request by the designated deadline.

WHAT IS THE FORMAT OF THE EXAMINATION?

The certification examination is composed of 200 multiple-choice questions that use the four-option format. No combination or "K" questions are used. Questions are designed as brief practice scenarios, and require you to decide what you should *do* based on your application of occupational therapy *knowledge*. You have 4 hours to complete the examination. Each item has the same weight in scoring, and every question on the examination has only one correct answer. There is not a penalty for guessing, so you should *never* leave a question unanswered. In fact, the computerized format allows you to "flag" questions you have difficulty answering, so that you can easily locate these questions later.

WHAT DOES THE EXAMINATION COVER?

The examination covers the following seven categories (additional information is available at www.NBCOT.org):

1. Evaluation

This portion comprises approximately 16% of the exam, or about 32 questions. These questions apply to tasks related to your ability to evaluate the individual, analyze the data, and identify problem areas. You must be familiar with multiple methods for collecting data, such as observation, chart review, screening, interviewing, and standardized and non-standardized assessments (although few will actually be identified by name). You will also need to understand how to prioritize strengths and weaknesses and document results. The scope of COTA involvement and ways in which the COTA and OTR collaborate in the evaluation process are important to know as well. This category corresponds to NBCOT's "Domain A."

When studying for this category, be sure to review a variety of methods for evaluating sensation, motor performance, cognition (especially Allen's Cognitive Levels), psychosocial performance, and development (both standardized and non-standardized). Familiarize yourself with the proper techniques for administering evaluations. Be certain to review normal and abnormal human development and pathological conditions. You should also review the effects and side effects of medications, and the basic sciences, including anatomy, kinesiology, psychology, and neuroscience. Finally, review features of the OT process and role delineation.

2. Treatment Planning

This portion comprises approximately 15% of the exam, or about 30 questions. These questions will test your ability to plan interventions based on evaluation results and theory. It will address tasks such as collaborating with the individual, caregivers, OTR, and team members, and selecting the *most appropriate* frame of reference and setting goals. It will test your ability to adapt or modify tasks or the environment, and to select and/or design occupation-based interventions that establish or restore function or prevent negative outcomes. You will also need to know how to select the *most appropriate* intervention, perform activity analysis, and select appropriate environments and contexts for treatment. Finally, this portion will test your ability to document treatment/intervention plans and write goals. This category corresponds to NBCOT's "Domain B."

Questions in this category will require you to design treatment for individuals of all ages who have a wide range of abilities and disabilities; therefore, familiarity with human development, pathology, and the basic sciences is important. Good clinical reasoning skills and knowledge of the basic tenets of occupational therapy will be critical for success in this section. You will need to be able to select and document the *best* theory-based treatment plan and project the outcomes. Knowledge of a wide range of therapeutic media, purposeful activities, and relevant precautions and contraindications will be essential.

3. Treatment Implementation

This portion comprises approximately 45% of the exam, or about 90 questions—more than any other category. These questions apply to tasks related to providing occupation-based interventions for individuals and/or their caregivers once the treatment plan has been developed. You will need to show you know when, where, and how to provide treatment, while applying good therapeutic use of self, and effective communication skills. You will need to recognize when and how to grade and adapt activities and environments, and be able to select, construct, and provide the *most appropriate* devices, including adaptive equipment, splints, and technology. These questions will also test you on your ability to instruct individuals and others on subjects such as joint protection, time management, and care of assistive devices. There will also be questions related to documenting intervention. This category corresponds to NBCOT's "Domain C."

Review for this category will also require familiarity with the basic sciences, pathology, and human development. You will need to be familiar with a wide range of therapeutic media, adaptive equipment, splints and splinting methods, and some physical agent modalities and technology. You will also need to understand group theories, how groups develop and function, and how to lead groups. The emphasis in this portion is on how you can *most effectively* implement occupation-based treatment, your therapeutic use of self, how to respond to various behaviors, and your ability to assess the individual's response to the intervention and react as needed.

4. Effectiveness of Treatment and Discharge Planning

This category comprises approximately 12% of the exam, or about 24 questions. These questions apply to tasks associated with monitoring and modifying the treatment plan and discharge planning. Questions in this category will address the task of evaluating and re-evaluating continuously to determine if goals and treatment methods are appropriate and realistic, and revising the treatment plan when necessary. This category also deals with discharge planning and its associated tasks, such as identifying the need for, and selecting the *most appropriate* follow-up services, recommending equipment for home use, and developing and instructing the individual and others in home programs. This area will also cover discharge documentation and timely and appropriate termination of services. This category corresponds to NBCOT's "Domain D."

Study for this portion of the examination is similar to the three categories previously identified. In addition, you should be familiar with service delivery models available to individuals after discharge, such as home health, outpatient services, and other community resources.

5. Occupational Therapy for Populations

This category comprises approximately 5% of the exam, or about 10 questions. These questions apply to provision of occupational therapy to groups of people rather than individuals—often under-served, at-risk, or well populations—through preventive, supportive, or remediative services in select settings. Examples of such settings include adult day programs, schools, homeless shelters, and work environments. Questions in this category address tasks such as assessing the needs of the organization or population, recommending and implementing interventions, measuring outcomes, and consulting. This category corresponds to NBCOT's "Domain E."

Study for this portion is similar to the first three categories previously identified. In addition, you should be familiar with community service delivery models, consultation skills, and the characteristics and needs of under-served, at-risk, and well populations.

6. Service Management

This category comprises approximately 5% of the exam, or about 10 questions. Questions in this section apply to tasks relating to management and service delivery, such as developing, coordinating, and promoting occupational therapy services; program evaluation; and supervision of staff and students. This category corresponds to NBCOT's "Domain F."

Study for this portion will involve basic principles of supervision, program evaluation, and risk management. Review of AOTA documents such as the *Standards of Practice and Occupational Therapy Roles*, and documents related to supervision of OT and non-OT personnel is recommended. You also need to know methods for evaluating services, such as quality assurance and utilization review. Finally, it is important to understand how provision of OT services varies from one setting or service delivery model to another.

7. Professional Practice

This category comprises approximately 2% of the exam, or about 4 questions. Questions in this section apply to tasks relating to practicing competently, legally, ethically, and professionally. You may be asked about promoting occupational therapy to the public, applying and engaging in research, presenting and publishing, and fieldwork education. This category corresponds to NBCOT's "Domain G."

Study for this category will require familiarity with AOTA documents such as the *OT Code of Ethics and Standards of Practice*. You should also review concepts related to licensure, methods for maintaining competency, laws that affect the practice of OT, and role delineation between OTRs and COTAs. Because the exam is designed for a national audience, no state-specific information is included.

THE DAY OF THE EXAMINATION

At the time of this writing, little information is available about the computer-delivered examination. However, the following checklist should help you on the day of the examination:

[ ] Double check the date and time.

[ ] Know where you are going, how to get there, and where you will be able to park.

[ ] Bring your admission ticket.

[ ] Bring two forms of identification, including one photo ID with signature.

[ ] Bring a watch to help you stay on schedule during the 4-hour test. A clock option is available on each computer, but some find it distracting and prefer to turn it off.

Food and drinks, dictionaries, cell phones, and many other items are not permitted. Special permission is even required for bottled water.

WHAT HAPPENS AFTER THE EXAMINATION?

Test results are mailed approximately 4 weeks after the certification examination. Of the U.S. graduates taking the test for the first time in October 2001, about 84% passed. A score of 450 or higher is required to pass the certification examination. A grievance process is outlined in the NBCOT Candidate Handbook. If you experience difficulty with the testing conditions, or have any other complaints about your experience taking the examination, you must report it *immediately* to NBCOT.

Candidates can request that results be sent to the licensing agency of the state(s) in which they plan to practice. There is a fee for each report you request—no reports are sent free of charge. Almost all states require a copy of the report. It is recommended that the candidate complete an application for state licensure before taking the examination. Often, these applications require a notarized copy of transcripts from an accredited occupational therapy program, letters of reference, a picture identification, and so forth. Depending on the state licensure laws and facility requirements, COTAs may or may not be able to work with a temporary permit until examination results are received. Candidates should contact the licensing agency as soon as they know the state in which they plan to practice. Candidates should learn as early as possible what information will be necessary for licensure and when applications should be submitted.

Candidates who fail the examination must retake the entire examination. There is no limit on the number of times an individual may take the examination.

HOW TO USE THIS WORKBOOK

This workbook has five complete 200-question sample tests that simulate the actual examination by asking questions in a four-option, multiple-choice format. Questions in the first three tests are organized to allow you to assess your performance in each of the seven categories. Questions in the fourth test are grouped by population, allowing you to assess your competence with various age groups and diagnostic categories. The sequence of questions in the fifth test is randomized, simulating the format of the NBCOT examination. This format can be more difficult because the topic and item areas change frequently. The final examination enables you to evaluate how well you have retained and been able to implement the techniques recommended in this workbook. The mix of questions in each test covers the range of entry-level occupational therapy practice, thus providing a general review of the profession.

A complete set of answers follows each examination. In order to help the test taker, the workbook provides a complete rationale for each answer, which explains both correct and incorrect answers. Hence, each question-answer unit is actually a mini-lesson on not one, but four concepts. In addition, each answer provides the test taker with a reference from which further information may be obtained on the subject matter. A complete reference list is located at the end of the workbook.

The section on test-taking tips will help you to identify your strengths and weaknesses and organize and set priorities for study time. A guide for developing a study plan is provided at the end of this section.

WHERE DO I BEGIN?

Viewed as one task, preparing to take the examination can seem overwhelming. Breaking the process into smaller parts makes it more manageable. The personal study plan chart following this section can help you with the first step, identifying your areas of strength and weakness. Once you have completed this step, the second step is to complete your study plan. The final step is to pull all of the information together and take the practice examinations. It may be helpful to review the test-taking tips occasionally.

TEST-TAKING TIPS

Test-Taking Tip 1

Visit the NBCOT web site periodically. You can access the Candidate Handbook and other vital information about the examination at the NBCOT web site (**www.NBCOT.org**). It is essential that you read the Candidate Handbook thoroughly and more than once – you will pick up something new each time you read it. This web site has the most current information regarding test dates and locations and is updated frequently. This site also has details about how the examination was developed and how it is scored.

Test-Taking Tip 2

Using this book to create a personal study plan. The question most frequently asked by students preparing for the examination is, "How do I start?" This guide will help you put all your educational preparation together and organize your study time. It will also make you comfortable with multiple-choice questions. All students preparing for the examination should have their coursework at their fingertips, including books, notes, handouts, etc. Once you have assembled the stacks of information you have accumulated over the years, the question arises, "Where do I start?"

One way to use this workbook is to develop a study plan based on your performance on the simulation examinations. Start by taking simulation Examination 1 and record how many correct answers you score in each category compared to the number of questions that will be on the certification examination in this category.

This will give you some idea of the categories for which you need more concentrated review and study. The next step is to define your strengths and weaknesses. To do this, choose a category and then go through all the component parts of that category as well as the background knowledge areas suggested for review. Classify the areas in which you are weakest as "D," and those in which you are strongest as "A." Assign "B" or "C," with "B" being stronger than "C," to the remaining practice areas. Within each letter grouping, identify the weakest subject with the number 4, and sequentially number through to the strongest subject—the higher the number, the higher your study priority. Once this has been completed, your individualized studying needs have been organized and priorities set for accomplishment.

After completing simulation Examinations 2 and 3, record the numbers of your correct answers for each category. This will further indicate areas for which you still need review.

Now that you have set your priorities for studying, set target dates for completing your review of each area or subject. For instance, you may choose to work on category #1 (evaluation) during the month of January. Another individual may choose to review evaluation the first week of January, treatment planning (category #2) the second week of January, and so forth. Design your study plan to meet your needs. Set target dates that are realistic and attainable.

When the planning is complete, it is time for the study to begin. Start with the area listed as "D4" (high priority for review) and work your way through to the last "D." Once this is finished, continue with the "C," "B," and "A" items. When you have reviewed all areas, you may choose to begin again at D4, or to reset priorities for your studying needs. The easiest part of this task will be defining the time frame in which to study specific topics. The toughest challenge will be implementing the examination review plan!

Table 1. STUDY PLAN OF CATEGORIES FOR CERTIFICATION EXAMINATION #1 - EVALUATION

Percentage of items on certification examination - 16% Number of questions in each simulation examination - 32	Self-Rating
Questions in this category test the ability to apply knowledge to the following kinds of tasks:	
• Identification of the role of the COTA within the occupational therapy evaluation process as performed under the supervision of, and in cooperation with, the occupational therapist • Methods for reviewing and using preliminary data from persons, records, and charts • Performance of skilled clinical observations of persons and environments • Interview styles and formats used to gain information, and related communication skills • Knowledge of the screening process, including selection, administration, scoring, and analysis of results • Standardized and non-standardized assessment selection, administration, and analysis of results • General evaluation procedures for sensory, motor, cognitive and psychosocial performance components • Assessment tools and methods for performance areas, including ADL, work and productive activities, play, and leisure • Assessment of developmental status • Interpretation of assessment findings to determine and prioritize needs for OT services • Development of documentation and reports based on assessment findings	
Background knowledge to review for the evaluation category:	
• Basic science knowledge underlying performance; anatomy, kinesiology, psychology, neuroscience • Normal and abnormal human development • Progression of skill development in performance areas of ADL, work and productive activities, play, and leisure • Pathological conditions and resulting sensorimotor, cognitive, and psychosocial impairments • Impact of disability and injury in terms of the individual's roles and occupational performance • Impact of disability and injury on the individual's caregivers, family, and sociocultural environment • Influence of the context, such as physical and social environments, and temporal factors on human performance • Effects and side effects of medications **Your score on practice exam 1 _____/32___** **Your score on practice exam 2 _____/32___** **Your score on practice exam 3 _____/32___**	

#2 - TREATMENT PLANNING

Percentage of questions from this category - 15% Number of questions in each examination - 30	Self-Rating
Questions in this category test the ability to apply knowledge to the following kinds of tasks:	
• Identification of the role and tasks of the COTA within the treatment planning process • Using principles of clinical reasoning • Utilizing collaborative skills with individuals, caregivers, and team members in the treatment planning process • Demonstration of familiarity with theories, models of practice, and selection of appropriate frames of reference and treatment approaches to address needs identified in evaluation • Development and documentation of measurable goals based on evaluation findings • Development and documentation of treatment plans reflecting intervention priorities • Selection of intervention methods and strategies from a wide range of restorative, compensatory, adaptive, preventive, and education-based treatment options • Identification of relevant precautions and intervention contraindications • Recommendations for frequency, amount, and duration of treatment • Analysis of individual potential based on clinical judgment	
Background knowledge to review for the treatment planning category	
• Basic science knowledge underlying performance; anatomy, kinesiology, psychology, neuroscience • Normal and abnormal human development • Progression of skill development in performance areas of ADL, work and productive activities, play, and leisure • Pathological conditions and resulting sensorimotor, cognitive, and psychosocial impairments • Impact of disability and injury in terms of the individual's roles and occupational performance • Impact of disability and injury on the individual's caregivers, family, and sociocultural environment • Influence of the context, such as physical and social environments, and temporal factors on human performance • Effects and side effects of medications	
Specific areas to review:	
• Elements of a treatment plan, including construction of long- and short-term goals • Models of practice, theories and frames of reference underlying intervention for sensorimotor, cognitive, and psychosocial performance components and for performance areas • Rationales for theory and intervention selection • Process of activity analysis and activity grading relative to performance areas, components, and contexts. • Adaptation possibilities for tasks, objects, and environmental factors affecting performance **Your score on practice exam 1** _____ **/30** **Your score on practice exam 2** _____ **/30** **Your score on practice exam 3** _____ **/30**	

#3 - TREATMENT IMPLEMENTATION

Percentage of questions from this category - 45% Number of questions in each examination - 90	Self-Rating
Questions in this category test the ability to apply knowledge to the following kinds of tasks:	
• Communication and collaborative skills used in presenting treatment plans to individuals, family, team members, and others • Selection and implementation of activities, modalities, and media to achieve therapeutic goals • Adaptation and grading of activities • Selection and implementation of compensatory and adaptive methods to achieve therapeutic goals • Implementation of interventions to prevent or limit further impairment, disability, or dysfunction • Training, teaching, and instructional methods for use with adults and children of varying developmental and cognitive abilities • Revision of intervention based on continued monitoring of progress toward goal achievement	
Specific areas to review (in addition to background knowledge also noted for categories #1 and 2 above)	

• Interventions typically used with specific pathological conditions
• Therapeutic use of self and motivational strategies to maximize treatment effectiveness
• Interventions to address occupational performance deficits in ADL, work and productive activities, and play and leisure
• Principles and application of compensatory strategies, including the use of assistive technologies, assistive and adaptive devices, environmental modification, and assistance from others
• Training, teaching, and instructional methods for use with adults and children of varying developmental and cognitive abilities, and for caregivers and supervised personnel
• Specific approaches and techniques to address sensorimotor performance deficits, including:
 	
    use of physical agent modalities
    splinting, orthotics, and prosthetics
    therapeutic exercise program and manual techniques
    sensory re-education and sensory processing techniques
    motor learning, neurodevelopmental frames of reference, and positioning strategies
    wheelchair selection and management
    adaptive device selection, adaptation, and training
    occupation-based activities
    environment-based interventions
 	
• Specific approaches to address cognitive performance deficits, including:
 	
    cognitive rehabilitation techniques, such as dynamic interactional and functional approaches
    training techniques and methods of assisting and cueing
    compensatory methods used in dementia such as task-breakdown
    Allen's cognitive disabilities
    perceptual rehabilitation techniques
 	
• Specific approaches to address psychosocial performance deficits, including strategies for dealing with behavioral issues of specific psychiatric conditions, organic brain disorders, and substance abuse in children, adolescents, and adults, including:
 	
    therapeutic use of self and individual treatment approaches
    group leadership skills and intervention techniques based on application of group process	

interventions, which address living skills, coping skills and stress management, pre-vocational exploration, and work readiness

- Knowledge of intervention possibilities in various settings and service delivery models and resources in the community and elsewhere that can support occupational performance
- Incorporation of relevant precautions and contraindications into treatment considerations
- Clinical problem solving related to individual client/patient response to intervention and reassessment
- Recording of treatment process and documentation of progress
- Selection and implementation of methods to monitor outcome effectiveness of intervention

Your score on practice exam 1 _____ /90
Your score on practice exam 2 _____ /90
Your score on practice exam 3 _____ /90

#4 - EFFECTIVENESS OF TREATMENT AND DISCHARGE PLANNING

	Self-Rating
Percentage of questions from this category - 12% Number of questions in each examination - 24	
Questions in this category test the ability to apply knowledge to the following kinds of tasks:	
• Methods of reevaluation for monitoring treatment plan effectiveness and progress made by the individual • Revision of goals and modification of treatment plans on the basis of individual response to intervention • Planning for timely service termination • Initiating and completing the discharge planning process in collaboration with the individual • Prioritizing needs and making recommendations and referrals for follow-up services • Developing home programs and recommendations for strategies to maximize performance in expected discharge environment • Providing discharge related information and instruction to individuals, caregivers, team members, and other professionals • Selecting and recommending adaptive devices, equipment, and modifications • Documenting the OT services provided, and writing discharge summaries and reports	
Background knowledge to review for the effectiveness of treatment and discharge planning category is similar to that of categories #1, #2, and #3	
• Basic science knowledge underlying performance; anatomy, kinesiology, psychology, neuroscience • Normal and abnormal human development • Progression of skill development in performance areas of ADL, work and productive activities, play, and leisure • Pathological conditions and resulting sensorimotor, cognitive, and psychosocial impairments • Impact of disability and injury in terms of the individual's roles and occupational performance • Impact of disability and injury on the individual's caregivers, family, and sociocultural environment • Influence of the context, such as physical and social environments, and temporal factors on human performance • Effects and side effects of medications	
Specific areas to review:	
• Service delivery models available to individuals following discharge, such as home health, outpatient services, and community resources	

	Self-Rating
• Factors that indicate the need for further services for children and adults in a variety of practice settings and performance contexts **Your score on practice exam 1** _____ /24 **Your score on practice exam 2** _____ /24 **Your score on practice exam 3** _____ /24	

#5 - OCCUPATIONAL THERAPY FOR POPULATIONS

	Self-Rating
Percentage of questions from this category - 5% Number of questions in each examination - 10	
Questions in this category test the ability to apply knowledge to the following kinds of tasks:	
• Identification and assessment of populations at risk for occupational performance deficits • Identification and assessment of under-served populations • Identification and assessment of well populations who may benefit from occupation-based services • Development of intervention recommendations for preventive, supportive, or remediative services • Implementation of programming for populations • Providing information, education, and training to others to implement population-based programs	
Background knowledge to review for the effectiveness of treatment and discharge planning category is similar to that of categories #1, #2, #3, and #4	
Specific areas to review:	

• The significance of occupation in maintaining health and well-being
• The role of occupation as intervention for chronic health problems and in prevention of disability
• Adaptation of tasks, objects, and environments to enhance occupational performance and safety for groups
• Injury prevention methods and wellness strategies to promote health
• Strategies to support occupational performance at developmental stages throughout the life span
• Service delivery models benefiting from population-based programs, including:
 	
    community settings, such as senior centers and homeless shelters
    early intervention settings, schools, and other training or educational programs
    elderly care environments, such as adult day programs and assisted living centers
    work and industrial environments
    wellness settings	

• The role of the consultant and consultation skills • Methods of monitoring effectiveness of population-based interventions and programs **Your score on practice exam 1** _____ /10 **Your score on practice exam 2** _____ /10 **Your score on practice exam 3** _____ /10	

#6 - SERVICE MANAGEMENT

	Self-Rating
Percentage of questions from this category - 5% Number of questions in each examination - 10	
Questions in this category test the ability to apply knowledge to the following kinds of tasks:	
• Coordination of occupational therapy services	

• Management and coordination of resources and personnel • Promotion and marketing of occupational therapy services • Supervision of staff and students • Maintaining professional development and competence of staff • Identifying safety issues and implementing policies and procedures to minimize risk • Evaluation of service effectiveness, outcomes, and quality, using program evaluation methods	
Specific areas to review:	
• Provision of services in diverse systems and delivery models, and how services vary in different settings • Standards of practice • Roles and expectations of various occupational therapy personnel • Principles of leadership, marketing, financial management, and budgeting • Principles and standards of supervision and interpersonal management skills • Methods of service assessment and improvement, such as quality assurance, outcomes monitoring, and utilization review **Your score on practice exam 1** _____ /10 **Your score on practice exam 2** _____ /10 **Your score on practice exam 3** _____ /10	

#7 - PROFESSIONAL PRACTICE

	Self-Rating
Percentage of questions from this category - 2% Number of questions in each examination - 4	
Questions in this category test the ability to apply knowledge to the following kinds of tasks:	
• Compliance with lawful regulations that govern the practice of occupational therapy • Adhering to ethical codes and applying ethical principles to the practice of occupational therapy • Engaging in presentations and publications that add to the professional knowledge base • Engaging in research activities and applying knowledge gained from research to practice • Contributing to the education of occupational therapy practitioners, students, and others • Promotion and advancement of occupational therapy to the public • Maintaining professional competence through professional development activities	
Specific areas to review:	
• Standards of Practice • OT Code of Ethics • Roles, responsibilities, and scope of practice of OTRs and COTAs • The process of accreditation and certification • National requirements for credentialing and governing occupational therapy practice • National laws and policies that impact the practice of the profession • Basic elements in the design and implementation of research studies • Procedures of data collection for use in outcome and other evaluative studies • Methods for maintaining competence **Your score on practice exam 1** _____ /4 **Your score on practice exam 2** _____ /4 **Your score on practice exam 3** _____ /4	

Test-Taking Tip 3

Be prepared. The more prepared you are to take the examination, the more comfortable you will feel during the examination. Preparation includes studying the knowledge base of occupational therapy, getting a good night's sleep, and coming prepared to the examination. Although the examination is computerized, candidates do not need to have advanced computer skills. When studying is complete, most of the preparation is complete. However, when asked to identify the single most important part of preparing for the examination, a graduating class of students agreed that the answer is getting a good night's sleep. Plan to arrive at the test site 20 to 30 minutes before the examination. Arriving early will give you time to register and acclimate yourself to the environment.

Test-Taking Tip 4

Prepare your body as well as your mind! Eating a well-balanced breakfast can actually help your performance on the examination. A breakfast high in carbohydrates and low in fat will increase your energy and will not produce a sluggish feeling. Avoid caffeine the day of the examination because caffeine will ultimately make you tired and drowsy. Finally, wear comfortable clothing in layers to allow you to adjust as necessary to the temperature of the room.

Test-Taking Tip 5

Pace yourself. The test is to be completed within 4 hours. Within this time frame, you have to answer 200 multiple-choice questions. Begin by familiarizing yourself with the computer test program. One technique for pacing the examination is to divide the test into four equivalent 50 question sections. You should aim to complete each of the four sections within 50 minutes to 1 hour. Understanding the format of the test and budgeting your time will help you work through the questions more efficiently, and enable you to complete the examination in the time allotted. Another pacing technique is to use a watch or the clock provided by the computer test program, and at the end of every 15 to 20 questions, briefly glance at the time to maintain a sense of your pace. If you have completed all the questions and have time left, go back to see if you can answer any of the questions you "flagged." If questions still remain incomplete within the last 10 minutes of the examination, select one letter and fill in all of the remaining questions with that letter. *Remember, there is no penalty for guessing—only for leaving questions unanswered!* Another method is to wear a watch that can be set to signal on the hour. When the examination begins, set the watch for 12:00. Between 12:00 and 4:00, the watch will signal each hour; therefore, you can check your pace without having to "watch the clock." The goal is to complete at least 25% of the examination, or 50 questions per hour. Avoid wasting time by looking frequently at your watch. If you find the computer test program clock too distracting, you have the option of turning it off.

Test-Taking Tip 6

When you use the same letter for more than three answers in a row, double check the questions to verify each answer. Test writers usually break up strings of four or more of the same letter or answer. The multiple-choice format is generally set so that three consecutive answers of the same letter is the maximum. If you have selected four or more of the same letters consecutively, it may be beneficial to recheck the answers. *Save this task for the end of the examination!*

Test-Taking Tip 7

Use key techniques to help select the correct answer.
1. ***Follow your instincts when answering questions.*** The first answer chosen is usually the correct one. Change an answer only if you later realize your first answer was definitely not correct.
2. ***Ask, "What is this question about?"*** Try to decipher what the question is testing by selecting the key terms in the questions, trying not to become distracted by peripheral information. By identifying what the question is testing, you may be more likely to select the correct answer.
3. ***Anticipate the answer.*** Many times you may anticipate an answer while reading a question. If so, look for the anticipated answer among the options. However, it is important to read and consider all of the options to verify that the anticipated answer is the correct answer.
4. ***Use logical reasoning.*** A commonly used technique is the process of deduction-eliminating answers that are incorrect. Doing this allows you to concentrate on the options that remain.

As you complete the questions on the examination, remember these techniques and practice using them when you have difficulty answering a question.

Test-Taking Tip 8

There are no trick questions. Questions are designed to test entry-level, not advanced, knowledge and reasoning. Be careful not to read too much into the questions. However, most questions will have two answers that appear to be correct. Many questions will ask for the "first" action the therapist should take, or the "best" or "most appropriate" choice. Make sure to note the qualifiers to help you determine the best answer.

Test-Taking Tip 9

Use the computer test program to your advantage. The computer test program allows you to "flag" a question so that you can go back to it later. It also allows you identify unanswered questions and to change answers right up to the time you finally submit the test.

SIMULATION EXAMINATION 1

Directions: Circle the correct answer to the following questions. When you have completed this examination, check your answers against the answer key that follows. As you will see, an explanation is given for each answer along with a reference for further study. The book author is listed as well as the chapter author. See the bibliography for complete references. Study the areas in which your comprehension was low, then test yourself again by taking Simulation Examination 2.

Evaluation

1. **In assessing the dressing skills of a 5-year-old child, the COTA observes that the child is able to put on a jacket, zip the zipper, and tie a knot in the draw string, but needs verbal cueing to tie a bow. The COTA would MOST likely determine that the child's dressing skills are:**
   A. age appropriate.
   B. delayed.
   C. advanced.
   D. limited.

2. **In administering an assessment of fingertip pinch strength, the OT practitioner would instruct the individual being tested to place his or her fingers in which position?**
   A. Thumb against the tip of the index finger
   B. Thumb against the side of the index finger
   C. Thumb against the tips of the index and middle fingers
   D. Thumb against the tips of all the fingers at once

3. **The OT treatment approach that will MOST likely meet the overall needs experienced by individuals with substance abuse problems is to:**
   A. assist with skill development in the areas of leisure, self-expression, and ADLs.
   B. educate the family members about making safety modifications to the kitchen area.
   C. encourage Alcoholics Anonymous involvement, address personal appearance, and issues of loss.

   D. make aftercare arrangements for vocational counseling and AA; provide time management education for self-care activities.

4. **A COTA observes that a 10-month-old child is able to sit alone by propping himself forward on his arms, but consistently loses his balance when reaching for a toy. This behavior MOST likely indicates:**
   A. a developmental delay.
   B. unintegrated primitive reflexes.
   C. normal development.
   D. advanced development.

5. **An individual demonstrates the ability to pick up a penny from a flat surface. This represents which of the following prehension patterns?**
   A. Lateral
   B. Palmar
   C. Tip
   D. Three-jaw chuck

6. **When conducting a structured interview, it is MOST important for the OT practitioner to:**
   A. rephrase the interview questions in his or her own words.
   B. ask questions that he or she thinks are pertinent to this patient.
   C. ask the questions as they are stated on the interview sheet.
   D. ask additional questions (other than those listed) to gain further insight into the patient.

7. **A 3-year-old child demonstrates the ability to use the toilet independently except for wiping and readjusting clothing afterward. This behavior indicates the child is performing at which of the following levels?**
   A. Significantly below age level
   B. Slightly below age level
   C. At age level
   D. Above age level

8. **The COTA is observing dressing skills in an individual with COPD. While putting on his shirt, the individual becomes short of breath and stops to rest before finishing with the shirt and going on to his trousers. This behavior MOST likely indicates a deficit in:**
   A. postural control.
   B. muscle tone.
   C. strength.
   D. endurance.

9. **An individual with the goal of increasing attention span is frequently observed watching the person next to her instead of performing her assigned task. This behavior MOST likely indicates a problem with:**
   A. memory.
   B. spatial operations.
   C. generalization of learning.
   D. distractibility.

10. **In screening a child who has been referred to OT, the PRIMARY goal of the OT practitioner is to:**
    A. obtain necessary information for an occupational therapy consultation with teachers or parents.
    B. test a wide variety of developmental behaviors.
    C. establish an information base for the occupational therapy treatment plan.
    D. determine the need for further evaluation.

11. **A COTA is working with an individual who is unable to name or demonstrate the use of common household objects. This behavior MOST likely indicates:**
    A. apraxia.
    B. stereognosis.
    C. visual agnosia.
    D. alexia.

12. **When reporting data collected to the OTR, it is MOST important for the COTA to:**
    A. observe everything the patient said and did during the interview and provide extensive notes for the OTR to read.
    B. provide the OTR with a comprehensive treatment plan based on the results of the evaluation.
    C. provide a summary of observations of the patient's behavior, including what the patient said and did during the interview.
    D. provide an interpretation of how the patient behaved during the interview.

13. **A child is observed grabbing toys from others, becoming easily frustrated, and is unable to sit still. This behavior MOST likely indicates:**
    A. ADHD.
    B. mood disorder, manic episode.
    C. conduct disorder.
    D. anxiety disorder.

14. **An individual who had a stroke is copying a picture of a clock. The drawing appears as a lopsided circle with a flat side on the left. The numbers one through eight are written in numerical order around the right side of the clock. The hands are correctly drawn on the clock to represent three o'clock. The individual's performance appears to demonstrate:**
    A. right hemianopsia.
    B. left unilateral neglect.
    C. cataracts in the left eye.
    D. bitemporal hemianopia.

15. **An individual alternately exhibits laughing and crying throughout a treatment session. This behavior should be documented as:**
    A. mania.
    B. emotional lability.
    C. paranoia.
    D. denial.

16. **Evaluation of a school-age child diagnosed with moderate mental retardation should generally focus on:**
    A. positioning and communication skills.
    B. communication, self-care, and social skills.
    C. ADLs and IADLs.
    D. feeding and personal hygiene.

17. **An individual who uses a wheelchair is being discharged from a rehabilitation**

facility to home. In determining accessibility of the interior home environment, the area the COTA should be MOST concerned with is:

A. location of telephones and appliances.
B. arrangement of furniture in bedrooms.
C. steps, width of doorways, and threshold heights.
D. presence of clutter in the environment.

18. A woman experienced repeated sexual abuse by her father as a child. She now describes her father's abusive actions as being caused by his stress of being fired from a job because of new management. The defense mechanism she is MOST likely to be using is:

A. identification.
B. projection.
C. denial.
D. rationalization.

19. A child has considerable difficulty with problem solving when playing with Lego blocks and becomes frustrated and gives up easily. This MOST likely indicates a problem in which area of play?

A. Sensorimotor
B. Imaginary
C. Constructional
D. Game

20. An OT practitioner is making a home visit to an elderly client who lives alone. The client exhibits severe hand weakness. When addressing safety in the home, the MOST important area to assess is the individual's ability to:

A. work locks and latches on doors and windows.
B. use built-up utensils while eating.
C. use energy conservation techniques.
D. manipulate fasteners on clothing.

21. A supermarket employee with obsessive-compulsive disorder takes an hour to stock 24 soup cans on the shelf. He reports that once he has placed all the cans on the shelf, he removes them all and starts over because "all the labels were not lined up exactly in the same direction." Which of the following methods would MOST effectively evaluate this individual's work performance?

A. Functional assessment of work-related skills, such as carrying and opening cartons and shelving items

B. Cognitive assessment using the Allen's Cognitive Levels evaluation
C. Verbal interview focusing on the requirements of the individual's job
D. Task evaluation using a "clean" medium like a puzzle

22. Which of the following assessment methods would an OT practitioner MOST likely choose in order to learn about a family's values and priorities?

A. Interview
B. Skilled observation
C. Inventory
D. Standardized test

23. A person with functional limitations in shoulder abduction and external rotation is performing self-care activities. Which of the following is MOST essential for the COTA to assess?

A. Buttoning a shirt
B. Combing the hair
C. Tucking in a shirt in the back
D. Tying a shoe

24. A COTA is scheduled to interview an individual with a head injury about her home environment, and family and child care responsibilities. Knowing the individual has an attention span of 10 to 15 minutes, which of the following should the COTA do FIRST?

A. Schedule a 30-minute treatment session.
B. Obtain as much information as possible from the chart.
C. Interview the individual using appropriate verbal and nonverbal communication.
D. Perform the interview in an environment where distractions can be minimized.

25. During the interview with the parents of a 3-year-old child with mild CP, the OT practitioner learns that the child is regularly fed by his grandmother and does not have any independent feeding skills. The FIRST issue the OT practitioner needs to explore further is:

A. the degree of abnormal muscle tone in the UEs.
B. the possibility of developmental delay.
C. the cultural context and family interaction patterns.
D. the need for adapted equipment.

26. A method that an OT practitioner can use to document total finger flexion

without recording the measurement in degrees would be to measure the:

A. passive flexion at each joint and total the numbers.
B. distance from the fingertip to the distal palmar crease with the hand in a fist.
C. active flexion at each joint and total the measurements.
D. distance between the tip of the thumb and the tip of the fourth finger.

27. A COTA needs to report the results of an ADL evaluation to the supervising OTR. The OTR, who is on her way to the cafeteria for lunch, states she has to leave immediately after lunch to go to another facility. Which is the BEST method for the COTA to use to communicate the evaluation results to the OTR?

A. With a phone call
B. In a written report
C. During discussion at lunch in the cafeteria
D. During discussion in the OT office

28. When evaluating sensation of an individual with hemiplegia, the COTA should FIRST:

A. apply the stimuli distally to proximally.
B. test the involved area then the uninvolved area.
C. present test stimuli in an organized pattern to improve reliability during retesting.
D. apply the stimuli to the uninvolved area proximally to distally in a random pattern.

29. When assessing the sense of proprioception at an individual's joint, movement within the range would BEST be performed:

A. until pain is elicited.
B. until the stretch reflex is elicited.
C. at the end ranges of the joint.
D. at the midrange of the joint.

30. An individual who attends a day program for adults with developmental disabilities has difficulty participating in group activities because of extreme anxiety related to being around others. The BEST way to determine whether the individual is experiencing anxiety during group sessions would be to:

A. observe the individual's body language during group sessions.
B. ask the individual to complete a questionnaire rating her anxiety level after each session.

C. have group members provide feedback to the individual and COTA about her anxiety level.
D. allow the individual to select two other clients she feels she'd be comfortable with in a small group.

31. Infants and preschool children with musculoskeletal disorders require ongoing examination of their upper extremity strength, coordination, and functional abilities. The OT practitioner will obtain the majority of assessment information during infancy and preschool through:

A. assessments related to the specific diagnosis that determine hand function.
B. dynamometer and pinch meter function.
C. observation of play and hand function.
D. functional independence measures.

32. An individual is able to complete full range of shoulder flexion while in a side-lying position during an evaluation. However, against gravity, the client is not quite able to achieve 50% of the range for shoulder flexion. This muscle should be graded as:

A. good (4).
B. fair (3).
C. fair minus (3-).
D. poor plus (2+).

33. The mother of a 3-month-old infant recently returned to her job as a bookkeeper on a part-time basis. She reports that she has difficulty concentrating at work because she keeps thinking about the baby, and that when she's at home, she is distracted because she feels she should be at work. This PRIMARILY indicates a problem in the area of:

A. parenting skills.
B. attention span.
C. assertiveness.
D. role performance.

Treatment Planning

34. The treatment goal for a 4-year-old child with hypotonia is to improve grasp. Which of the following activities would be BEST for preparing the child's hand for grasp activities?

A. Dropping blocks into a pail
B. Placing pegs on a pegboard
C. Weight-bearing on hands

D. Holding and eating a cookie

35. An older adult with diabetes is working on a macramé project as a way of increasing standing tolerance. The MOST relevant safety factor for the COTA to take into consideration is the:

A. length of the cords she will start with.
B. thickness of the cords she will be using.
C. texture of the cords she will be using.
D. type of surface she will be standing on.

36. The treatment goal that BEST addresses the psychosocial skill of self-expression is:

A. the client will identify and pursue activities that are pleasurable to the self.
B. the client will use facial expressions and gestures that are consistent with stated emotions during assertive, passive, and aggressive role-play situations.
C. the client will recognize his or her own behavior and possible negative and positive consequences.
D. the client will identify his or her own assets and limitations after an art or movement group.

37. In planning a therapeutic dressing intervention for a first-grade child who is mentally retarded, the COTA's FIRST consideration should be the need for:

A. adaptive equipment.
B. adaptive clothing.
C. proper positioning.
D. adapted teaching techniques.

38. A COTA is fabricating a resting pan splint for a client with extremely fragile skin. Which of the following areas will the COTA have to inspect most carefully for signs of skin breakdown?

A. Metacarpal heads, pisiform, and, trapezium
B. Volar PIP joints, medial fifth digit, and thumb MP joint
C. Ulnar styloid, distal head of radius, and thumb CMC joint
D. Thumb PIP joint, pisiform, and hamate

39. The COTA needs to identify an activity that will address psychosocial goals by (1) allowing the individual to experience success using a messy process, and (2) requiring the individual to delay gratification. The activity process that is BEST for providing this experience is:

A. working in a group with three other individuals.
B. selecting the design pattern for a tile trivet.
C. applying grout to a tile trivet and waiting for it to dry.
D. encouraging the individual to clean off the table at the end of the group session.

40. A school-age child demonstrates aggressive and disruptive behavior in school as a result of a low sensory threshold. Which of the following suggestions would be MOST useful to discuss with the teacher regarding an upcoming class bus trip to the zoo?

A. Review the bus rules with the child and apply consequences consistently.
B. Let the child sit at the front of the bus and use a tape player with earphones.
C. Give the child the responsibility of monitoring classmates as "bus patrol."
D. Let the child set the criteria for a successful trip, and provide a reward if the criteria are met.

41. Which of the following interventions is MOST appropriate for an individual who has recently been diagnosed with rheumatoid arthritis and is in the acute stage of the disease?

A. Strengthening with resistive exercises
B. Positioning, adaptive equipment, and patient education
C. Discharge planning
D. Preparing the patient for surgical intervention

42. A COTA is working with an individual who was admitted to an inpatient psychiatric program for major depression. This individual is also diagnosed with stage 4 AIDS. The BEST general focus of treatment at this point would be to:

A. restore and maintain performance of self-chosen occupations that support performance of valued occupational roles.
B. increase physical endurance and maintain desired self-care tasks.
C. facilitate resolution of current and anticipated losses through the grieving process.
D. restore and maintain functional performance of the individual's primary work role.

43. A fifth-grade child with significantly low muscle tone caused by Duchenne's muscular dystrophy is losing trunk control when sitting. Which of the following

frames of reference should the COTA consider when planning the treatment program?

A. Neurodevelopmental treatment
B. Sensory integration
C. Biomechanical
D. Visual perceptual

44. **A COTA is planning a program for an individual who needs to increase shoulder strength, range of motion, and endurance. Which of the following activities is MOST suitable for periodic upgrading?**

A. Blowing up and tying balloons of various sizes
B. Playing a game of balloon darts
C. Painting faces on balloons
D. Playing balloon volleyball

45. **A sales executive is participating in a time-management program. Which of the following would be the expected outcome for the client?**

A. To control anxiety when arriving late for a meeting
B. To take responsibility when late with reports
C. To cope with feelings of inadequacy when missing a deadline
D. To arrive at work on time consistently

46. **The COTA is selecting activities for an 8-year-old child with Duchenne's muscular dystrophy. Which of the following developmental issues is MOST important to consider when identifying activities for this child?**

A. Establishment of basic trust
B. Freedom to use his initiative
C. Development of self-identity
D. Reinforcement of competence

47. **Which individual would benefit the MOST from using a wrist-driven flexor hinge splint during a prehension activity?**

A. A client with a C1 injury
B. A client with a C3 injury
C. A client with a C6 injury
D. A client with a T1 injury

48. **An individual with a history of depression and social isolation is hospitalized for the third time due to suicidal ideation. Completion of an interest checklist indicates interests in crafts, cooking, and participation in social activities. In planning treatment for a short hospitaliza-** tion, which of the following activities would be MOST appropriate for this individual?

A. Identify social opportunities using a local phone book.
B. Scan a craft catalogue to identify possible leisure interests.
C. Implement writing in a personal log on a daily basis.
D. Look through a recipe book to develop cooking as a leisure activity.

49. **A COTA who is beginning treatment for a child with athetoid CP is concerned about the child's inability to control flexion and extension of the arm when reaching for a toy. The child flexes or extends too much, which makes placement of the hand very difficult. The MOST appropriate goal for this type of problem in hand function would be to improve the:**

A. ability to isolate movement.
B. ability to grade movement.
C. ability to control how fast movement occurs.
D. bilateral integration of arm movements.

50. **A COTA is working with a patient recovering from a hand injury who complains of pain when any sensation is felt on the affected hand. In planning a program of desensitization training for the patient, the MOST appropriate sequence for grading the sensory stimuli that will be applied to the patient's hand is from:**

A. soft to hard to rough.
B. tap to rub to touch.
C. light to medium to heavy.
D. rough to hard to soft.

51. **A COTA is conducting an ongoing assertiveness training group. Which of the following strategies would be MOST helpful in the development of group cohesion?**

A. Define assertiveness, passivity, and aggression for the group members.
B. Allow and encourage all group members to release their aggressive feelings physically and verbally toward inanimate objects.
C. Demonstrate commonly used assertiveness techniques to the group members.
D. Encourage group members to share similar experiences and reactions with each other.

52. **A school-age child with multiple handicaps is beginning to develop some con-**

trolled movement in the upper extremities. It would be MOST appropriate to introduce switch operated assistive technology when the child:

A. develops tolerance of an upright sitting posture.

B. can reach and point with accuracy.

C. demonstrates any reliable, controlled movement.

D. develops isolated finger control.

53. A COTA is working with an individual with amyotrophic lateral sclerosis who is no longer able to ambulate for kitchen or home management activities. Which of the following interventions BEST addresses the goals of independence in meal preparation for this individual?

A. Meal preparation techniques using a wheelchair

B. Training in the use of adapted cooking equipment

C. Simple cooking activities while standing at the counter for gradually increasing amounts of time

D. Beginning with cold meals and progressing to hot meals

54. In carrying out inpatient treatment groups for individuals with schizophrenia, the COTA should routinely:

A. use projective media, such as clay, to facilitate expression of feelings.

B. allow an individual group member to work in an isolated area away from the group.

C. use simple and highly structured activities.

D. discuss the individuals' delusions with them.

55. A child with behavioral problems has difficulty with peer interactions. Which of the following aspects of the treatment plan is MOST important?

A. Provide activities in an authoritarian environment.

B. Allow the child the opportunity to develop basic social skills on his own.

C. Provide enjoyable activities in a safe and accepting environment.

D. Strictly enforce rules for group play.

56. A long-term goal for a client following a hip arthroplasty is independence in lower extremity dressing. The MOST relevant short-term goal for the COTA to work on would be that the:

A. client will increase standing tolerance to 10 minutes.

B. client will increase hip flexion to 90 degrees.

C. client will demonstrate appropriate hip precautions.

D. client will apply energy-conservation techniques during dressing activities.

57. A COTA is planning a craft activity for an adolescent who has been hospitalized following a suicide attempt. An interest checklist indicates experience with fiber arts. Which of the following activities would be considered MOST appropriate for this individual?

A. Leather wallet with single cordovan lacing

B. Macramé choker

C. Ceramic beads

D. Decoupage wooden key fob

58. A 9-year-old child with sensory integration problems has not developed a preferred hand for printing or writing. Which intervention option would MOST likely result in eventual development of a preferred hand to use in writing activities?

A. Develop right-handed skills because most children are right-handed.

B. Wait a few more years until the child decides which hand is preferred.

C. Let the child's teacher decide on a preferred hand.

D. Consider and treat underlying sensory integration problems as a possible cause.

59. A COTA is preparing a work conditioning program for a patient who has decreased endurance. The COTA's FIRST step in developing a work conditioning program for this patient would be:

A. implementing, adapting, or modifying work activities.

B. creating nonspecific job-simulated work tasks.

C. implementing job-specific work tasks.

D. creating a simulated work environment.

60. A COTA is planning a collage activity task group for several clients with depression. The PRIMARY purpose of using an OT task group with these clients is to:

A. provide opportunities to evaluate areas of function.

B. focus the group on a topic that is common

to all of the members and can be discussed by the members.

C. encourage here-and-now explorations of member behaviors and issues, while promoting learning through doing.

D. encourage the members to develop sequentially organized social interaction skills with the other members.

61. The COTA reviews various functional activities that are being incorporated into her client's hand rehabilitation program. The COTA explains to the client that functional activities may include:

A. active range of motion and self range of motion techniques.

B. crafts, games, and self-care tasks.

C. cone stacking, pegs, and pulleys.

D. mild, moderate, and resistive theraband exercises.

62. A COTA who works in an outpatient facility recommends that clients with Parkinson's disease be treated in a therapeutic group. The COTA is MOST likely to select group treatment for these clients because:

A. it is more effective in preventing motor problems associated with Parkinson's disease.

B. it provides social interaction and support, as well as activity.

C. it is an effective way to present therapeutic exercise activities.

D. it requires less therapist time because the therapist can leave once the group has started.

63. A COTA is planning a meal preparation activity for an adult client with attentional and organizational deficits secondary to alcohol abuse. The treatment goals address the client's difficulties in properly sequencing tasks. The most appropriate activity to use FIRST is:

A. setting the table.

B. planning an entire meal.

C. baking cookies using a recipe.

D. preparing a shopping list.

Treatment Implementation

64. When teaching children with moderate mental retardation to feed, groom, and dress themselves, the COTA is MOST likely to use which technique?

A. Chaining

B. Practice and repetition

C. Demonstration

D. Role modeling

65. An individual with an IV drug abuse problem has developed AIDS. The OT evaluation revealed that the individual's major problems are with daily tasks, self-esteem, physical deconditioning, and anxiety. Which of the following approaches would be MOST beneficial to the client?

A. Have the patient practice stress reduction using meditation, yoga, and energy conservation techniques.

B. Have the patient participate in aerobic activities to combat deconditioning.

C. Provide video lectures on AIDs to educate the client about the disease process.

D. Incorporate energy conservation techniques and daily aerobic activities into the client's ADLs.

66. An individual with an anxiety disorder feels so overwhelmed he cannot get himself from his room to OT group each morning. Which of the following strategies will be MOST helpful?

A. Reduce distractions and keep the lights low.

B. Provide a stimulating environment with real life opportunities.

C. Give him a tour of the OT department and a schedule of activities.

D. Leave doors open and avoid being alone with the individual.

67. The COTA is attempting to increase playfulness with a 7-year-old girl with sensory integrative dysfunction. The child experiences difficulties with motor tasks and often complains that no one likes her. After establishing rapport with the child, the COTA would MOST likely introduce which of the following?

A. Playing a game of "Go Fish"

B. Playing a game of checkers

C. Jumping rope

D. Role playing a tea party with "Barbie" dolls

68. A patient with a short below-elbow amputation is lacking sensation in the residual limb. The MOST appropriate intervention would be for the COTA to teach the patient:

A. techniques of tapping, rubbing, and application of textures to the residual limb.

B. to routinely inspect the skin closely for signs of skin breakdown.

C. to perform deep massage on the residual limb.

D. the necessary procedures of proper skin hygiene.

69. **A COTA is running a discharge planning group in which individuals discuss their personal feelings and concerns about returning to the community. Which of the following would be the BEST method to facilitate this process?**

A. Patients write fears and concerns on index cards and then the COTA collects and reads the cards to the group for discussion.

B. Patients write fears and concerns on index cards and then take turns reading their cards to the group.

C. Patients each take a turn verbalizing their fears and concerns to the group.

D. The psychologist speaks to the group about discharge fears in general.

70. **A COTA is working with a child whose poor visual attention is affecting his ability to perform school work. An adaptation of the sensory environment that would BEST improve attention during a visual task is to have the child:**

A. work with lively background music to increase competing sensory input.

B. work against a patterned background to increase competing visual input.

C. use headphones during work to reduce competing sensory input.

D. use dim lighting to reduce the visual input.

71. **A COTA is treating a client with Parkinson's disease whose primary functional problems are caused by a shuffling gait. The MOST relevant environmental recommendation the COTA could make to address a potential safety hazard in the home is to:**

A. increase illumination in hallways.

B. screen out distracting stimuli in the environment.

C. place door locks higher or lower than eye level.

D. remove scatter rugs throughout the house.

72. **After a 30-year hospitalization, an individual with mental illness has been discharged to a community group home. She is used to being told what to do and**

where to go. **Which of the following would be the BEST approach to take for this individual's first meal preparation group?**

A. Have the individual plan the menu for the following group session.

B. Give the individual one task to do such as making drinks.

C. Ask the individual what she would like to do.

D. Suggest that the individual just observe the group.

73. **The COTA is observing a 3-year-old child during tooth brushing. The child demonstrates good bilateral upper extremity/ hand strength, but decreased dexterity. Which piece of equipment would the COTA MOST likely encourage the child to use during brushing?**

A. A small soft bristle toothbrush

B. A velcro strap attached to a toothbrush

C. An electric toothbrush

D. A soft sponge-tipped toothette

74. **An individual with chronic obstructive pulmonary disease and low endurance is taught to modify his bathing techniques for carryover after discharge. The COTA should recommend which of the following as the BEST bathing method?**

A. Tub bathing with hot water

B. Standing for a quick shower

C. Using a bath chair and a hand-held shower with tepid water

D. Tub bathing using lukewarm water

75. **An individual consistently confuses white glue with white grout during a tile activity. Which of the following actions would the COTA implement to remain consistent with an activity adaptation approach?**

A. Review the difference between glue and grout with the individual.

B. Replace the white glue with blue glue.

C. Avoid the use of white tiles.

D. Complete the last step of the activity (applying grout) for the individual until they have learned how to apply grout successfully.

76. **A sixth grader with a diagnosis of athetoid cerebral palsy needs an adapted computer for communication. Her upper extremity control is poor because of fluctuating muscle tone. The COTA suggests that the BEST way for her to operate her computer is to use a:**

A. single pressure switch, firmly mounted within easy reach.
B. lightweight keyboard placed at midline.
C. low-resistance mouse and pad.
D. mercury switch headband set to respond to minimal movement.

77. **A COTA is instructing a person with arthritis how to maintain range of motion while performing household activities. Which of the following activities would the COTA MOST likely recommend to accomplish this?**

A. Use short strokes with the vacuum cleaner.
B. Keep elbow flexed when ironing.
C. Keep lightweight objects on low shelves.
D. Use a dust mitt to keep fingers fully extended.

78. **An individual with mental retardation lives in a group home and is expected to participate in laundry activities. The individual is usually successful with routine performance of daily tasks, is able to recognize whether clothing is clean or dirty, demonstrates sequencing skills, and is independent in most self-care activities. What advice should the COTA provide to the group home staff to enable the individual to perform laundry activities at the HIGHEST level of independence possible?**

A. The staff will probably need to instruct the individual to place dirty items in the hamper and remove sheets from the bed.
B. The staff should encourage problem solving when obstacles arise.
C. The individual will be independent in use of a washer and dryer, but the staff may need to demonstrate the use of new products.
D. The staff may only need to monitor water temperature and the amount of soap being used.

79. **A child with athetoid CP is working in OT to develop self-feeding skills. The COTA observes that when the child attempts to pick up food, it slides off the plate. Which adaptation does the COTA provide to solve this problem?**

A. A swivel spoon
B. A nonslip mat
C. A mobile arm support
D. A scoop dish

80. **A patient who had a CVA has difficulty using his left upper extremity for reaching activities because of fluctuating muscle tone. According to the Neurodevelopmental Treatment approach, one of the MOST effective ways to teach a person to normalize high muscle tone in affected extremities prior to functional activities is by:**

A. placing a weighted cuff on the extremity.
B. weight bearing through the upper extremity in sitting or standing.
C. using the unaffected arm for all reaching activities.
D. "forced use" of the affected extremity.

81. **An individual with memory and attention deficits exhibits poor table manners and is working to address this in an ADL group. Which method is MOST appropriate for this individual?**

A. Role plays that include practicing good table manners.
B. Reward the individual with dessert when he uses good manners.
C. Instruct group members to remind him when he forgets his good manners.
D. Reinforce use of good manners with praise and rewards.

82. **Which of the following would a COTA MOST likely introduce to a group of 10-year-old children with paraplegia?**

A. "Simon Says"
B. Imaginative/role playing group with dolls and stuffed animals
C. "Duck, duck, goose" and "Hot Potato"
D. A tabletop air hockey competition

83. **The goal for an elderly person with Parkinson's disease is to dress herself independently. The BEST adaptation to compensate for this person's physical deficits would be:**

A. Velcro closures on front opening clothing.
B. large buttons on front opening clothing.
C. larger clothing slipped on over the head with no fasteners.
D. stretchy fabric clothing with tie closures in the back.

84. **A client is participating in an assertiveness training group within a work setting. The expected outcome of this intervention is that the client will MOST likely improve the ability to:**

A. engage in relevant conversations with coworkers.

B. use appropriate facial expressions when disagreeing with coworkers.

C. express disagreement with coworkers in a productive manner.

D. use courteous behavior when disagreeing with coworkers.

85. **A young child exhibits tactile defensiveness with all dressing tasks. Which of the following would the COTA recommend as the MOST effective handling method for this child?**

A. Tickle him prior to dressing and undressing.

B. Play loud music when undressing him.

C. Lightly stroke the child's arms and legs while dressing him.

D. Hold him firmly when picking him up and dressing him.

86. **An individual who is being discharged after participating in an inpatient pulmonary rehabilitation program for chronic obstructive pulmonary disease, is given a list of tips from the COTA to use in the home to promote function. Which of the following items will the COTA MOST likely recommend?**

A. Perform pursed-lip breathing when doing activities.

B. Use a long-handled sponge while in the shower.

C. Take hot showers to reduce congestion.

D. Avoid air conditioned rooms during warm months.

87. **A COTA is organizing a group picnic outing to a park. The most important precaution for the COTA to implement for those group members taking neuroleptic medications is to:**

A. encourage the use of PABA-free sunblock and hats.

B. encourage members to move slowly when changing positions from sitting to standing.

C. encourage members to use an antiperspirant and wear light colored clothing.

D. take along low-calorie snacks such as carrot and celery sticks.

88. **A COTA is positioning a child with low muscle tone and postural instability into a prone stander to develop head righting. The child rapidly shows fatigue and associated reactions. How can the COTA**

BEST adjust the stander to decrease these reactions while continuing to address the goal of head righting?

A. Place the child in prone on the floor.

B. Position the stander at 45 degrees from the floor.

C. Position the stander at 75 to 90 degrees from the floor.

D. Position the child upright in a prone or supine stander.

89. **During a stress management group, an individual recently diagnosed with multiple sclerosis complains that his teenage children are resistive to helping with chores that were previously his responsibility (e.g., mowing the lawn and taking out the trash). Which of the following stress management techniques would the COTA MOST likely recommend to address this client's concerns?**

A. Using effective communication skills

B. Applying time management techniques

C. Deep breathing

D. Laughter

90. **An individual with a history of depression and low self-esteem has just begun to participate in a home management group. This individual had previously identified cooking as a leisure interest that he is good at. Which of the following approaches will MOST effectively promote individual growth and self-confidence?**

A. Praise the cooking skills of the individual in front of the group.

B. Have the individual plan and demonstrate a cooking activity to the entire group.

C. During a meal preparation activity, have the individual demonstrate a step that he is familiar with to two or three group members.

D. Incorporate cooking activities only after the individual expresses a desire to participate in them.

91. **The COTA is working with the family of a 3-year-old child who lacks sitting balance in the bathtub. The family is requesting an alternative to a shower bench, because the child seems to enjoy submersing herself in the warm bathtub water, and their insurance does not cover durable medical equipment costs. Which of the following would the COTA MOST likely recommend?**

A. Place a foam-lined plastic laundry basket in the tub.

B. Place a horseshoe-shaped inflatable bath collar around the child's neck while bathing.

C. Utilize a bath hammock in the tub while bathing.

D. Suggest that the child shower in a standing position instead of bathing in the tub.

92. **A resident of a long-term care facility is receiving OT because of difficulties with eating. The FIRST step of intervention the COTA performs with this resident at mealtime is to:**

A. provide skid-proof placemats, plate guard, and utensils with built-up handles.

B. observe for swallowing after each bite of food.

C. instruct the caregivers about a special eating setup for the resident.

D. position the person in an upright posture, making sure head is flexed slightly and in midline.

93. **Which of the following is MOST important when using a remotivation approach with a group of elderly individuals?**

A. Use pictures, music, and discussion to encourage discussion of memories.

B. Discuss an upcoming holiday and base an activity on that holiday.

C. Adapt the environment to maximize independent functioning.

D. Focus on group activities designed to enhance interpersonal skills.

94. **A child with quadriplegia complains of frequently slumping to the side when sitting in a wheelchair. The COTA would MOST likely recommend which of the following to enable the child to maintain optimal wheelchair positioning?**

A. A reclining wheelchair

B. An arm trough

C. Lateral trunk supports

D. Lateral pelvic supports

95. **An individual with a C6 spinal cord injury is unable to button his shirt. The COTA would be MOST likely to select which type of adaptive equipment to assist this client with buttoning?**

A. A buttonhook with an extra long, flexible handle

B. A buttonhook with a knob handle

C. A buttonhook on a 0.5 inch diameter, 5 inch long wooden handle

D. A buttonhook attached to a cuff that fits around the palm

96. **An individual diagnosed with borderline personality disorder tells a COTA that she is the only one she can trust. The next day she accuses the COTA of lying to her. The best way for the COTA to respond is to:**

A. tell the individual her feeling have been hurt.

B. remain matter of fact and consistent in approach.

C. ask the individual how she has felt when lied to in the past.

D. apologize and try to determine how the misunderstanding occurred.

97. **A teenager with fine motor incoordination reports difficulty with self-care. Which of the following options would this individual find MOST beneficial?**

A. Wash mitt

B. Spray deodorant

C. Toothpaste with a flip-open cap

D. Toothbrush with a built-up handle

98. **A COTA is working with a group of patients who have orientation deficits resulting from head injuries. Using an adaptive or compensatory approach, the MOST appropriate intervention would be to:**

A. provide verbal cues, external aids such as calendars and family pictures, and opportunities to practice using the external aids.

B. reduce the number of distractions by moving the group to a quiet room.

C. present information in short units, spaced with time between each segment.

D. connect new information to previously learned knowledge and skills.

99. **A COTA instructs a client with chronic neck pain to use psychosocial pain management techniques. Which of the following strategies should the COTA implement to assist in the management of this individual's chronic pain?**

A. Biofeedback, distraction, and relaxation techniques

B. Specific skill training

C. Strength and endurance building techniques

D. Cognitive retraining techniques

100. The parent of an infant with hypertonia reports that dressing the child is extremely difficult. When teaching this parent how to put shoes and socks on the child, the COTA should recommend FIRST flexing the child's:

A. hips.
B. knees.
C. ankles.
D. toes.

101. A COTA is treating a restaurant worker with carpal tunnel syndrome. The MOST important instruction for the COTA to give the client is to avoid or modify activities that encourage:

A. increased wrist extension, such as carrying dishes.
B. prolonged wrist flexion, such as scrubbing pots and pans.
C. tasks that increase ulnar deviation, such as wiping tables.
D. increased radial deviation, such as screwing and unscrewing and filling sugar, salt, and pepper containers.

102. When working with an individual who is severely depressed and demonstrates psychomotor retardation, it is MOST important to:

A. encourage more rapid responses.
B. provide extensive visual and auditory sensory stimulation.
C. give simple directions and patiently wait for responses.
D. provide activities involving large groups.

103. A child diagnosed with ataxic CP exhibits tremors in the upper extremities. When she feeds herself, the tremors cause most of the food to fall off her spoon before it can reach her mouth. Which of the following adaptations should the COTA recommend?

A. Replace the spoon with a blunt-ended fork.
B. Build up the handle of the spoon.
C. Give the child a swivel spoon.
D. Bend the spoon handle 45 degrees.

104. A client is having difficulty getting around her home as a result of low vision. The MOST appropriate strategy the COTA can recommend to improve accessibility would be to:

A. instruct the client to sit while performing ADL.
B. provide strong color contrast at key areas to identify steps, pathways, etc.
C. recommend the client arrange to get assistance from another person when moving within her home.
D. recommend training in white cane use, for identifying obstacles in the home.

105. A COTA has been working on laundry skills with an adult with developmental disabilities who lives at home with her aging parents. Although the client is able to use the washer and dryer successfully with only verbal cues, her mother continues to do her laundry. The COTA should:

A. explain to the mother that it is critical to allow the client to do her own laundry in order to achieve independence.
B. discuss the meaning and value of the client's doing her own laundry with the mother and client.
C. ask the father to intercede to stop the mother from doing the client's laundry for her.
D. acknowledge that independence in laundry skills may not be an appropriate goal for this client.

106. An early intervention COTA is working with a toddler whose significant physical disabilities have limited the child's ability to explore the environment. The BEST "low tech" assistive technology play aid to allow the child to experience cause and effect and some control over an aspect of his or her environment would be:

A. a tape recorder for the child to listen to music.
B. a switch-adapted battery-operated toy car that knocks down a block tower.
C. storybook software for use on a computer.
D. a powered wheelchair.

107. The BEST way to instruct an individual with hemiparesis to button a shirt is to:

A. button all the buttons before putting the shirt on.
B. get the shirt all the way on, then line up the buttons and holes, and begin buttoning from the top.
C. get the shirt all the way on, then line up the buttons and holes, and begin buttoning from the bottom.
D. use a buttonhook with a built-up handle.

108. A young man with a history of depression constantly makes negative statements about himself. The goal set for him in the task group is to increase self-esteem. After several sessions, he is showing more self-confidence and asks the COTA for her phone number because "you're so nice to me." The MOST appropriate response is for the COTA to:

A. give him her phone number and tell him to call when he is feeling depressed.

B. ignore the request, but remind him he's doing a good job.

C. tell him she has a boyfriend.

D. in private, explain the nature of the client-therapist relationship.

109. A child is unable to bring her hand to her mouth for feeding because of weakness in supination. The MOST helpful adapted utensil for this child would be a:

A. spoon with an elongated handle.

B. "spork."

C. spoon with a built-up handle.

D. swivel spoon.

110. In a work-hardening program, a COTA is teaching a warehouse worker with low back pain how to lift objects from the floor and place them on a shelf. Before doing this, the COTA should FIRST review:

A. energy conservation techniques.

B. work simplification strategies.

C. home maintenance activities.

D. proper body mechanics.

111. An individual has demonstrated competence in heating canned soup. The COTA recommends modifying the treatment plan and upgrading the cooking activity to:

A. baking brownies.

B. making an apple pie.

C. making toast.

D. making a fresh fruit salad.

112. The mother of a physically disabled 3-year-old has a goal that her child will be walking independently around the house. This is an unrealistic goal for the child but one that would be helpful to the mother who is finding her child difficult to lift. The BEST way to assist in the development of family-centered intervention for this child would be to:

A. support and work on the parent's goal as is.

B. suggest an alternative, realistic OT goal of improving sitting balance for playing.

C. propose a modified goal that still meets the parent's needs.

D. empower the child to set her own goals.

113. An individual with Guillain-Barré syndrome demonstrates poor to fair strength throughout the upper extremities. Which is the most appropriate approach for the COTA to use in the EARLY stages?

A. Gentle, nonresistive activities

B. Progressive resistive exercise

C. Fine motor activities

D. Active range of motion against moderate resistance

114. A COTA is planning a community living program for clients who are to be discharged after an average of 25 to 30 years of hospitalization. One of the goals of this program is to train the clients to effectively manage their money. Which of the following activities should be used FIRST?

A. Provide each client with $25 to spend during a group trip to the local shopping center.

B. Provide samples of coins and paper money.

C. Use a board game to introduce the concept of receiving and spending money.

D. Establish a hospital-based community store where the clients can buy clothing.

115. A COTA is working with a group of children in an early intervention program. All of the children in the group are able to sit independently on the floor except for one child with cerebral palsy. The child has told the COTA that he wishes to sit on the floor like his peers and not in his wheelchair. The COTA would MOST likely recommend that the child use a(n):

A. hammock.

B. floor sitter.

C. adapted wheelchair insert.

D. prone stander.

116. An individual with complete C7 quadriplegia demonstrates fair plus (3+) strength in the wrist extensors. Which of the following interventions would the COTA introduce to MOST effectively increase strength in the wrist extensors?

A. A craft activity using increasingly heavy hand tools
B. Mildly resistive activities that are halted as soon as the individual begins to fatigue
C. Electric stimulation to the wrist extensors
D. Moderate resistance during AROM to the wrist

117. **A COTA is using leather stamping as part of a group activity but feels the need to increase the problem solving processes within the group. The BEST approach for encouraging problem solving in a craft media group is to:**
   A. begin with activities that have obvious solutions and high probabilities of success, and then gradually increase the complexity.
   B. begin with activities that require gross motor responses and progress to activities that require fine motor responses.
   C. structure the number and kinds of choices available.
   D. gradually increase the time used in the activity by 15-minute increments.

118. **The COTA and physical therapist are attempting to order a wheelchair for a child with severe cerebral palsy who will most likely never ambulate. The child has no cognitive limitations and frequently expresses the desire to be independent in mobility, especially within the school setting. The COTA and physical therapist will MOST likely recommend that the family order a:**
   A. power wheelchair.
   B. standard wheelchair.
   C. caster cart.
   D. prone scooter.

119. **An individual with ALS and mild dysphagia becomes extremely fatigued at breakfast, lunch, and dinner. Which is the FIRST intervention the COTA should consider recommending?**
   A. Speak with the physician about tube feedings.
   B. Sit in a semireclined position during meals.
   C. Eat six small meals a day.
   D. Substitute pureed foods for liquids.

120. **A COTA is working with an elderly woman with a diagnosis of depression and dementia during the clean-up portion of a cooking activity. The patient begins to dry the plates and utensils she has already dried. The COTA should:**

A. tell the client that the same dishes and utensils are being redried.
B. put the dried dishes away and begin to hand her wet dishes.
C. ask the client to stop the activity because it seems too difficult.
D. ask the client to describe what she is doing.

121. **An 8-year-old boy with conduct disorder is disruptive, uncooperative, and occasionally combative during therapy. From a behavioral point of view, the MOST appropriate strategy to use to address the child's conduct would be to:**
   A. allow the child to express his anger without restraint for a short period to vent his frustration.
   B. ignore the behavior and continue with therapy with or without the child's cooperation.
   C. attempt to reason with the child to get his cooperation.
   D. set clear expectations for behavior and enforce consequences, such as a time-out, if the child looses control.

122. **An individual with left upper extremity flaccidity is observed sitting in a wheelchair with his left arm dangling over the side. The FIRST positioning device the COTA should introduce to the client is a(n):**
   A. lap tray.
   B. wheelchair armrest.
   C. arm sling.
   D. arm trough.

123. **A very confused nursing home resident is frequently found in the rooms of other residents in the middle of the night. Which of the following environmental adaptations would MOST effectively prevent wandering?**
   A. Apply wrist restraints after the client has fallen asleep.
   B. Keep hallways clear of obstructions to prevent injury.
   C. Disguise the bedroom door with wallpaper so it blends in with the surroundings.
   D. Suggest the night shift staff provide closer supervision.

124. **Of the following, which is the BEST activity a COTA could offer a preschooler to develop letter recognition skills?**
   A. Using flashcards
   B. Forming letters out of clay
   C. Matching cut-out letters to a sample

D. Coloring large letter outlines

125. An unmarried patient with a spinal cord injury is on a rehab unit and constantly flirts with a COTA. The MOST appropriate action for the COTA to take would be:

A. firmly reject the patient's advances.
B. acknowledge the patient's actions and mildly flirt back in order to protect the patient's self-esteem.
C. request the supervising OTR discuss the effects of SCI and sexual functioning with the patient.
D. set personal boundaries appropriate to the therapist–patient relationship.

126. A COTA is working with an individual who is unable to complete the multiple steps that are necessary to brush his teeth. In response to this, the practitioner modifies the activity by having the client perform the task one step at a time while gradually adding more steps with each success. The COTA is attempting to employ which of the following?

A. Repetition
B. Cueing
C. Rehearsal
D. Chaining

127. A COTA working in the school system is adapting a chair for a student with extensor tone. Which of the following should the COTA recommend to the teacher in order to inhibit the child's extensor tone, while maintaining a functional seated position in the classroom?

A. Provide lateral trunk supports to the seat.
B. Place a seatbelt at a 45-degree angle at the hips.
C. Insert a wedge-shaped seat that is higher in the front.
D. Install a lapboard.

128. During a cooking evaluation, an individual with a history of traumatic brain injury exhibits moderate upper extremity incoordination. Which of the following recommendations would be MOST beneficial for this individual?

A. Use built-up utensil handles.
B. Use heavy utensils, pots, and pans.
C. Use a high stool to work at counter height.
D. Place the most commonly used items on shelves just above and below the counter.

129. Task-specific training is being used to train an individual with severe cognitive limitations to put on a tee shirt. This training will be MOST effective if it takes place:

A. in the individual's bedroom.
B. in the OT department.
C. at least twice a week.
D. when the client is feeling cooperative.

130. A COTA is working with a child with a developmental disability who frequently bites his siblings and parents. Which of the following would the COTA MOST likely recommend?

A. Encourage the parents to use verbal feedback, and explain to the child that biting is inappropriate.
B. Tell the parents to enforce time-out periods for each biting incident.
C. Encourage the child to wear a necklace with chewable objects attached.
D. Tell the parents that the child will eventually stop biting when one of his siblings bites him back.

131. An individual with joint changes that limit finger flexion would be MOST comfortable using utensils with:

A. regular handles.
B. weighted handles.
C. a universal cuff attachment.
D. built-up handles.

132. A client with severe depression and suicidal ideation stops the COTA as she is about to leave the inpatient unit at the end of the day and asks her to accept her favorite necklace as a gift of thanks. Which of the following responses is MOST important?

A. Explain that the "Code of Ethics" prevents her from accepting gifts.
B. Accept the gift so as not to imply rejection.
C. Report the incident to the client's physician.
D. Ask the client about her reasons for wanting to give her a gift.

133. A COTA works in a public elementary school. Which of the following activities should the COTA suggest to promote prewriting skills for a child in kindergarten?

A. Maneuvering through obstacles and focusing on making turns
B. Having the child create his or her own books on specific topics

C. Rolling clay into a ball
D. Drawing lines and shapes using shaving cream, sand, or finger paints

134. When treating individuals in the acute phase of cardiac rehabilitation, it is important for the COTA to FIRST select activities that:
A. can be accomplished without causing fatigue.
B. decrease the effects of prolonged inactivity.
C. promote strength, ROM, and endurance.
D. can be carried out independently after discharge.

135. A client with paranoia prefers to stay away from the group, working alone at another table. The BEST action for the COTA to take is to:
A. encourage the client to join the group.
B. tell the client he is required to sit with the group.
C. tell the client it is okay to work where he is until he feels comfortable in joining the group.
D. stay with the client until he is ready to join the group.

136. A COTA is preparing for the discharge of a preadolescent child with limited strength and endurance. Which of the following home adaptations is MOST important to recommend?
A. Mount lever handles on doors and faucets.
B. Remove all throw rugs.
C. Install nonskid pads on steps.
D. Mount a table top easel for written homework.

137. An individual with a high level spinal cord injury is returning home. Which type of adaptive technology would the client MOST likely require to ensure safety in the home?
A. An environmental control unit
B. A call system for emergency and nonemergency use
C. A remote control power door opener
D. An electric page turner

138. Which of the following is the MOST effective way for a COTA to structure the intervention environment for a patient who exhibits seductive or sexual acting out behavior?
A. Provide a stimulating environment that of-

fers options for engagement in real life activities.
B. Provide a large area of personal space, where the person is protected from physical contact with others.
C. Provide a quiet, relaxed environment, but not isolated from other people.
D. Provide an environment where all possible distractions have been removed or reduced.

139. A student has been working on learning to activate a switch for a communications device needed in the fourth grade classroom. The switch is mounted on the wheelchair tray, but the student is having difficulty operating it because of excessive muscle tone. Despite practicing for extended periods of time, the student is not making any progress. The COTA decides to:
A. work on coordinated reach in a sidelying position first and then transfer the skill to sitting position.
B. passively stretch the student's upper extremity to increase range of motion.
C. use a brightly colored switch to increase visibility.
D. use systematic behavioral reinforcement through shaping.

140. While participating in activities to improve strength, an individual with multiple sclerosis who was recently admitted to the hospital complains of fatigue. Which of the following actions is the MOST appropriate for the COTA to take?
A. Instruct the individual to work through the fatigue to complete the session.
B. Instruct the individual to work through the fatigue for another 5 to 10 minutes.
C. Discontinue strengthening activities.
D. Give the individual a rest break.

141. A COTA is leading a craft media group with adolescents diagnosed with schizophrenia. Which of the following is the BEST method to use to facilitate problem solving?
A. Begin with activities that have obvious solutions and a high probability of success, and then gradually increase the level of complexity.
B. Begin with activities that require gross motor responses, and then gradually progress to fine motor responses.

C. Select activities that require interaction with others, and then provide opportunities to discuss and analyze how the group went.

D. Gradually increase the time used in the activity by 15-minute increments.

142. The MOST appropriate device a COTA can recommend to a child's parents to promote the development of upper lip control while feeding is a:

A. straw.

B. "spork."

C. deep spoon.

D. shallow spoon.

143. An OTR/COTA team is performing an assistive technology intervention with a client who has severe limitations of motor function resulting from CP. The FIRST function of the OTR/COTA team in this process is to:

A. identify the most appropriate commercially available forms of assistive technology.

B. identify the abilities, needs, and life goals of the client.

C. select the appropriate method of accessing the technology.

D. modify the assistive technology device to meet the needs of the client.

144. Prior to discharging a client from the hospital, the OTR requests that the COTA instruct a patient in some quick and easy to learn stress management techniques. Which of the following should the COTA review FIRST?

A. Autogenic training

B. Meditation

C. Deep breathing and verbalization

D. Work simplification and energy conservation

145. The COTA is working with a child who has insufficient thumb opposition. This position makes it difficult for the child to write efficiently. The COTA recommends that the child practice opposition by:

A. placing a universal cuff on the child's hand.

B. using the pointer finger only when working on a keyboard.

C. using a weighted writing utensil holder.

D. pulling tiny objects out of clay.

146. An individual complains of perspiration, which is causing his resting hand splint to be uncomfortable. The BEST action for the COTA to take is to:

A. recommend putting talcum powder in the splint.

B. line the splint with moleskin.

C. fabricate a new resting hand splint with perforated material.

D. provide a stockinette sleeve for the individual to wear inside the splint.

147. A client with schizophrenia begins to experience hallucinations while participating in a life skills group led by a COTA. Which environmental strategy would be BEST to minimize the hallucinations?

A. Leave the person in the same environment.

B. Isolate the person completely from other people.

C. Move the person to a more stimulating environment.

D. Move the person to a quieter, less stimulating environment.

148. A second-grade child has a diagnosis of muscular dystrophy. The child operates a manual wheelchair, but his mobility is slow because of muscle weakness. The COTA should consider discussing a powered wheelchair with the OTR when the:

A. child starts junior high school and will be expected to switch classrooms several times daily.

B. child's speed over long distances becomes less than that of a walking person.

C. child's home can be made accessible for a power wheelchair.

D. child becomes unable to propel a manual wheelchair.

149. The spouse of a patient with a progressive disease has come into the OT department to learn how to help the spouse perform functional activities at home. The COTA should FIRST instruct the family member regarding:

A. methods for motivating the patient to perform ADLs.

B. techniques on how to analyze activities to solve problems.

C. methods used to provide cues to the patient.

D. techniques on how to perform activities safely.

150. An individual attending an adult day program has expressed interest in obtaining employment. In groups, however, the individual grabs tools from others, frequently acts out of turn, and has diffi-

culty accepting feedback. Participation in which one of the following interventions is MOST appropriate for addressing this individual's limitations and preparation for a work environment?

A. Operating the photocopy machine in a clerical group
B. Handing out trays and utensils in a food service group
C. Placing books back on the shelves in a library group
D. Balancing the books at the end of the day in a thrift store group

151. A first-grade child with a diagnosis of attention deficit disorder, hyperactivity type, is receiving OT to increase his attention span. Keeping this in mind, the COTA introduces a construction activity. When blocks were placed in front of the child, the child swept many of them onto the floor and started throwing the remaining ones around the room. How can the COTA MOST effectively restructure the activity to facilitate a successful experience for this child?

A. Use soft foam blocks.
B. Provide blocks of one color only.
C. Use interlocking blocks.
D. Present only a few blocks at a time.

152. A COTA is applying PNF techniques for weight shifting during an activity that requires an individual to use their right hand to remove groceries from a bag on the floor to the right. The MOST benefit would be gained from this activity by then placing the groceries:

A. on the counter directly in front.
B. on the counter to the left side.
C. in the upper cabinet to the right side.
D. in the upper cabinet to the left side.

153. A COTA is leading a discussion with a group of individuals who are diagnosed with major depression. The MOST helpful approach for the COTA to take is to:

A. be upbeat, positive, and cheerful when encouraging the individuals to discuss their feelings.
B. offer even-tempered acceptance, reflecting back what is heard without agreeing that the situation is hopeless.
C. remain silent and still while the individuals are describing their feelings.
D. allow the individuals to structure and lead the group discussion.

Effectiveness of Treatment and Discharge Planning

154. A child who has difficulty with visual perception of "position in space" will soon be discharged from an outpatient OT program. Of the following, which would be the BEST activity to recommend to the child's classroom teacher and parents?

A. Identifying letters on a distracting page
B. Finding geometric shapes scattered in a box
C. Following directions about objects located in front, in back, and to the side
D. Making judgments about moving through space

155. An individual with ALS swims three times a week to maximize strength and endurance. Initially able to swim for only 10 minutes, the individual is now able to swim 20 minutes without becoming fatigued. The NEXT step is to:

A. continue the program of swimming 20 minutes, three times a week.
B. decrease swimming frequency to two times a week.
C. increase swimming time to 25 minutes or to tolerance.
D. provide adaptive equipment that will enable the individual to swim using less energy.

156. A client with a history of anger self-control issues has met the goals of independently identifying stressors in his home and work life, which tend to provoke his anger, and identifying his typical behaviors when dealing with anger provoking situations. The COTA's NEXT action should be to:

A. begin instruction in anger management strategies, such as relaxation.
B. change the focus of treatment to developing self-assertiveness skills.
C. provide activities, such as hammering, that provide outlets for anger.
D. recommend discontinuation of services to the OTR.

157. Which of the following is the MOST important precaution to emphasize to parents when discharging a child with lower extremity paralysis as a result of myelomeningocele?

A. Practice regular skin inspection.

B. Avoid feeding the child chewy foods that may cause choking.

C. Monitor apnea episodes.

D. Avoid situations that can stimulate tactile defensiveness.

158. A 45-year-old client with COPD has the long-term goal of being able to shop independently for groceries. The client has achieved the short-term goal of going to a convenience store and purchasing three items. Which statement is the BEST revised short-term goal for this client?

A. Client will purchase 10 items at the supermarket with supervision.

B. Client will cook a one-dish meal with items purchased at the supermarket.

C. Client will identify food items needed for developing a shopping list.

D. Instruct client in energy conservation techniques that apply to grocery shopping.

159. A COTA is working on laundry skills with an adult with cognitive disabilities. Initially, the OT practitioner recommended that the group home staff work with the individual for 2 months on how to recognize when clothing is dirty and needs to be laundered. After 2 months, however, the individual continues to wear soiled garments. The OT practitioner determines that the individual is unable to recognize or judge when clothing is dirty. What is the NEXT step that should be taken to maximize the individual's independence in doing laundry?

A. Instruct the individual to wear clothes for 2 days and to then launder those items.

B. Assess the individual's ability to recognize dirty clothing.

C. Recommend that the individual take clothes for dry cleaning rather than wash them at home.

D. Recommend to the staff that they do the individual's laundry from now on.

160. Direct OT services are being discontinued for a student with attention deficit disorder, but consultation will be provided to help the child adjust to the new classroom. Which recommendation can the COTA make to help the teacher adapt the environment to promote optimal learning without affecting other students?

A. Use dim lighting and reduce glare by turning down lights.

B. Remove all posters and visual aids to reduce visual distractions.

C. Provide a screen to reduce peripheral visual stimuli.

D. Restructure classroom activities into a series of short-term tasks.

161. A patient with poor visual acuity is about to be discharged after completing a rehabilitation program following a total hip replacement. The MOST appropriate environmental adaptation to ensure that the client can go up and down stairs safely is:

A. installing a stair glide.

B. installing handrails on both sides of the steps.

C. marking the end of each step with high contrast tape.

D. instructing the patient to take only one step at a time when going up or down.

162. A COTA is working with an individual who has identified alcohol abuse as a contributing factor to the depression that he has been experiencing. At discharge, the MOST appropriate type of group to recommend to this individual is a(n):

A. advocacy group.

B. self-help group.

C. support group.

D. psychotherapy group.

163. A 12-year-old student will be discharged after receiving treatment for anxiety disorder. Which would be the MOST appropriate recommendation for an extracurricular school activity?

A. Competitive gymnastics team

B. Debating club

C. School newspaper

D. Basketball team

164. An individual with lower extremity paralysis uses a standard manual wheelchair and is ready to be discharged to home. During the home evaluation, the COTA notes that the entrance to the bathroom is 32 inches wide and the toilet is 15 inches high. Which of the following recommendations will BEST facilitate use of the bathroom for this individual?

A. Widen the doorway.

B. Raise the toilet.

C. Widen the doorway and raise the toilet.

D. Widen the doorway and lower the toilet.

165. An individual with Alzheimer's disease has difficulty following multiple-step instructions. Which method will the COTA instruct the caregiver to use when presenting instructions?

A. Give frequently repeated one- or two-step instructions.

B. Provide three-step instructions with gestures for demonstration.

C. Write instructions down for the individual that are over three steps.

D. Have individual verbally repeat instructions after the therapist gives them.

166. A COTA is formulating a home program of play activities for the parents of a child with developmental delay. The type of activities that would be BEST for development of symbolic play skills would be:

A. building blocks.

B. board games.

C. craft kits.

D. doll house and dress-up clothes.

167. A COTA has completed patient education with an individual who has just received a splint for carpal tunnel syndrome. When documenting this session, the COTA will indicate that the patient was instructed in precautions, splint wearing schedule, and care of a:

A. wrist cock-up splint.

B. thermoplastic splint.

C. resting hand splint.

D. dynamic MP flexion splint.

168. A patient who sustained a mild head injury is about to be discharged to his home and return to work. He is still having difficulty with memory, particularly remembering appointments and activities. External memory devices that the COTA could recommend to assist this patient would be:

A. visual imagery techniques.

B. calendars.

C. mnemonics.

D. repetition.

169. During OT treatment, a child has a seizure. The MOST important actions for the OT practitioner during the seizure are to:

A. check breathing and administer mouth-to-mouth resuscitation if necessary.

B. attempt to restrain the child's movements to prevent injury.

C. ease the child to a lying position, remove or pad nearby objects, and loosen clothing.

D. take no action except observation of the child.

170. A COTA in an acute care hospital is using the SOAP note format to document information about an individual with dementia. Which statement would the COTA place in the subjective section of the note?

A. The therapist will establish a daily self-feeding routine using verbal and physical cues to encourage the individual to open containers on the lunch tray.

B. The individual has been able to identify closed liquid beverage containers on the meal tray for four out of six presentations.

C. The individual is able to identify and drink liquids presented in cups without lids, but leaves beverages in closed containers untouched.

D. The individual asks for more beverages during meals, but appears surprised when the therapist indicates beverages in closed containers are on the meal tray.

171. An individual about to be discharged from an inpatient psychiatric unit asks, "when I apply for jobs, what should I put down when the application asks if you have been hospitalized in the past 6 months?" The therapist's response should include strategies that address:

A. developing assertiveness.

B. improving self-esteem.

C. anger management.

D. managing stigma.

172. A preteen with a diagnosis of spastic cerebral palsy is enjoying computer-assisted learning while making significant progress in written communication, but he complains of general fatigue, body aches, and eye strain. To adapt the computer activity to decrease fatigue, which aspect of the activity should the COTA consider first?

A. The time he spends at the computer

B. The size of the computer screen

C. The challenge level of the learning program

D. His control of the keyboard

173. **The COTA is instructing a carpenter recovering from a work injury in the proper use of body mechanics. Which of the following statements in the discharge note would MOST likely indicate that the patient was using proper body mechanics?**

    A. Patient worked a full day without becoming fatigued.
    B. Patient reinstalled a door without reinjury.
    C. Patient used power tools without reports of upper extremity pain.
    D. Patient was able to hammer continuously for a sustained period of time.

174. **A COTA needs to document the following statement, "patient states she is frightened by the anger she feels when doing ceramics." In which portion of a SOAP note would the COTA place this information?**

    A. Subjective section
    B. Objective section
    C. Assessment section
    D. Plan section

175. **A COTA is leading a discussion on relapse prevention for a group of clients about to be discharged. The MOST useful strategy for the COTA to stress for preventing relapse in persons with mental health disorders is to:**

    A. get adequate physical exercise.
    B. self-monitor signs of illness and seek help if signs occur.
    C. maintain personal hygiene.
    D. make life changes (e.g., new job, going to school).

176. **A patient with quadriplegia was unable to grasp a toothbrush with a built-up handle, using tenodesis, at the time of her initial evaluation. After working on upper extremity strengthening and grooming skills for 2 weeks, the COTA needs to determine the degree of progress that has been achieved in this area. The BEST way to determine progress using a functional method of evaluation, is for the COTA to:**

    A. measure the patient's grip strength with a goniometer.
    B. measure the patient's pinch strength with a pinch meter.
    C. assess the patient's ability to hold the toothbrush with a built-up handle.
    D. assess the patient's ability to hold the toothbrush using a universal cuff.

Occupational Therapy for Populations

177. **When a COTA is employed as an activities director in a nursing home, efforts should PRIMARILY be directed toward:**

    A. promoting ADL independence for as many residents as possible.
    B. insuring that services are reimbursable by Medicare when possible.
    C. individual assessment and intervention for occupational performance deficits.
    D. providing a variety of physical, creative, productive, and educational activities.

178. **The OT staff of a psychiatric hospital recognize the need to develop a transition program to help their clients with chronic mental illness successfully re-enter and remain in the community. Which of the following activities should come FIRST in a predischarge program for individuals who have experienced long-term hospitalization, and do not feel ready to leave the hospital?**

    A. Visit the day program the individual will be attending, and introduce the client to other clients and staff.
    B. Collaborate with clients on developing goals they need to achieve in order to live in the community successfully.
    C. Introduce and discuss concepts of community living, and give clients an opportunity to voice their concerns.
    D. Evaluate skills related to community living such as money management, personal safety, and self-care.

179. **A COTA is involved with a parenting skills group for teenage mothers who have HIV and for their children. Which of the following is MOST important when working with the mothers of infants?**

    A. Activities that promote mother-child communication and foster attachment
    B. Modeling and discussing appropriate disciplinary techniques
    C. Activities that promote language development and cognitive skills
    D. Peer interaction for both mothers and babies

180. **The administrator of an assisted living facility has asked a COTA to help implement programming that will decrease the number of residents needing to move from the ALF to nursing homes. The**

MOST important area for the COTA to address is:

A. adaptive equipment needs.
B. fall prevention.
C. meaningful use of leisure time.
D. balancing work, leisure, and rest.

181. An OT practitioner is planning to provide a program to address the needs of persons with Alzheimer's disease, and their families, as part of a hospital outreach program. One of the areas of intervention which would be MOST beneficial to maintaining safety and supporting function at home in the advanced stages of Alzheimer's is:

A. strength and endurance activities.
B. cognitive rehabilitation techniques.
C. environmental modification.
D. assertiveness skills.

182. An OT practitioner working for the school system has identified a general need to enhance the fine coordination skills of elementary school students to facilitate better writing skills. The BEST intervention to treat this population would be to:

A. screen students for writing problems, and provide in-depth assessment of those identified.
B. provide remedial activities for those students identified as having fine coordination deficits.
C. recommend activities to develop fine coordination that teachers can incorporate into classroom programming.
D. recommend additional OT staff to provide direct services for students.

183. An OT practitioner is working to reduce the application of restraints for the population of a long-term care facility. The MOST appropriate form of intervention for the OT practitioner to provide is:

A. identifying legal issues related to restraint reduction.
B. providing staff education, recommendations, and support for restraint alternatives.
C. investigating incidents of resident abuse related to restraint reduction.
D. assessing the level of risk and liability involved with restraint use.

184. Which of the following is the MOST appropriate emphasis of a cooking group for young women with eating disorders?

A. Increasing knowledge of a variety of weight-loss techniques
B. Information on the caloric content of different foods
C. Preparing and consuming nutritional and normal-size portions of food
D. Preparing healthy and appealing-looking meals

185. Which of the following activities would be MOST appropriate for vocational skills training for high school students with severe learning disabilities?

A. Stocking the shelves at a local grocery
B. Packaging items in a local sheltered workshop
C. Cleaning the school cafeteria after lunch
D. Reading help wanted ads and role playing interviews

186. An OT practitioner wishes to assess the results of a life skills training program provided to individuals at a shelter for abused women. Which of the following methods would be the MOST comprehensive method for obtaining this information?

A. Final evaluation of each client involved
B. Client satisfaction survey
C. Program evaluation
D. Utilization review

Service Management

187. An individual has accepted his first job as a COTA. What would be the most appropriate level of supervision for this individual?

A. Daily, direct contact at the site of work
B. Direct contact with supervision available on an as needed basis, at least once a month
C. Minimal supervision provided on an as needed basis, and it may be less than once a month
D. Direct contact at least every seven days at the site of work

188. An OT practitioner is leading a grooming group for female clients in a psychosocial treatment setting. Which of the following options BEST complies with universal precautions?

A. Use disposable cotton swabs and have clients bring their own cosmetics.

B. Use disposable gloves when combing client's hair.

C. Wash and dry makeup brushes between uses.

D. Avoid bringing cosmetics in glass containers to the group.

189. **An OTR with expertise in hand rehabilitation is assessing a COTA's service competency in hand function assessment. At what point is service competency established?**

A. When the COTA consistently obtains the same results as the OTR

B. After the COTA passes the NBCOT examination

C. When the COTA has obtained a specified number of continuing education credits in hand rehabilitation

D. After the COTA has practiced for a minimum number of years, as specified by state licensure

190. **An OT practitioner providing services to a community mental health program has been asked to examine the effectiveness of the OT groups that have been provided over the past 6 months. Which of the following procedures should be used to accomplish this goal?**

A. Quality assurance

B. Peer review

C. Utilization review

D. Program evaluation

191. **One week after a COTA begins a new job, half of the OT department is out with the flu, including the COTA's supervisor. The COTA observes an aide carrying out an ADL training session with a patient who is scheduled for discharge the next day. Which of the following actions should the COTA take?**

A. Allow the aide to finish so the patient will be prepared for discharge.

B. Take over the session and terminate the aide.

C. Bring the issue to the attention of the facility administrator.

D. Discuss the observations with an OTR who is present.

192. **A COTA has expressed interest in taking on some administrative duties in an OT department. Which of the following du-**
ties would be MOST appropriate for the COTA to assume?

A. Development of a quality assurance program

B. Supervision of entry-level OTRs and COTAs

C. Supervision of noncertified personnel

D. Development of marketing strategies to promote a new program

193. **A COTA is preparing to lead a cooking group. He is new to the facility, and uncertain of the facility's policies and procedures relating to food storage and handling. Which of the following actions would be MOST appropriate for the COTA to take?**

A. Read the facility's infection control plan.

B. Contact the dietary department for clarification.

C. Read the facility's risk management plan.

D. Use only canned food for the group activity this time.

194. **During a group community re-entry outing, one individual complains of chest pain. The COTA monitors the client's heart rate and blood pressure. The client's resting heart rate is 120 bpm, and blood pressure is 220/180 mm Hg. The MOST appropriate action for the COTA to take is to:**

A. continue the community re-entry outing.

B. immediately return the patients to the hospital.

C. help the patient lie down and wait until his vital signs return to normal.

D. call 911.

195. **While documenting the week's OT sessions in an individual's chart, a COTA notices that a progress note from 2 weeks ago was not completed. The COTA recalls providing treatment that week and how the patient responded. The ONLY appropriate action for the COTA to take is to:**

A. complete the note using the original date.

B. document services provided, and date the note as a late entry.

C. leave the chart as is without documenting services provided.

D. write a brief note stating that documentation was not completed for the specified dates.

196. **A COTA recently hired by a hand rehabilitation center is required, as part of the**

job description, to perform paraffin treatments with designated patients. Which of the following actions must the practitioner take in order to comply with this requirement?

A. Obtain the necessary theoretical and technical background on paraffin treatment.
B. Practice providing paraffin baths with an experienced OTR present for an adequate period of time.
C. Ensure that an experienced OTR is on-site whenever paraffin is used.
D. Demonstrate service competency in the use of paraffin.

Professional Practice

197. An instructor from a local nursing school has asked a COTA to speak about OT to a class of first year nursing students. The COTA feels uncertain about giving the lecture because of a lack of resources. The MOST appropriate action for the COTA to take is to:

A. recommend that the nursing course instructor call AOTA and obtain public relations information to share with the nursing students.
B. decline to do the in-service, but send information to the instructor.
C. decline to do the in-service and find an OTR to do the lecture.
D. use brochures, posters, videotapes, and films available from the AOTA to enhance the presentation.

198. An OT practitioner is asked by administration to complete billing early by projecting therapy time for patients that are yet to be seen. One of these patients later refuses therapy because of medical illness. What is the BEST course of action to take?

A. Contact administration to let them know of the unforeseen change in service delivery and make appropriate adjustments to billing.

B. Leave the billing "as is", but document that services were attempted but not provided.
C. Strongly encourage the patient to attempt to participate in treatment and consider the associated time and effort as billable activity.
D. Make no changes to billing, but try to make the time up during subsequent treatment sessions.

199. A COTA working with an elderly client in a skilled nursing facility determines that the client appears to have met all of her goals. The client is not scheduled for discharge until the following week. The MOST appropriate plan of action is for the COTA to:

A. discharge the client from therapy.
B. continue to see the client for therapy until otherwise instructed by the OT.
C. collaborate with the OTR to determine discharge options and actions.
D. place the client on "hold" until the anticipated date of discharge.

200. An OT practitioner spends 15 minutes reviewing a new patient's chart and talking to the nurse, who indicates that the patient is preoccupied with finances. As the OT practitioner enters the room, the patient states that he does not want to be seen by any of the therapists because his insurance has run out and he cannot afford to pay for the treatment. Which of the following actions would be MOST appropriate for the OT practitioner to take?

A. Treat the individual per the physician's order and notify the nurse that the man's preoccupation with finances continues.
B. Based on his refusal, do not treat the individual and document the interaction in the chart.
C. Treat the individual, but do not charge or document the services.
D. Do not treat the individual and only charge for the time spent completing the chart review.

ANSWERS FOR SIMULATION EXAMINATION 1

1. (A) age appropriate. The child being observed is performing dressing activity which is age appropriate for a 5-year-old child. A typical child at this age can dress unsupervised and is able to tie and untie knots, but generally does not know how to tie a bow independently. See reference: Case-Smith (ed): Shepherd, J: Self-care and adaptations for independent living.

2. (A) Thumb against the tip of the index finger. The correct position for tip pinch is the thumb against the tip of the index finger. The thumb against the side of the index finger (answer B) describes the position for lateral pinch. The thumb against the tips of the index and middle fingers (answer C) describes the test position for three-jaw chuck, or palmar pinch. The thumb against the tips of all the fingers (answer D) is not a standard test position. See reference: Trombly (ed): Trombly, CA: Evaluation of biomechanical and physiological aspects of motor performance.

3. (A) assist with skill development in the areas of leisure, self-expression, and ADLs. In general, the areas of focus with OT intervention for individuals identified with substance abuse problems are alternative leisure time use, improved expression of feelings, and the acquiring of social and occupational roles. The approach described in answer B addresses the cognitive disability frame of reference approach. Answers C and D may address specific needs of the patient, but not the overall needs of this population. See reference: Early: Understanding psychiatric diagnosis: The DSM-IV.

4. (A) a developmental delay. Typically developing children (answer C) should be able to sit unsupported for several minutes by the age of 8 to 9 months; therefore, this child demonstrates delayed development (answer A). The ability to sit while propped forward on his arms indicates primitive reflexes have been integrated (answer B). Sitting unsupported earlier than 8 months could indicate advanced development (answer D). See reference: Case-Smith (ed): Case-Smith, J: Development of childhood occupations.

5. (C) Tip. Tip prehension is accomplished by flexing the IP joint of the thumb, and the PIP and DIP joints of the finger, and bringing the tips of the thumb and finger together. This type of prehension is used to pick up objects such as a pin, nail, or coin. Lateral prehension (answer A) is formed by positioning the pad of the thumb against the radial side of the finger. This prehension pattern is used for holding a pen, utensil, or key. Palmar prehension (answer B), also known as three-jaw chuck (answer D), is formed by positioning the thumb in opposition to the tips of the index and middle fingers, forming a pad-to-pad opposition. This form of prehension is commonly used to

lift objects from a flat surface and to tie a shoelace. See reference: Pedretti and Early (eds): Belkin, J and Yasuda L: Orthotics.

6. (C) ask the questions as they are stated on the interview sheet. A structured interview requires following the procedure, order, and wording of the questions to be asked. Answers A, B, and D are appropriate for semistructured interviews (e.g., in pursuit of more details and information). See reference: Early: Data collection and evaluation.

7. (C) At age level. At 3 years of age, a child is expected to know when he or she has to use the toilet and be able to get on and off the toilet. Three-year-old children may need assistance to cleanse themselves effectively and to manage fasteners or difficult clothing. Complete independence in using the toilet (answer D) is usually achieved by the age of 4 to 5 years. By the age of 2 years (answer B), most children have daytime control over elimination, with occasional accidents, so they still need to be reminded to go to the toilet. One-year-old infants (answer A) indicate discomfort when wet or soiled. See reference: Case-Smith (ed): Shepherd, J: Self care and adaptations for independent living.

8. (D) endurance. A deficit in endurance is demonstrated by the individual's inability to sustain cardiac, pulmonary, and musculoskeletal exertion for the duration of the activity. Answer A, a deficit in postural control, would be correct if the client had been unable to maintain his balance while putting on the shirt. A deficit in muscle tone (answer B) would have been evident if the client had demonstrated spasticity while putting on the shirt. Inability to push his arms through the resistance created by the shirt sleeve would demonstrate a deficit in strength (answer C). See reference: AOTA: Uniform Terminology for Occupational Therapy, ed 3.

9. (D) distractibility. Distractibility involves losing one's focus because of other stimuli. Memory (answer A) is the ability to recall knowledge and past events. Problems with spatial operations (answer B) are generally observed when individuals attempt to fit objects into specific spaces. Generalization of learning (answer C) may be observed by asking the client to use existing knowledge in a new situation. See reference: Early: Responding to symptoms and behaviors.

10. (D) determine the need for further evaluation. The purpose of screening is to determine whether further assessments are needed and, if so, which tests would be appropriate for that child. A screening test is not designed for planning programs (answer C) or consultation (answer A), and they do not test any skills (answer B) in a comprehensive way. See reference: Solomon (ed): Peralta,

AM and Kramer, P: General treatment considerations.

11. (C) visual agnosia. Visual agnosia is the inability to recognize common objects and demonstrate their use in an activity. Apraxia (answer A) is the inability to perform purposeful movement on command. A person with alexia (answer D) is unable to understand written language. Stereognosis (answer B) is the ability to identify an object by manipulating it with the fingers without seeing it. See reference: Trombly (ed): Quintana, L: Evaluation of perception and cognition.

12. (C) provide a summary of observations of the patient's behavior, including what the patient said and did during the interview. An observation summary should present a concise and accurate picture of what happened so that the OTR can understand almost as well as if they were present during the interview. It is a summary, and should not include extensive descriptions (answer A) or interpretations of the interview (answer D). A treatment plan (answer B) should be developed collaboratively with the OTR. See reference: Early: Data collection and evaluation.

13. (A) ADHD. This behavior exemplifies the excessive fidgeting and restlessness, inattention, and impulsiveness characteristic of ADHD. Although some of the symptoms of overactivity and impulsiveness are part of a mood disorder of the manic type (answer B), there are also usually symptoms of grandiosity and inflated self-esteem. A child with a conduct disorder (answer C) would exhibit interference with the basic rights of other children or societal rules. A child with anxiety disorder (answer D) would show signs of uneasiness, apprehension, or dread associated with anticipation of danger. See reference: Neistadt and Crepeau (eds): Florey, L: Psychosocial dysfunction in childhood and adolescence.

14. (B) left unilateral neglect. This is the inability to respond or orient to perceptions from the left side of the body. Evidenced as left unilateral neglect (answer B), this deficit is also apparent in the draw-a-man test, flower-copying test, house test, and completing a human figure or face puzzle. Unilateral neglect is contralateral to the side of a brain lesion, therefore, left unilateral neglect would result from right-sided brain damage. Left neglect occurs most commonly in right hemisphere lesions. A cataract (answer C) would cause a visual impairment with detail on both sides of a page. Bitemporal hemianopia (hemianopia is also referred to as hemianopsia), also known as "tunnel vision," occurs when the individual's peripheral vision lost (answer A). The individual would still be able to cross midline with cataracts or bitemporal hemianopia (answer D). A right neglect would not see the right side, and this type of patient would draw all the figures on the left side of the page. Visuospatial deficits are an important factor

influencing functional independence outcomes. Visuospatial ability should be taken into account when establishing treatment goals as well as during discharge planning. See reference: Trombly (ed): Quintana, L: Evaluation of perception and cognition.

15. (B) emotional lability. Emotional lability is the rapid shifting of moods. Emotional lability may be one of the symptoms observed in individuals experiencing mania (answer A). Paranoia (answer C) describes enduring beliefs about being harmed. Denial (answer D) is not acknowledging the presence of information. See reference: Early: Responding to symptoms and behaviors.

16. (B) communication, self-care, and social skills. Children with moderate mental retardation are likely to require some support for ADLs and IADLs, and can usually communicate either verbally or nonverbally. They are likely to have deficits in the areas of academic performance, communication, self-care, and social skills. Individuals with profound mental retardation are dependent on others for nearly all their needs, and often have neuromuscular, orthopedic, or behavioral deficits. Evaluation of these individuals should focus on positioning and communication skills (answer A). Individuals with mild mental retardation have the potential for independence in ADLs and IADLs (answer C), may achieve academic performance at the third to seventh grade level, and may eventually obtain employment. Individuals with severe mental retardation may be able to learn habitual activities, such as feeding and personal hygiene (answer D). Functional potential is often determined by physical limitations. They may learn to communicate verbally or nonverbally, and will require significant support to engage in most tasks. See reference: Solomon (ed): Newman, D: Mental retardation.

17. (C) steps, width of doorways, and threshold heights. The first area of evaluation would be the steps, width of doorways, and presence and height of door thresholds to determine whether the wheelchair user will be able to enter or exit interior spaces in the wheelchair or whether structural modifications are required. Answers A, B, and D reflect areas that will also need to be evaluated, however, they are not as critical to initial interior access. See reference: Pedretti and Early (eds): Foti, D: Activities of daily living.

18. (D) rationalization. Making excuses for, or justifying, the behavior of others that is generally considered to be unacceptable, is called rationalization. Identification (answer A) occurs when one takes on the characteristics of another person. Projection (answer B) is the blaming of other people for performing the behaviors. Denial (answer C) is refusing to acknowledge that the behavior occurred. See reference: Christiansen and Baum (eds): Bonder, B: Coping with psychological and emotional challenges.

19. (C) Constructional. Constructional play involves building and creating things. It is in this area of play that children develop a sense of mastery and problem-solving skills. Sensorimotor play (answer A) generally develops a child's body awareness and sensory experience. Imaginary play (answer B) involves manipulating people and objects in fantasy as a prelude to dealing with reality. Game play (answer D) requires the ability to learn and apply rules in play. See reference: Kramer and Hinojosa (eds): Luebben, AJ, Hinojosa, J, and Kramer, P: Legitimate tools of pediatric occupational therapy.

20. (A) work locks and latches on doors and windows. The ability to manipulate the locks and latches is a safety concern because the individual may be unable to open them to let family members into the home or close them to keep intruders from entering. Built-up handles (answer B), energy conservation techniques (answer C), and adaptations to clothing fasteners (answer D) are not safety issues. See reference: Trombly (ed): Feinberg, JR and Trombly, CA: Arthritis.

21. (A) Functional assessment of work-related skills, such as carrying and opening cartons and shelving items. Observation of the individual performing actual job responsibilities will provide more objective and measurable information about the individual's strengths and weaknesses in the area of job performance than a verbal interview (answer C) or task evaluation (answer D). Although a "dirty" medium may be contraindicated when initially working with an individual with OCD of the washing type, it would not be an issue for this individual because his OCD is of the checking type. There is nothing to indicate the individual has cognitive deficits, therefore a cognitive evaluation (answer B) would not be indicated. See reference: Early: Data collection and evaluation.

22. (A) Interview. Interviews provide "an opportunity for the parents to identify their values and priorities about the skills being evaluated by the therapist" (p. 207). Open-ended questions are best for eliciting information regarding the family's feelings about the intervention. Answers B, C, and D are structured observation methods, through which information on specific skills or functional levels is collected. See reference: Case-Smith (ed): Stewart, KB: Purposes, processes, and methods of evaluation.

23. (B) Combing the hair. An individual normally abducts and externally rotates the shoulder to comb his or her hair; therefore, the individual is more likely to have difficulty in this area than any of the others. Shoulder abduction is not required for buttoning a shirt (answer A) or tying a shoe (answer D). Tucking in a shirt in the back (answer C) requires shoulder abduction and internal rotation. Tying shoelaces (answer D) is less dependent on shoulder motion than

on hip and spine flexibility. See reference: Pedretti and Early (eds): Foti, D: Activities of daily living.

24. (B) Obtain as much information as possible from the chart. By reviewing the individual's medical records before the interview, the COTA can determine what information has already been obtained. This will enable the COTA to make the best use of the available time, and to avoid asking the individual to answer the same questions twice. With such a limited attention span, it would probably be more efficient to schedule two 15-minute sessions rather than one 30-minute session (answer A). Answers C and D are both essential to good interview technique, but would occur at the time of the actual interview, after collecting data from the chart. See reference: Early: Data collection and evaluation.

25. (C) the cultural context and family interaction patterns. Cultural expectations may determine behavior standards and the expression of family roles. Continued feeding of a young child with a handicap may be the expression of nurturing and caring. Such an expression may be viewed as more important than the promotion of independence and self-reliance. Answers A, B, and D may be valid issues as well, but should be addressed after the OT practitioner has familiarized himself or herself with the cultural and familial context of the feeding process. See reference: Case-Smith (ed): Case-Smith, J and Humphry, R: Feeding intervention. Shepherd, J: Self care and adaptations for independent living.

26. (B) distance from the fingertip to the distal palmar crease with the hand in a fist. The distance from the fingertip to the distal palmar crease with the hand fisted may be measured in either inches or centimeters. This measures how close the fingertip comes to the palm. A person who has full flexion would have a measurement of zero. Answers A and C are incorrect as actively or passively measuring the flexion at each joint and totaling them are measurements taken with a goniometer and recorded in degrees. Answer D, measuring the distance between the tip of the thumb and the fourth phalanx, is incorrect because it is a measurement of opposition. See reference: Hunter, Schneider, Mackin, and Bell (eds): Cambridge, C: Range of motion measurements of the hand.

27. (B) In a written report. The OTR can read the written report at her leisure. Confidential information about an individual must be respected by OT practitioners and should not be discussed in public places (answer C). A phone call (answer A) and a discussion in the OT office (answer D) would both require time the OTR does not have available. See reference: Early: Data collection and evaluation.

28. (D) apply the stimuli to the uninvolved area proximally to distally in a random pattern. The general guidelines for sensation testing are that the person's vision should be occluded, the stimuli should be randomly applied intermingled with false stimuli, a practice trial should be performed before the test, and the unaffected side or area should be tested before the affected side or area. Also, the amount of time a person has to respond should be established. See reference: Trombly (ed): Bentzel, K: Evaluation of sensation.

29. (D) at the midrange of the joint. Proprioception (or position sense) is demonstrated when an OT practitioner passively positions the joint being tested and the individual is able to imitate the position with the opposite extremity. The joint should not be moved through range to an extent that would elicit a stretch or pain response (answers A and B), which would be at the end ranges of the joint. Movement should be at a rate of approximately 10 degrees per second to prevent the stretch reflex from being elicited. The end points of the range (answer C) are used as the starting positions from which proprioception testing is initiated, because it is in these positions that the stretch or pain response would occur. See reference: Trombly (ed): Bentzel, K: Evaluation of sensation.

30. (A) observe the individual's body language during group sessions. By observing an individual's body language for behaviors such as fidgeting, nail biting, toe tapping, etc., the COTA can determine whether an individual is experiencing anxiety during the group activity. Completion of a questionnaire (answer B) and feedback from group members (answer C) may not be practical or reliable alternatives for an individual with cognitive deficits. Answer D is an adaptive strategy, not a method for assessing anxiety. See reference: Early: Responding to symptoms and behaviors.

31. (C) observation of play and hand function. The observation of play and hand function is the most appropriate way to obtain assessment information during infancy and preschool ages. "Much of the assessment, during infancy and preschool, centers around observation of play and hand function" (p. 609). Answers A, B, and D are all appropriate choices after the child is old enough for formal assessment. See reference: Neistadt and Crepeau (eds): Atkins, J: Orthopedic and musculoskeletal problems in children.

32. (C) fair minus (3-). The definition of fair minus (3-) is the grade given when an individual moves a part through incomplete range of motion (< 50%) against gravity, or through complete range of motion with gravity eliminated against slight resistance. A grade of good (4), answer A, indicates ability to move through full range of motion against gravity and to take moderate resistance. A fair grade (3), answer B, would be the ability to move through the full range of motion against gravity but not take any additional resistance. A grade of poor plus (2+), an-

swer D, would move through full range of motion with gravity eliminated and take minimal resistance before suddenly relaxing. See reference: Trombly (ed): Trombly, CA: Evaluation of biomechanical and physiological aspects of motor performance.

33. (D) role performance. Role performance is "identifying, maintaining, and balancing functions one assumes or acquires in society (e.g., worker, student, parent, friend, religious participant)" (p. 462). This individual is having difficulty balancing the roles of worker and mother, and is feeling stressed and conflicted. This stress may result in difficulty maintaining attention (answer B). Evaluation by an OT could include assessment of parenting and assertiveness skills (answers A and C) to determine if these are areas of need, and, if so, interventions could be designed to address these areas to support successful role performance. See reference: Early: Psychosocial skills and psychological components.

34. (C) Weight-bearing on hands. Weight-bearing on hands (answer C) is the only activity that will facilitate hand function in the preparation phase. Weight-bearing on the hands gives deep pressure to the surface of the hand. It facilitates wrist and arm extension, as well as shoulder cocontraction, to prepare the arm for reach, and stabilization of the hand for grasping. Answers A, B, and C provide different types of grasp activities that could be used as therapy. See reference: Case-Smith (ed): Exner, CE: Development of hand skills.

35. (C) texture of the cords she will be using. Coarse materials like jute may shred and give splinters or injure the skin on hands and fingers. This is particularly important for individuals with diabetes who frequently have poor sensation and circulation in their extremities. Skin damage must be avoided because healing is compromised. The length of the cord (answer A) would be significant for an individual with limited range of motion. The thickness of the cord (answer B) would be significant for an individual with limited hand function. The type of surface the individual stands on (answer D) would be important to an individual with back pain. See reference: Reed and Sanderson (eds): Diabetes mellitus—type II.

36. (B) the client will use facial expressions and gestures that are consistent with stated emotions during assertive, passive, and aggressive role-play situations. Self-expression is the use of a variety of styles and skills to express thoughts, feelings, and needs. It is also the ability to vary one's expressions, thoughts, feelings, and needs. Being able to vary one's expression during role playing of three different styles of expressing feelings is an example of this. Identifying pleasurable activities (answer A) will help to develop interests. Recognition of one's behaviors and consequences (answer C) relates to self-control. Identifying one's own assets and limitations (answer D) is related to self-concept. See reference: AOTA: Uniform Terminology for Occupational Therapy, ed 3.

37. (D) adapted teaching techniques. Answer D is correct because a child with this type of disability characteristically has learning problems that require teaching methods such as "chaining" or behavior modification. Answers A, B, and C are of secondary importance, because physical coordination may be impaired, or there may be other physical limitations, such as abnormal muscle tone or significant problems with balance could also be present. These additional problems may require adaptive equipment, clothing, or techniques. However, all aspects of dressing depend on the child's ability to learn procedures of dressing; therefore, it is necessary to consider task analysis and teaching approach first. See reference: Case-Smith (ed): Shepherd, J: Self-care and adaptations for independent living.

38. (C) Ulnar styloid, distal head of radius, and thumb CMC joint. The ulnar styloid, distal head of the radius, and thumb CMC joints are the most common sites for pressure because of their overt bony prominences. Answers A, B, and D are also areas that could potentially be susceptible to skin breakdown, but are not primary sites of pressure when fabricating a resting pan splint. See reference: Pedretti and Early (eds): Belkin, J and Yasada, L: Orthotics.

39. (C) applying grout to a tile trivet and waiting for it to dry. Applying grout to a tile trivet and waiting for it to dry (answer C) provides a variety of opportunities for therapeutic gains. The process of grouting a tile trivet involves covering the individual's tile design with grout mixture, which is a messy step. The individual then sees that the tile pattern is emphasized with the addition of the grout. Waiting for the grout to dry requires an individual to delay gratification. Answer A, working in a group of three, would address social and interpersonal interaction skills, but not the goals related to experiencing success and delaying gratification. Answer C, selecting the design pattern, and answer D, encouraging clean-up, would also address other goals. See reference: Neistadt and Crepeau (eds): Crepeau: Activity analysis, a way of thinking about occupational performance.

40. (B) Let the child sit at the front of the bus and use a tape player with earphones. A child who is seated in the front of the bus will experience less jostling by peers, resulting in less tactile and visual stimulation. Also, the earphones will reduce auditory overload. The method described in answer B addresses the underlying problem of the child's low tolerance for sensory stimulation. Answers A, C, and D are behavioral management techniques that do not take the child's hypersensitivity into account. See reference: Case-Smith (ed): Cronin, AF: Psychosocial and emotional domains.

41. (B) Positioning, adaptive equipment, and patient education. Positioning and adaptive equipment are necessary to maintain the integrity of the musculoskeletal system and to prevent deformity. Patient education about the disease and ways of dealing with its effects can also be started at this stage. Resistive exercises (answer A) are not appropriate if there is joint swelling and inflammation, and are always used cautiously with individuals with RA because of the potential for tissue damage. Discharge planning would be more relevant at a later time (answer C). Surgical intervention (answer D) would not be needed in the early stages of rheumatoid arthritis. It may be offered later as a corrective measure for long-standing deformities. See reference: Pedretti and Early (eds): Buckner, WS: Arthritis.

42. (A) restore and maintain performance of self-chosen occupations that support performance of valued occupational roles. The individual's depression is likely to be in reaction to the AIDS disease and major loss of functioning at stage 4. Stage 4 of AIDS generally means severe physical and neurologic changes. Because the change of function can be broad, answer A is the most comprehensive approach. Answers B and C are too restrictive to be a "major focus." Answer D, restoration of work, is typically unrealistic at stage 4 of AIDS. See reference: Neistadt and Crepeau (eds): Pizzi, M and Burkhardt, A: Occupational therapy for adults with immunological diseases.

43. (C) Biomechanical. According to Colangelo, "The biomechanical frame of reference is applied when a person cannot maintain posture through appropriate automatic muscle activity because of neuromuscular or musculoskeletal dysfunction" (p. 257). This child's physical status has changed with decreasing postural control. Adaptive support devices need to be considered, and a biomechanical frame of reference provides this approach. Answer A is not correct because the neurodevelopmental treatment frame of reference is concerned with improving posture and movement, and supportive equipment is prescribed for that purpose. Answer B is not correct because the sensory integration frame of reference is concerned with sensory input in relation to posture and movement in children with sensory integration disorders, whereas Duchenne's disease is a neuromuscular disorder. Answer D is not correct because the visual perceptual frame of reference is concerned with guiding and compensating for visual perceptual problems, not postural delays. See reference: Kramer and Hinojosa (eds): Colangelo, CA: Biomechanical frame of reference.

44. (D) Playing balloon volleyball. An activity such as balloon volleyball may be graded for improving strength by adding resistance to the arm in the form of weights. Endurance may be improved by adding more repetitions of the movement. Raising the height of the net can increase the range of motion required. Blowing up and tying balloons (answer A), and painting faces on balloons (answer B) are primarily fine motor activities. An individual who throws darts at balloons (answer C) would be able to increase the resistance needed for shoulder strengthening by adding weight to the arms or using balloons with thicker rubber. However, this activity is less suitable to increase the number of repetitions, because the repeated loud noise associated with bursting the balloons would be annoying. See reference: Pedretti and Early (eds): Breines, E: Therapeutic occupations and modalities.

45. (D) To arrive at work on time consistently. Time management mandates the importance to "recognize one's values and priorities, structure a daily routine, schedule one's time, and organize tasks efficiently" (p. 467). Answers A, B, and C are ways of coping with being late, not strategies for the time management goal of being on time. See reference: Early: Psychosocial skills and psychological components.

46. (D) Reinforcement of competence. According to Erikson, an 8-year-old child is usually at the stage of industry versus inferiority, during which time he or she develops a sense of competency. For a client who is expected to lose motor function gradually, a treatment plan that will provide an ongoing sense of competence (possibly in other areas) is especially relevant. Answers A, B, and C describe other developmental issues identified by Erikson that are typically achieved at other ages: basic trust (answer A) in infancy; initiative (answer B) during the toddler years; and self-identity (answer C) during adolescence. See reference: Case-Smith (ed): Law, M, Missiuna, C, Pollock, N, and Stewart, D: Foundations of occupational therapy practice with children.

47. (C) A client with a C6 injury. An individual with C6 quadriplegia has some use of the abductor pollicis longus, extensor pollicis longus, extensor digitorum communis, and extensor carpi ulnaris. The extensor tone of the muscles in conjunction with the splint will operate the power for prehension force. Individuals with CI or C3 injuries (answers A and B) have higher level lesions and lack the wrist extension strength needed to operate the wrist-driven flexor hinge splint. An individual with a T1 injury (answer D) is able to grasp and manipulate utensils without difficulty or need for assistance. See reference: Trombly (ed): Hollar, LD: Spinal cord injury.

48. (A) Identify social opportunities using a local phone book. With the interest checklist already completed, the COTA can help the individual identify one or two choices that promote socialization in the community. The COTA can coach the individual on pertinent questions to ask (e.g., hours, cost, directions) and help the individual make these calls prior to discharge. While craft and cooking books (answers B and D) are useful materials to help improve new or existing skills, cooking and craft activities are fairly isolating in nature. A personal log (answer C) is a good way to encourage self-expression, but would not be helpful in developing outlets for socialization. See reference: Early: Leisure skills.

49. (B) ability to grade movement. The grading of movement goal (answer B) best addresses the difficulty with control of the midrange of a movement pattern (common in children with athetosis). Answer A is incorrect, because this goal would be appropriate for a child who cannot break up a flexion or extension pattern during a movement. Answer C is not correct, because this goal is appropriate for a child who has difficulty with an arm or hand movement being too fast or too slow (graded movements are also too fast). Answer D is also incorrect, because this goal is appropriate for a child who has difficulty bringing both arms to midline and using them effectively together. See reference: Case-Smith (ed): Exner, CE: Development of hand skills.

50. (A) soft to hard to rough. The desensitization process involves applying a sequence of graded texture and force stimuli to the skin to reduce tactile hypersensitivity. Texture begins with soft, progresses to hard, and moves to rough stimuli. Answer B is incorrect because the force of the stimuli begins at the level of touch, progresses to rub, and moves to tapping as tolerance for sensation increases. Light, medium, and heavy (answer C) do not specify what the texture and force of the stimuli would be during training. Answer D is incorrect because a person with hypersensitivity would be unable to tolerate stimuli beginning with a rough texture. See reference: Trombly (ed): Bentzel, K: Remediating sensory impairment.

51. (D) Encourage group members to share similar experiences and reactions with each other. Answer D is a strategy designed to develop cohesiveness among members. Many people have reported that recognizing one's similarities with other people is a very valuable experience. Answers A and C are designed to impart information. Answer B is an example of catharsis, which may not be helpful to all members. Moreover, the OT practitioner must be aware of, and understand, the precautions necessary for the use of catharsis. See reference: Early: Group concepts and techniques.

52. (C) demonstrates any reliable, controlled movement. As long as the child can produce any reliable, controlled movement, switches can be adapted to meet positioning and mobility needs. Accurate reach and pointing (answer B) or isolated finger control (answer D) are not necessary to use simple pressure switches. An upright sitting position (answer A) would not be required if the child needed to be positioned in a reclining or sidelying position. See reference: Case-Smith (ed): Swinth, Y: Assistive technology: Computers and augmentative communication.

53. (A) Meal preparation techniques using a wheelchair. As the disease progresses, individuals with ALS lose the strength required for ambulation and, therefore, begin to use wheelchairs. The development of meal preparation skills using a wheelchair, such as transportation of items, addressing work heights, using adaptive equipment (answer A encompasses answer B), and safety issues, is therefore the best answer. Gradually increasing standing tolerance (answer C) is not appropriate for this individual because motoric function will continue to deteriorate. Developing competence in preparing cold meals before advancing to hot meals (answer D) is more appropriate for individuals with cognitive or perceptual deficits. See reference: Dutton: Rehabilitation postulates regarding intervention.

54. (C) use simple and highly structured activities. Projective media, isolation, and discussing delusions are all contraindicated for people with schizophrenia. Projective activities (answer A) are most useful for encouraging expression of feelings. It may be appropriate to separate individuals (answer B) who are violent or unable to tolerate the presence of others nearby, but this would not be part of the regular group routine. Discussing delusions (answer D) is undesirable because it is likely to reinforce them. See reference: Early: Responding to symptoms and behaviors.

55. (C) Provide enjoyable activities in a safe and accepting environment. Children who learn to enjoy activities alone will be more likely to cooperate with peers in a group activity. It is unlikely that the child will initiate and develop social interaction in an environment that inhibits independence (answer A). Children with peer interaction problems need to be taught some basic social skills (unlike answer B) in order to increase successful peer interaction. Children will more likely learn and accept rules and limits established by their group than by an authority figure (answer D). See reference: Kramer and Hinojosa (eds): Olson, LJ: Psychosocial frame of reference.

56. (C) client will demonstrate appropriate hip precautions. The ability to stand for 10 minutes (answer A) or to increase hip flexion to 90 degrees (answer B) is not necessary for independence in dressing. Use of appropriate hip precautions (answer C), however, is mandatory. Energy-conservation techniques (answer D) are appropriate for individuals who demonstrate very low endurance levels, which is not an issue for most individuals following hip replacement surgery. See reference: Sladyk, K and Ryan, SE (eds): Gower, D and Bowker, M: A plumber and golfer with total hip arthroplasty.

57. (D) Decoupage wooden key fob. A wooden key fob with a decoupage finish is the safest craft choice because it is free of sharp, toxic and cordlike materials. A ceramic object (answer C) could be broken into sharp pieces that an individual could use to harm him or herself. Craft projects that contain rope or cordlike materials that could be used in hanging (answers A and C) should also be avoided. Although macramé is related to the fiber arts and may be of interest to this individual, it would not be considered a safe choice because of the cords involved. See reference: Early: Safety techniques.

58. (D) Consider and treat underlying sensory integration problems as a possible cause. Often children's sensory integration problems interfere with the development of hand dominance. The cause could be deficits in motor planning, decreased ability to cross the body midline, poor sensory perception in the arms and hands, delayed integration of reflex patterns, and so forth. Answers A, B, and C are incorrect because they do not address possible underlying causes for poorly established hand dominance. See reference: Case-Smith (ed): Parham, LD and Mailloux, Z: Sensory integration.

59. (B) creating nonspecific job-simulated work tasks. Nonspecific job-simulated work tasks such as carrying, pushing, and pulling are appropriate examples of work conditioning. Answer C, job-specific work tasks, are representative of a work-hardening goal. Answers A and D are examples of intervention (work hardening), that are implemented after the client achieves success in the area of work conditioning. See reference: Neistadt and Crepeau (eds): Festoon, S and Gagman, P: Treatment of work and productive activities: Functional restoration, an industrial approach.

60. (C) encourage here-and-now explorations of member behaviors and issues, while promoting learning through doing. The purpose of task groups, as developed by Fidler, is to focus on the here-and-now; involve learning through doing, activity, and processing; and involve the development of daily living skills and work skills. Answer A describes an evaluative group, and answer B describes a topical discussion group, rather than a task group. Answer D describes the purpose of developmental group levels proposed by Mosey. See reference: Cole: A psychoanalytic approach.

61. (B) crafts, games, and self-care tasks. Crafts, games, and self-care tasks can best be described as functional activities that should be a component of hand rehabilitation. Answers A, C, and D are all considered to be adjunct activities that may be implemented as a precursor to functional activities. See reference: Pedretti and Early (eds): Kasch, MC and Nickerson, E: Hand and upper extremity injuries.

62. (B) it provides social interaction and support, as well as activity. Parkinson's disease frequently causes social isolation because of decreased mobility and communication, therefore group treatment is particularly valuable for these clients. Answer A is incorrect because group treatment is not necessarily better for addressing motor problems. Presenting exercise activities (answer C) can be effective in groups, but it would not be the primary reason to select a therapeutic group for clients with Parkinson's. Answer D is incorrect because the therapist is responsible for leading a therapeutic group and would not leave until the group session has concluded. See reference: Trombly (ed): Newman, EM, Echevarria, ME, and Digman, G: Degenerative diseases.

63. (C) baking cookies using a recipe. This is a well delineated meal preparation activity that provides structure with a specific sequence of tasks. Setting a table or preparing a shopping list (answers A and D) do not necessarily require sequencing of tasks. Planning a meal (answer B) involves a great deal of organizational ability, and would not be an appropriate choice for an initial activity to address goals relating to sequencing tasks. See reference: Early: Responding to symptoms and behaviors.

64. (A) Chaining. Chaining with the child who demonstrates a cognitive disability shows the entire process of a task with all sequences. Initially, the child performs only the beginning or end of a task. Thus, the child concentrates on only a small part of the task, but gradually increases participation in all sequences in their correct order. Answers B, C, and D are other methods that can be used, but forward and backward chaining are particularly successful instructional methods for individuals who are mentally retarded. See reference: Early: Medical and psychological models of mental health and illness.

65. (A) Have the patient practice stress reduction using meditation, yoga, and energy conservation techniques. Individuals with AIDS should implement a form of exercise to provide mobility and reduce stress, without draining his or her physical resources, in addition to using energy conservation techniques during ADL. It would not be appropriate for an individual to participate in an aerobics program (answers B and C), because of the high energy demands. Video lectures (answer C) would provide information about AIDS, would but not necessarily address physical deconditioning and self-esteem issues. See reference: Reed and Sanderson (eds): Immunologic disorders.

66. (C) Give him a tour of the OT department and a schedule of activities. Becoming familiar with an environment in advance and knowing what to expect can help reduce anxiety. Reducing distractions and keeping lights low (answer A), may be useful environmental adaptations for individuals with mania or hyperactivity. Providing a stimulating environment and real life activities (answer B), is recommended for in-

dividuals experiencing delusions. OT practitioners should leave doors open and avoid being alone (answer D) with individuals who are hostile or violent. See reference: Early: Responding to symptoms and behaviors.

67. (D) Role playing a tea party with "Barbie" dolls. Answer D, role playing with dolls, is the most appropriate choice because the COTA is encouraging the child to partake in pretend play. "Playfulness, like play, encompasses intrinsic motivation, internal control, and freedom to suspend reality" (p. 296). Role playing is focused primarily on the activity at hand, rather than the end product, such as in answer A (playing a game of "Go Fish") and answer B (playing a game of checkers). Answer C, jumping rope, might frustrate the child secondary to her difficulty with motor tasks. The end goal of an occupational therapy treatment would be to increase the child's play skills in the hopes that the child will begin to interact more comfortably within the home, school and peer environment. See reference: Solomon (ed): Clifford-O'Brien, J: Play.

68. (B) to routinely inspect the skin closely for signs of skin breakdown. Teaching a patient with a residual limb to compensate for the lack of sensation with visual inspection, is essential to prevent injury from skin breakdown. Answer A is incorrect because tapping, rubbing, and application of textures is used when a residual limb is hypersensitive. Answer C, deep massage, is a technique used to loosen and prevent scar adhesions. Answer D, teaching procedures of skin hygiene, is important, but would not, by itself, prevent skin breakdown, which is the primary concern when the residual limb lacks sensation. See reference: Pedretti and Early (eds): Keenan, DD and Rock, LM: Upper extremity amputations.

69. (A) Patients write fears and concerns on index cards and then the COTA collects and reads the cards to the group for discussion. This method allows for anonymity by having each patient write down their concerns without including their names, thereby eliminating any fear of embarrassment. Answers B and C require the patients to make public their concerns, which might prevent complete openness when attempting to express their concerns and fears. Although there are certain concerns that might be common to a large number of patients, and having a team member address these concerns in general would be helpful (answer D), this approach would not address the specific concerns of the patients in this group. See reference: Early: Group concepts and techniques

70. (C) use headphones during work to reduce competing sensory input. Reducing competing sensory input is helpful in increasing visual attention. Increasing competing input (answers A and B), or reducing the amount of visual input (answer D), may reduce the ability to attend to visual stimuli. See reference: Case-Smith (ed): Schneck, CM: Visual perception.

71. (D) remove scatter rugs throughout the house. The greatest safety hazard would be from the presence of scatter rugs in the house, which could cause the client with a shuffling gait to trip and fall. Individuals with Parkinson's disease are at high risk for falls. Answer A, increasing illumination in hallways, would be more important if the client had low vision. Answer B, screening out distracting stimuli, and answer C, placing door locks higher or lower than eye level, are safety adaptations made for individuals with cognitive deficits, rather than motor deficits. See reference: Neistadt and Crepeau (eds): Griswold, LA: Community-based practice area.

72. (B) Give the individual one task to do such as making drinks. Having the individual start with one of the components of the activity addresses decision-making and problem-solving skills without overwhelming her. Planning a menu (answer A) requires a high level of decision making and is too challenging. Asking the individual what she would like to do (answer C) is too open-ended, and would be too overwhelming. Limiting the individual to an observer role (answer D) would alienate her from the group process. See reference: Early: Analyzing, adapting, and grading activities.

73. (C) An electric toothbrush. According to Case-Smith, "for the child who independently brushes, an electric toothbrush enables more thorough cleaning. This is a good solution for children with limited dexterity, although for children with weakness, an electric toothbrush may be too heavy to manage" (p. 516). Answer A, using a soft bristle brush, would most likely assist a child with tongue thrust, while answer B, attaching a velcro strap to the toothbrush, would assist a child who has decreased grip strength in the hand. Answer D, encouraging the child to use a soft sponge-tipped toothette, is typically indicated in the child with oral hypersensitivity or defensiveness. See reference: Case-Smith (ed): Shepherd, J: Self-care and adaptations for independent living.

74. (C) Using a bath chair and a hand-held shower with tepid water. The best bathing method for a person with COPD considers the energy demands of the task, as well as the effect of water temperature, in light of the person's functional status. A person with COPD has difficulty breathing when the environment is hot or humid, or when there is a high degree of steam. Answer A is incorrect because of the energy demand of transferring into a tub, and the use of hot water may cause difficulty breathing. Answer B, standing for a quick shower, is also incorrect because even if brief, standing would be more energy demanding than sitting, and an overhead shower can increase humidity. A lukewarm tub bath (answer D) would provide lower humidity by using the coolest

water temperature, but the need to transfer in and out of the tub may make the task very energy demanding. See reference: Trombly (ed): Atchison, B: Cardiopulmonary disease.

75. (B) Replace the white glue with blue glue. Activity adaptations enable an individual to become more functional in his or her task performance. Reviewing the difference between glue and grout (answer A) would be a cognitive approach. Avoiding the use of white tiles (answer C) could be a solution if the problem were figure-ground related. Completing the last step of the activity for the individual (answer D) reflects a forward-chaining approach. See reference: Early: Analyzing, adapting, and grading activities.

76. (A) single pressure switch, firmly mounted within easy reach. A child with fluctuating muscle tone lacks stability and demonstrates extraneous movement, therefore, deliberate motor action is most effectively executed on a securely mounted device using simple movement patterns. Answers B, C, and D involve devices that would respond to slight touch, and would therefore not be effective for a person with extraneous movement and difficulty grading motor action. See reference: Case-Smith (ed): Swinth, Y: Assistive technology: Computers and augmentative communication.

77. (D) Use a dust mitt to keep fingers fully extended. Using dust mitts prevents prolonged finger flexion and allows the fingers to remain straight while dusting. Pushing the vacuum (answer A) forward by straightening the elbow completely, then pulling it back close to the body utilizes long strokes and promotes good elbow and shoulder range of motion. When ironing (answer B), trying to get the elbow into full extension helps to maintain elbow range of motion. Keeping lightweight objects (answer C) on high shelves encourages reaching, which helps maintain shoulder range of motion. See reference: Pedretti and Early (eds): Buckner, WS: Arthritis.

78. (D) The staff may only need to monitor water temperature and the amount of soap being used. This individual is functioning within the level 4 range of Allen's Cognitive Levels. Because this individual can recognize whether items are clean or dirty, cueing to place dirty items in the hamper (answer A) is not necessary. Independent use of the washer and dryer (answer C) and problem solving (answer B) are more appropriate for individuals functioning at level 5, in which the individual demonstrates flexibility in response to change. See reference: Allen, Earhardt, and Blue: Analysis of activities.

79. (D) A scoop dish. A scoop dish is a plate with a high rim that provides a surface against which to push the food. The child would have less difficulty with controlling movement of food because the sides of the scoop dish would provide a shape that aids scooping of food onto the spoon. A swivel spoon (answer A) helps primarily when supination is limited. A nonslip mat (answer B) helps stabilize the plate itself, and a mobile arm support (answer C) positions the arm to help weak shoulder and elbow muscles to position the hand. See reference: Case-Smith (ed): Case-Smith, J and Humphrey, R: Feeding intervention.

80. (B) weight bearing through the upper extremity in sitting or standing. Weight bearing is the most effective way of normalizing tone, according to the NDT approach for adult hemiplegia. Placing a weighted cuff on the extremity (answer A) would have the effect of increasing muscle tone, making reaching more difficult. Answer C, using only the unaffected upper extremity, would accomplish the reaching task, but would not normalize muscle tone in the affected upper extremity. Answer D, "forced use," is a treatment concept used to encourage functional motor return in hemiplegic upper extremities, but is not a method designed to normalize muscle tone, nor is it a specific technique of the NDT approach. See reference: Pedretti and Early (eds): Davis, JZ: Neurodevelopmental treatment of adult hemiplegia: The Bobath approach.

81. (A) Role plays that include practicing good table manners. A cognitive approach is best for individuals with memory and/or attention deficits, for those who must learn to do situational problem solving, or when skills learned need to be generalized to other situations. Cognitive approaches include role playing, rehearsal, imagery and memory enhancement techniques. Behavioral approaches include cause-effect associations, shaping, reinforcement and behavior modification (answers B, C, and D). Behavioral approaches are recommended for individuals whose cognitive abilities are impaired by psychosis, who have normal attention span and memory abilities, or those living in a highly structured and consistent environment. See reference: Christiansen (ed): Leonardelli Haertlein, CA and Blodgett, MC: Self-care strategies in intervention for psychosocial conditions.

82. (D) A tabletop air hockey competition. Tabletop air hockey is the best choice because the rules of this type of game coincide with the developmental abilities of the child. This game would also be easily played at a wheelchair level. According to Case-Smith, "in middle childhood (6 to 10 years old) children play in cooperative groups and value interaction with their peers...In these peer groups, children learn to cooperate, but also to compete. They are now interested in achievement through play" (p. 91). Answers A and C ("Simon Says" and "Duck, duck goose") are activities that would be most appropriate for preschool or kindergarten age children, while answer B, role playing with toys, is more appropriate for children ages 3 to 4 years old. See reference:

Case-Smith (ed): Case-Smith, J: Development of childhood occupations.

83. (A) Velcro closures on front opening clothing. Velcro closures on front-opening clothing (answer A), would require the least amount of dexterity, which becomes increasingly difficult with Parkinson's disease. Large buttons on front opening clothing (answer B) might be easier than smaller buttons, but would still require more manipulation than Velcro closures. Clothing slipped on over the head with no fasteners (answer C) would eliminate the need for dexterity, but having to raise the arms would be problematic because of the rigidity and stiffness of the limbs that typically accompanies Parkinson's disease. Though clothing which stretches freely is easier to put on than tightly constructed clothing, the need to tie the closures in the back of the garment (answer D) would be difficult for a person with upper extremity rigidity. See reference: Trombly (ed): Newman, EM, Echevarria, ME and Digman, G: Degenerative diseases.

84. (C) express disagreement with coworkers in a productive manner. Assertiveness is the ability to express feelings in an appropriate and productive manner. Answers A, B, and D are examples of additional social interaction skills, however, they do not address an assertiveness component. Answers A and B are examples of actions taken when engaging in conversation, and answer D is an example of proper social conduct. See reference: Early: Psychosocial skills and psychological components.

85. (D) Hold him firmly when picking him up and dressing him. Holding the child firmly inhibits responses to light touch, which are usually uncomfortable for children with tactile defensiveness. Tickling (answer A), and light stroking (answer C), are also uncomfortable or intolerable for a child with tactile defensiveness. A strong stimulus such as loud music causes further discomfort during a time when the child is extremely vulnerable to the sensation of light touch (i.e., when clothing is being removed). See reference: Case-Smith (ed): Parham, LD and Mailloux, Z: Sensory integration.

86. (A) Perform pursed-lip breathing when doing activities. Pursed-lip breathing is a technique that narrows the passage of air during expiration. This technique helps individuals with COPD keep the airway open and improves breathing efficiency. The overall effect is improved endurance and tolerance for activities. Taking hot showers and avoiding air conditioning during warm weather (answers C and D) are incorrect in that both activities are contraindicated for individuals with COPD. Using a long-handled bath sponge (answer B) may be helpful, but is not the most likely tip to be on a home program for an individual with COPD. See reference: Neistadt and Crepeau (eds): Ferraro, R: Cardiopulmonary dysfunction in adults.

87. (A) encourage the use of PABA-free sunblock and hats. Individuals taking neuroleptic medications are prone to photosensitivity and need protection from the sun. A PABA-free sunblock is recommended because it reduces the chance of an allergic reaction to the sun. The precautions described in answer B are helpful to the individual experiencing postural hypotension, which can be a side effect of neuroleptic medication, but is not an issue for a picnic outing. Answers C and D are not linked to the side effects of neuroleptic medications. See reference: Early: Psychotropic medications and biological treatments.

88. (C) Position stander at 75 to 90 degrees from the floor. Answer C is correct because by adjusting the prone stander nearest to vertical (the least effect of gravity on the head or posture), the child will be able to tolerate working on head righting. Answer A is not correct because while working on the floor in prone, the head and neck are doing the most work against gravity. Answer D is not correct because the head and neck work the least against gravity in the standing or upright position. See reference: Kramer and Hinojosa (eds): Colangelo, CA: Biomechanical frame of reference.

89. (A) Using effective communication skills. Clarifying expectations, honestly defining needs, and providing tactful and constructive feedback are communication skills that promote understanding. Successful communication with the patient's children will most likely help them deal with their fears and concerns, increase their understanding of their father's condition, and elicit greater cooperation. Although time management techniques, deep breathing, and laughter (answers B, C, and D) are all useful and valid stress reduction techniques, they do not address the issue at hand, which is communication between the father and his children. See reference: Neistadt and Crepeau (eds): Giles, GM and Neistadt, ME: Treatment for psychosocial components: Stress management.

90. (C) During a meal preparation activity, have the individual demonstrate a step that he is familiar with to two or three group members. This is a good beginning toward increasing an individual's self-esteem. At this early stage, responsibility for planning the entire activity (answer B) is too challenging, but would be effective when self-esteem and confidence improve. While praise (answer A) may promote a positive self-image, praise alone is not enough. Waiting for the individual to initiate participation (answer D) may not provide the necessary encouragement and opportunities for growth that this individual needs. See reference: Early: Group concepts and techniques.

91. (A) Place a foam-lined plastic laundry basket in the tub. Answer A, a laundry basket with a foam-lined bottom, would be the most appropriate item for the COTA to recommend because this piece of equipment addresses both cost and positioning concerns. The laundry basket will also permit the child to continue to immerse herself in the tub, an activity that was stated as enjoyable to the child. Answer B, a horseshoe-shaped bath collar, would be indicated for a child with "severe motor limitations who is lying supine in shallow water" (p. 516). Whereas, answer C, a bath hammock, might be considered as an alternative choice for this child because "bath hammocks fully hold the body and enable the parent to wash the child thoroughly" (p. 516), this type of equipment would not be as cost effective as the laundry basket. Answer D, suggesting that the child stand in the shower versus showering, does not address the parent or child's immediate needs of bathing in the bathtub. If the child lacks sitting balance it is likely that they will also lack standing balance, thus indicating the need for durable medical equipment, such as a shower bench and/or grab bars. See reference: Case-Smith (ed): Shepherd, J: Self-care adaptations for independent living.

92. (D) position the person in an upright posture, making sure head is flexed slightly and in midline. Making sure that the resident is correctly positioned is the first step in addressing eating problems. Improper posture can result in difficulties with swallowing. Depending on the particular problems of the individual, providing adaptive devices (answer A) may or may not be helpful, but nontheless would not be the first step given without assessment of need. Observing for swallowing after each bite (answer B), and instructing caregivers as to proper setup (answer C) would also be important steps, but these would occur later in the intervention process. See reference: Larson, Stevens-Ratchford, Pedretti, and Crabtree (eds): Foti, D: Evaluation and interventions for the performance area of self-maintenance.

93. (A) Use pictures, music, and discussion to encourage discussion of memories. Remotivation approaches are used to encourage the expression of thoughts and feelings related to intact long-term memories. The topic should be linked to the group's past experiences and should be easy to understand. The reality orientation approach is designed to maintain or improve awareness of time, situation, and place, and often uses activities related to holidays and other temporal concepts (answer B). The environmental adaptation approach (answer C) promotes independence, but has no relevance to remotivation. Interpersonal skills (answer D) are most effectively addressed through role-playing and discussion groups. See reference: Early: Cognitive and sensorimotor activities.

94. (C) Lateral trunk supports. Lateral trunk supports (answer C) would help maintain correct alignment of the pelvis and trunk in the wheelchair. Answer A, a reclining wheelchair, would shift the child's weight posteriorly but would not prevent lateral shifting of the trunk. An arm trough (answer B) would probably contribute to lateral shifting, although bilateral arm troughs or a lapboard could help maintain a more centered trunk position. Lateral pelvic supports (answer D) would stabilize the pelvis and prevent it from shifting sideways, but would be too low to prevent the trunk from moving laterally. See reference: Pedretti and Early (eds): Adler, C and Tipton-Burton, M: Wheelchair assessment and transfers.

95. (D) A buttonhook attached to a cuff that fits around the palm. Individuals with C6 quadriplegia may have a tenodesis grasp or no grasp available to them. Therefore, a buttonhook that fits into the palm, or a buttonhook with a built-up handle, are the only appropriate choices. A buttonhook with a knob handle (answer B) or on a 5-inch dowel (answer C) is appropriate for an individual with a functional grasp, but limited dexterity. A buttonhook with an extra long, flexible handle benefits an individual with limited range of motion. See reference: Trombly (ed): Trombly, CA: Retraining basic and instrumental activities of daily living.

96. (B) remain matter of fact and consistent in approach. Individuals with borderline personality disorder demonstrate inconsistent behavior, have difficulty maintaining stable relationships, and have poor self image. Practitioners usually need to work hard to remain consistent and trustworthy to those individuals. It is important in this case that the OT practitioner recognizes this behavior as part of the pathology and not take it personally. Because the accusation is a result of pathology, the COTA has nothing to apologize for, and is unlikely to uncover any reasonable explanation for a misunderstanding (answer D). In addition, the practitioner should not complain of hurt feelings to a client (answer A). Delving into exploration of the individual's past (answer C) is not a recommended approach for occupational therapy. See reference: Neistadt and Crepeau (eds): Ward, JD: Psychosocial dysfunction in adults.

97. (C) Toothpaste with a flip-open cap. An individual with fine motor incoordination would be able to manage a toothpaste cap that flips open much more easily than a cap that must be removed completely from the tube. Also, toothpaste tubes with flip-open caps are larger in diameter, which make them easier to manage. A wash mitt (answer A), and a toothbrush with a built-up handle (answer D), are good options for those with weak grasp. Spray deodorant (answer B), has a small button to push, which would be difficult to operate for someone with incoordination. See reference: Pedretti and Early (eds): Foti, D: Activities of daily living.

98. (A) provide verbal cues, external aids such as calendars and family pictures, and opportunities to practice using the external aids. Verbal cues, external aids, and opportunities to practice using the external aids (answer A) would be most ap-

propriate for clients with deficits in orientation. Answer B, reducing distractions, and answer C, presenting information in short units, would be adaptive strategies to promote attention and information processing. Answer D, connecting new information to previously held knowledge and skills, is a technique to aid retrieval of information and improve memory. See reference: Unsworth (ed): Schwarzberg, S: Clinical reasoning with groups.

99. (A) Biofeedback, distraction, and relaxation techniques. Biofeedback, distraction, and relaxation techniques are all examples of psychosocial measures that can be introduced to manage pain. Answers B and C, specific skill training and endurance building, are not directly related to pain management techniques and are often associated with cognitive or motor limitations. Answer D, cognitive retraining techniques, are also not directly related to pain management techniques. See reference: Neistadt and Crepeau (eds): Engel, JM: Treatment for psychosocial components: Pain management.

100. (A) hips. Flexing the hips breaks up the extensor pattern and, combined with knee flexion, reduces tone in the lower extremities, thus facilitating dressing. Flexing more distal joints first (answers B, C, and D), is ineffective in reducing tone and may lead to excessive stress on the joints involved. See reference: Case-Smith (ed): Shepherd, J: Self-care and adaptations for independent living.

101. (B) prolonged wrist flexion, such as scrubbing pots and pans. Flexion at the wrist, especially while grasping or pinching (as in scrubbing pots), should be avoided or modified with a soft splint. Answer A, wrist extension, answer C, ulnar deviation, and answer D, radial deviation, do not tend to cause inflammation to the area surrounding the median nerve by repetitive compression or a static hold to that area of the wrist. See reference: Hunter, Schneider, Mackin, and Bell (eds): Baxter-Petralia, P: Therapist's management of carpal tunnel syndrome.

102. (C) give simple directions and patiently wait for responses. Severe depression can result in slowing of cognitive and motor functions, known as psychomotor retardation. The OT practitioner must not rush the individual (answer A), but should give her or him time to process information and respond. Too much stimulation (answers B and D) may cause the individual to withdraw even further. See reference: Neistadt and Crepeau (eds): Ward, JD: Psychosocial dysfunction in adults.

103. (A) Replace the spoon with a blunt-ended fork. For a child with incoordination and tremors, stabbing food with a blunt-ended fork is often more effective for feeding than using a spoon. The food will not fall off the fork, and the blunt tines will prevent any injury to the child. Building up the spoon handle (answer B) is more appropriate for a child with a weak grasp. A swivel spoon (answer C), and bending the handle 45 degrees (answer D), are more appropriate for a child with limited forearm and wrist motion. See reference: Case-Smith (ed): Case-Smith, J and Humphry, R: Feeding and oral motor skills.

104. (B) provide strong color contrast at key areas to identify steps, pathways, etc. Using contrast is a key environmental adaptation strategy for people with visual impairments. The more contrast, the easier it is to locate objects, steps, entrances, and pathways, thereby improving accessibility by maximizing remaining vision. Instructing the client to sit during ADL (answer A), or recommending human assistance (answer C), would not directly address accessibility. Answer D, recommending training in white cane use, is a method of improving mobility for a person who is blind. See reference: Larson, Stevens-Ratchford, Pedretti, and Crabtree (eds): Christenson, MA: Environmental design, modification and adaptation.

105. (B) discuss the meaning and value of the client's doing her own laundry with the mother and client. By discussing the intervention plan options with caregivers, the COTA can determine whether the goals and intervention are meaningful and relevant to the individuals involved. Unilaterally explaining the importance of independence to the mother (answer A), and asking the father to intercede (answer C), are actions that do not ascertain the value or significance of the goal, which, if not valued by the client and caregivers, is inappropriate. After speaking with the mother and client, the COTA may determine later that independence in laundry skills is not an appropriate goal (answer D). See reference: Early: Who is the consumer?

106. (B) a switch-adapted battery-operated toy car that knocks down a block tower. A switch-adapted battery-operated car would be most age appropriate activity that would allow a young child to experience how his or her actions affect the environment. Listening to music on a tape recorder (answer A), unless the tape recorder was specially adapted for the child to turn on, would be a passive activity. Storybook computer software (answer C) would facilitate early learning and a powered wheelchair is a high technology application for facilitating mobility. See reference: Angelo and Lane (eds): Lane, SJ and Mistrett, SG: Can and should technology be used as a tool for early intervention?

107. (C) get the shirt all the way on, then line up the buttons and holes, and begin buttoning from the bottom. It is easier to see the buttons and buttonholes at the bottom of the shirt (answer C) than at the top (answer B). Therefore, beginning to button from the bottom is more likely to result in success for the individual with motor or visual-perceptual deficits. Buttoning first (answer A) may result in

ripping off the buttons as the shirt is pulled over the head. A buttonhook with a built-up handle (answer D) would be more helpful for an individual with finger weakness or incoordination (e.g., quadriplegia). See reference: Pedretti and Early (eds): Foti, D: Activities of daily living.

108. (D) in private, explain the nature of the client-therapist relationship. It is inappropriate for the COTA to have more than a professional relationship with a client. While self-disclosing some information to clients can be a therapeutic tool, there is some information that would be misinterpreted or inappropriate (e.g., giving out personal information [Answer A]). Ignoring the client's request (answer B) constitutes avoidance on the COTA's part and is unprofessional. Though a difficult situation, the COTA looses an opportunity to provide valuable feedback to her client. Whether the COTA has a boyfriend or not (answer C), she should not use this as an excuse for not giving out her number. It is be an easy way out, but is unprofessional. See reference: Early: Therapeutic use of self.

109. (D) swivel spoon. A swivel spoon allows the head of the spoon to rotate as the child moves the handle into varying positions, thus compensating for poor supination. A child who is unable to reach her mouth due to limitations in shoulder or elbow flexion would benefit from a spoon with an elongated handle (answer A). A child who is unable to hold a spoon because of difficulty with grasp would benefit from a spoon with a built-up handle (answer C). A "spork" (answer B) is helpful for those who need to use one utensil as both fork and spoon. See reference: Trombly (ed): Feinberg, JR and Trombly, CA: Arthritis.

110. (D) proper body mechanics. Answer D, proper body mechanics is encouraged through didactic instruction and new learning, and remains part of the work-hardening program until discharge. The COTA should educate the individual regarding unwanted stress to the lumbar spine with lifting tasks. Answers A and B, energy conservation and work simplification, can be part of a work-hardening program, but tend to be indicated in cases where the individual demonstrates decreased endurance and fatigue with daily activities. Answer C, home maintenance activities, are typically introduced during inpatient or outpatient/home health OT interventions, not within the work-hardening setting. See reference: Pedretti and Early (eds): Burt, CM: Work evaluation and work hardening.

111. (A) baking brownies. A correctly sequenced progression of difficulty in meal preparation is access a prepared meal; prepare a cold meal; prepare a hot beverage, soup, or prepared dish; prepare a hot one dish meal; and prepare a hot multidish meal. Making a fresh fruit salad (answer D) is a less challenging activity, because no cooking is involved. Although both involve heating an item, preparing toast (answer C) is simpler than heating soup because opening a plastic bag is a less complex task than opening a can. Baking brownies (answer A) is slightly more complex, because of the progression from stove top to oven, and the addition of several ingredients that need to be mixed. Therefore, this would be the appropriate upgrade. Making an apple pie (answer B) requires a higher level of task performance and complexity than brownies, and would be an appropriate task after the individual demonstrates competence in the less complex task of baking brownies. See reference: Neistadt and Crepeau (eds): Rogers, JC and Holm, MB: Evaluation of activities of daily living (ADL) and home management.

112. (C) propose a modified goal that still meets the parent's needs. "In family-centered intervention the occupational therapist addresses the needs of the entire family rather than only concentrating on specific deficits in the child" (p. 722). Proposing a modified goal of functional mobility with an adaptive mobility device, would best address both the parent's need for decreased carrying, and the child's need to improve functional mobility within the environment. Agreeing to work on an unrealistic and possibly unachievable goal (answer A), would not meet the child's needs for developmentally appropriate intervention. Answer B, offering an alternative goal, would not be responsive to the problems identified by the family. Answer D is incorrect because this child is too young to establish her own goals, though this might be encouraged at later stages of therapy. See reference: Case-Smith (ed): Stephens, LC and Tauber, SK: Early intervention.

113. (A) Gentle, nonresistive activities. The initial phase of treatment for the individual with Guillain-Barré syndrome includes PROM and splinting, and positioning to protect weak muscles and prevent contractures. This should be followed by gentle, nonresistive activities and light ADL, as tolerated. Resistive exercises and activities (answers B and D) should be implemented after strength begins to improve. Activities within later treatment sessions should alternate between gross and fine motor (unlike answer C), and resistive and nonresistive types, to avoid fatigue. See reference: Pedretti and Early (eds): Lehman, RM and McCormack, GL: Neurogenic and myopathic dysfunction.

114. (C) Use a board game to introduce the concept of receiving and spending money. This activity provides an opportunity for the individuals to experience the value and purpose of money. Although it is important to introduce the actual value of coins and paper money, it is essential to combine this with concrete applications that a board game can supply. Answers A, B, and D are examples of graded activities to be used after the initial introduction of money concepts. See reference: Early: Activities of daily living.

115. (B) floor sitter. "A floor sitter may enable the child with cerebral palsy to play on the floor near his or her typically developing peers" (p. 725). Occupational therapy practitioners can recommend and provide appropriate adapted equipment and positioning devices when working in an early intervention setting. A hammock (answer A) would not allow the child to feel as if he "fits in." The child verbalized the desire to sit on the floor like his peers, whereas the hammock may make the child feel even more different then when he sits in his wheelchair. Hammocks are typically utilized in therapy to provide sensorimotor/vestibular input, and would not be indicated in this situation unless no other viable options were available. Introducing an adapted wheelchair insert and a prone stander (answers C and D), would be ignoring the child's desire to sit on the floor with his peers. Wheelchair inserts are often used for positioning a child in a wheelchair to permit increased trunk support and stability, thus allowing for more independent use of the upper extremities. A prone stander would allow a child to assume a standing or weight bearing position, but would not assist with positioning the child while sitting on a mat. See reference: Case-Smith (ed): Stephens, LC and Tauber, SK: Early intervention.

116. (A) A craft activity using increasingly heavy hand tools. Progressive resistive exercise is the most effective method for increasing strength in a muscle with fair plus strength. Mildly resistive activities that are stopped as soon as the individual begins to experience fatigue (answer B), are appropriate for maintaining or improving strength in individuals with conditions in which fatigue should be avoided (e.g., MS, ALS, and Guillain-Barré syndrome). Electric stimulation (answer C) is appropriate for increasing strength in very weak muscles. When performing resistive active range of motion with this individual, the COTA would use maximal resistance. In addition, a craft activity that can be performed against increasing resistance for prolonged periods of time, would be more effective than resisted active range of motion (answer D), which is usually only performed once or twice a day. See reference: Dutton: Biomechanical postulates regarding intervention.

117. (A) begin with activities that have obvious solutions and high probabilities of success, and then gradually increase the complexity. This strategy is effective in developing problem-solving skills. Gross and fine motor activities (answer B) can heighten awareness of self and develop coordination. Increasing the time spent on the activity (answer D) helps development of attention span. Structuring the number and kinds of choices (answer C) is a method for developing decision-making skills. See reference: Early: Analyzing, adapting, and grading activities.

118. (A) power wheelchair. A power wheelchair would be the most appropriate choice in this situation. According to Hays, "children without locomotion (i.e., the ability to move their body from one place to another)" (p. 340), can be placed in a specific functional group. One of these groups is that of "children who will never ambulate and need a power wheelchair, such as children who have severe cerebral palsy or spinal muscle atrophy" (p. 340). Answer B, a standard wheelchair, may be something the family would like to purchase in addition to the power wheelchair. Standard wheelchairs tend to be less expensive, lightweight, and portable. They are also convenient when a power wheelchair is in for repairs. Answers C and D (a caster cart and prone scooter) are not considered appropriate for the child with severe cerebral palsy, because adequate upper extremity function is required for use of the caster cart and scooter. See reference: Solomon (ed): Clayton, KS and Mathena, CT: Assistive technology.

119. (C) Eat six small meals a day. An individual with ALS who becomes fatigued eating three full meals a day should attempt eating six smaller meals a day before resorting to tube feedings or pureed diets (answers A and D). Eating regular food is usually more enjoyable and is therefore likely to enhance the quality of life. An upright position is optimal when feeding individuals with dysphagia. A semireclined position (answer B) can make swallowing more difficult or dangerous. See reference: Pedretti and Early (eds): Schultz-Krohn, W, Foti, D and Glogoski, C: Degenerative diseases of the central nervous system.

120. (B) put the dried dishes away and begin to hand her wet dishes. Compensating for mistakes helps to increase the sense of self-worth and integrity of individuals with dementia. This approach is preferable to drawing attention to errors, especially in situations in which safety is not an issue. Answers A, C, and D all draw attention to the individual's errors. See reference: Early: Responding to symptoms and behaviors.

121. (D) set clear expectations for behavior and enforce consequences, such as a time-out, if the child loses control. The behavioral frame of reference can be useful in helping children with maladaptive behavior to learn to modify their behaviors and to learn new more adaptive behaviors through the principle of reinforcement. To use this effectively, the child must clearly understand the expectations for behavior (or rules), and that there will be consistent consequences for behaviors that break the rules. Answers A and B, allowing the child to express his anger and ignoring the behaviors, would not help the child to learn new behaviors and could cause an increased loss of control. A child who is out of control and responding to impulses is not able to respond to an insight-based approach such as reasoning. See reference: Sladyk, K and Ryan, SE (eds): Florey, L: A second-grader with conduct disorder.

122. (D) arm trough. An arm trough would provide a stable surface that would keep the individual's arm in a safe and appropriate position. In addition, an arm trough approximates the humeral head into the glenoid fossa at a natural angle. If the individual has edema in his hand, a foam wedge may be placed in the trough to elevate the hand. A lap tray (answer A) would provide support, but is more restrictive than an arm trough, which should be attempted first. The fact that the individual's arm was seen dangling by the side of the wheelchair indicates that the wheelchair armrest alone (answer B) is inadequate. Answer C, an arm sling, would provide support for his arm, but would immobilize it in adduction and internal rotation. Current literature supports the use of slings only when necessary, such as during ambulation when a flaccid upper extremity may sublux or cause loss of balance. See reference: Pedretti and Early (eds): Gillen, G: Cerebrovascular accident.

123. (C) Disguise the bedroom door with wallpaper so it blends in with the surroundings. Decorating the door handle is also a good way to prevent the confused individual from recognizing the door. The 1987 Omnibus Budget Reconciliation Act mandated reduction in the use of chemical and physical restraints (answer A) with nursing home residents. Keeping hallways clear of obstructions (answer B) results in a safer environment for wanderers, but does not prevent wandering. Modifying the environment is preferable to increasing demands on nursing staff (answer D). See reference: Neistadt and Crepeau (eds): Toglia, JP: Cognitive-perceptual retraining and rehabilitation.

124. (B) Forming letters out of clay. Preschoolers learn best using a multisensory approach. Making letters out of such materials as clay, bread dough, chocolate pudding, or sandpaper uses the child's tactile, kinesthetic, and (in some cases) gustatory senses, as well as vision. In this way, new learning is reinforced through a variety of sensory channels. Flash cards (answer B), matching to sample (answer C), and coloring (answer D), are methods that rely primarily on visual processing, and cognitive skills and are better suited for strengthening existing skills in older children. See reference: Case-Smith (ed): Schneck, CM: Visual perception.

125. (D) set personal boundaries appropriate to the therapist–patient relationship. It is important to acknowledge the individual's need for sexual expression, while supporting the sense of self, and identifying acceptable relationships and behaviors. Setting boundaries while accepting the individual is the most appropriate therapeutic response. Outright rejection (answer A) may cause an individual to believe he or she is sexually undesirable or unlovable. Flirting back (answer B) may imply that a sexual relationship between COTA and the patient is acceptable. Although the individual may need to know how SCI affects sexual functioning (answer C), the behavior that requires a response is not about a lack of knowledge, but rather about how to appropriately express sexual interest and the need for reinforcement of a sexual identity. See reference: Pedretti and Early (eds): Burton, GU: Sexuality and physical dysfunction.

126. (D) Chaining. Chaining is frequently used when teaching a multiple step task because it is easier to teach one step at a time than it is to teach a complete activity. Repetition and rehearsal (answers A and C) involve repeating the whole activity until the activity is learned. Cueing (answer B) uses an external source to remind a person of the next step or part of that step. See reference: Pedretti and Early (eds): Sabari, JS: Teaching activities in occupational therapy.

127. (B) Place a seatbelt at a 45-degree angle at the hips. A seat belt correctly placed at a 45-degree angle to the child's hips would inhibit extensor tone. Answer A is incorrect because trunk support from lateral trunk supports is for sideward movement only. Although a wedge-shaped seat insertion (answer C) increases hip flexion more than 90 degrees and inhibits extensor tone, it is not the best choice because it could have the undesirable side effect of tightening hamstrings over time. Answer D is incorrect because, although it may contribute to holding a child in a chair, it does not affect the angle of the hip joint, which is necessary for decreasing extensor tone when sitting. See reference: Case-Smith (ed): Shepherd, J: Self-care and adaptations for independent living.

128. (B) Use heavy utensils, pots, and pans. Using heavy kitchen items (answer B) increases stability for individuals with incoordination. Other suggestions include using prepared foods, nonskid mats, easy open containers, serrated knives, and tongs. Built-up handles (answer A) are useful for individuals with limited grasp. A high stool (answer C) benefits those who fatigue easily. Placing the most commonly used items on shelves just above and below the counter (answer D) is a useful way to adapt the environment for individuals with limited reach. See reference: Pedretti and Early (eds): Foti, D: Activities of daily living.

129. (A) in the individual's bedroom. Because individuals who require task-specific training are unable to generalize learning to other situations (including other garments and other environments), it is important to train the individual in the environment where the task will be performed. This type of training should take place at least five times a week. See reference: Neistadt and Crepeau (eds): Toglia, JP: Cognitive-perceptual retraining and rehabilitation.

130. (C) Encourage the child to wear a necklace with chewable objects attached. "Excessive biting of inedible objects is a problem often encountered in

children with developmental disabilities…a chewy can be extremely helpful for children who bite excessively…the chewy can be worn as a necklace, attached to a belt, or even put in a pocket" (p. 227). Answers A, B, and D will most likely be ineffective when working with a young child with a developmental disability. Implementing answers A and B (verbal feedback and time-out periods) is unlikely to extinguish the behavior, while answer D (waiting until the child eventually gets bitten back) would be considered an ineffective and inappropriate solution to the problem. See reference: Solomon (ed): Jones, LMW and Machover, PZ: Occupational performance areas: Daily living and work and productive activities.

131. (D) built-up handles. Built-up handles, without adding extra weight, allow a comfortable grasp that regular utensils do not provide. A weighted handle (answer B) would cause more rapid fatigue and strain to the joints. An arthritic person most likely has adequate grasp and release with a built-up handle, making it easier to use than a universal cuff (answer C). See reference: Trombly (ed): Feinberg, JR and Trombly, CA: Arthritis.

132. (C) Report the incident to the client's physician. When an individual with depression and suicidal ideation gives away personal possessions, it may indicate she is considering suicide. The most important response is to notify the physician, although answers A, B, and D may all be appropriate. See reference: Early: Responding to symptoms and behaviors.

133. (D) Drawing lines and shapes using shaving cream, sand, or finger paints. The best activity to encourage prewriting would be drawing lines in different sensory media. Answer A, moving through an obstacle course with emphasis on making turns, would be a useful activity to focus on right-left discrimination. Answer B, having the child create his or her own books, is useful for increasing orientation to printed language. Answer C, rolling clay into a ball, is recommended for improving the ability to regulate pressure during hand activity. See reference: Case-Smith (ed): Amundson, SJ: Prewriting and handwriting skills. Exner, CE: Development of hand skills.

134. (B) decrease the effects of prolonged inactivity. Some of the main objectives of inpatient cardiac rehabilitation include decreasing the effects of prolonged inactivity, such as thromboembolism, orthostatic hypotension, and muscle atrophy; safely providing a program of monitored activity performance to maximize function; reinforcing cardiac precautions; and providing instruction in energy conservation techniques. It is acceptable and expected to encounter fatigue in this population after activity (answer A), however, activities that produce cardiac symptoms should be avoided. Activities that promote endurance and strength are beneficial, but ROM (answer C) is not usually an area of concern.

Most individuals do not need to relearn activities, other than applying energy conservation techniques, therefore, independent performance (answer D) is not a primary concern. See reference: Pedretti and Early (eds): Matthews, MM: Cardiac and pulmonary diseases.

135. (C) tell the client it is okay to work where he is until he feels comfortable in joining the group. The paranoid client frequently isolates themself from the rest of the group as a self-protective measure. Such a client should be allowed to do this until he or she feels comfortable in joining the group. Although it is a good idea to encourage this client to join the group (answer A), the COTA should not insist (answer B). The paranoid client may attempt to take control of an uncomfortable group situation by demanding that the COTA stay with him, away from the group (answer D). In this instance it is important to be supportive of the patient's need, but to remain with the group. See reference: Early: Responding to symptoms and behaviors.

136. (A) Mount lever handles on doors and faucets. For children with reduced strength and endurance, using less complex movements and less force results in energy conservation. Lever handles require less energy than knob handles on doors, faucets, and appliances. Answers B and C are environmental adaptations recommended to minimize the danger of slipping and falling for children with incoordination or postural instability. Answer D is contraindicated, because work at a vertical surface against gravity requires more energy than movement in a horizontal plane. See reference: Case-Smith (ed): Dudgeon, BJ: Pediatric rehabilitation.

137. (B) A call system for emergency and non-emergency use. A call system (answer B) is necessary for a person with a high level spinal cord injury to allow the caretaker to leave the room, but remains available to answer calls for assistance with daily needs or an emergency. This is frequently the first opportunity that a person with a spinal cord injury would have to control some part of his or her life, giving some feeling of independence or choice. An ECU (answer A) does allow independence in operating appliances, lights, and so on through the use of switches or voice control, but would not be a necessity for safety. A remote control power door opener that would allow a caretaker to enter would be useless if the individual is unable to call for assistance. An electric page turner (answer D) is useless without the ability to call for someone to position or replace reading material. See reference: Trombly (ed): Dow, PW and Rees, NP: High-technology adaptations to overcome disability.

138. (B) Provide a large area of personal space, where the person is protected from physical contact with others. Patients who exhibit sexual behaviors may be more likely to think about, and act on, their sexual impulses when they experience close physical contact with others. Answer A would be an appropriate intervention environment for individuals with delusional thinking. The environment described in answer C would be best for people experiencing hallucinations. An environment where all distractions are reduced as much as possible (answer D) is most relevant for individuals exhibiting manic behaviors. See reference: Early: Responding to symptoms and behaviors.

139. (A) work on coordinated reach in a side-lying position first and then transfer the skill to sitting position. The COTA should teach the skill with the child in the position in which they can most easily learn the skills and then teach how to transfer the skill to a more functional position. Answer B addresses a limitation in range of motion; answer C is a strategy for dealing with a visual impairment; and answer D pertains to behavioral and cognitive issues, none of which were mentioned as concerns for this child. See reference: Case-Smith (ed): Exner, CE: Development of hand skills.

140. (D) Give the individual a rest break. Fatigue may cause additional structural damage in the acute stage of MS so should be avoided. Rest breaks need to be scheduled to avoid fatigue. Strengthening activities (answer C) do not need to be discontinued, but should be designed to benefit the patient without causing undue fatigue. See reference: Dutton: Biomechanical postulates regarding intervention.

141. (A) Begin with activities that have obvious solutions and a high probability of success, and then gradually increase the level of complexity. Beginning with activities that have obvious solutions, that are usually successful, and gradually increase in complexity, is an effective method for developing problem-solving skills. Sensorimotor activities (answer B) in a group can facilitate self-awareness. Increasing the activity time (answer D) facilitates attention span improvement. Activities that require interactions with others (answer C) are useful for developing social conduct and interpersonal skills. See reference: Early: Analyzing, adapting and grading activities.

142. (D) shallow spoon. The use of a shallow spoon encourages the development of upper lip control because it makes it easier for the lip to remove all of the food on the spoon. It would be more difficult for the child to get food out of a deep spoon (answer C). Straws (answer A) can be used to develop sucking. A "spork" (answer B) is a device that combines the qualities of a fork and a spoon and is useful if the child can only manage one utensil. See reference: Case-Smith (ed): Case-Smith, J and Humphry, R: Feeding intervention.

143. (B) identify the abilities, needs, and life goals of the client. Identifying the abilities, needs, and life goals of the client should occur before any other steps in the process in order to make a match between the client's abilities, environmental demands, and the appropriate technology to carry out desired daily occupations. Answers A, C, and D are steps which would come later in the process. See reference: Christiansen and Baum (eds): Trefler, E and Hobson, D: Assistive technology.

144. (C) Deep breathing and verbalization.
"Deep (diaphragmatic) breathing involves slowly inhaling and exhaling to reduce tension in the shoulders, trunk, and abdomen...deep breathing is relatively easy to learn, requires no equipment and can be done anywhere" (p. 462). In addition to this, the act of verbalization, simply talking with friends regarding one's stress, can reduce stress levels. "Friends can offer different perspectives, new suggestions, and support, all of which are helpful in extricating a person from feeling stuck with a problem situation" (p. 463). Answers A and B, autogenic training and meditation, are useful stress management techniques, but both require a considerable amount of time and practice in order to successfully implement. Answer D, work simplification and energy conservation, typically impact endurance and the performance of an actual task. See reference: Neistadt and Crepeau (eds): Giles, GM and Neistadt, ME: Treatment for psychosocial components: Stress management.

145. (D) pulling tiny objects out of clay. By pulling tiny objects such as coins or pegs out of clay or putty, the child can work on increasing his ability to oppose his thumb to his digits. Answer A, a universal cuff, would most likely be used by a child who lacks grasp or digit strength. Answer B, using the pointer finger only when working on a keyboard, would not facilitate opposition between the thumb, unless use of the thumb with the space bar was encouraged. Answer C, using a weighted writing utensil, would be indicated for a child with decreased proprioception. See reference: Solomon (ed): Jones, LMW and Machover, PZ:Occupational performance areas: Daily living and work and productive activities

146. (D) provide a stockinette sleeve for the individual to wear inside the splint. A stockinette liner worn inside the splint will keep perspiration from irritating the skin by absorbing it through the liner. Stockinette also keeps the body part from direct contact with the plastic surface of the splint. Stockinette is inexpensive and can be washed easily with soap and water. Answer A, putting talcum powder in a splint, assists with odor control as a result of prolonged splint wear, but does not typically address the perspiration issue. In addition, it often requires frequent cleaning due to the accumulation of powder within the splint. While moleskin as a liner (answer B), may be comfortable, it does not clean well, hence it usually is removed because of the tendency to become soiled and odorous. Answer C, perforated ma-

terial, will assist with ventilation, but the patient will typically continue to perspire, thus indicating the need to utilize alternative or additional methods to keep the splint from See reference: Sladyk, K and Ryan, SE (eds): West-Frasier, J: Basic splinting.

147. (D) Move the person to a quieter, less stimulating environment. "Many of those who hallucinate do so when they are under stress, especially in environments that are too stimulating for them" (p. 251). Moving a person to a calmer, and less distracting environment, can help to decrease hallucinations if this type of stress is the precipitating factor. Answer A, leaving the person in the same environment would not help. Answer B, completely isolating the person from others, is not recommended because interpersonal contact can have the effect of reinforcing reality and reducing hallucinations. Answer B, moving the person to a more stimulating environment could have the effect of increasing hallucinations. See reference: Early: Responding to symptoms and behaviors.

148. (B) child's speed over long distances becomes less than that of a walking person. A child should be considered for a power wheelchair when the current means of locomotion proves less efficient and slower than locomotion by walking. Because the child will be experiencing progressive muscle weakness, energy conservation is of primary importance. Answers A and C address valid environmental considerations to be made after determining the general need for a powered chair. Waiting until the child becomes unable to propel the wheelchair (answer D), would make the transition more difficult and prevent the child from getting around independently in the meantime. See reference: Case-Smith (ed): Wright-Ott, C and Egilson, S: Mobility.

149. (D) techniques on how to perform activities safely. Instructing caregivers in methods that will promote safe performance of functional activities, such as locking the wheelchair brakes before standing up, and using proper body mechanics, is the first focus for caregiver training. Answers A, B, and C are also useful areas of caregiver instruction, however, safety is the first priority. See reference: Neistadt and Crepeau (eds): Hom, MB, Rogers, JC and James, AB: Treatment of activities of daily living.

150. (B) Handing out trays and utensils in a food service group. This individual demonstrates limitations in the area of interpersonal skills. Handing out trays and utensils requires minimal interaction, and would provide an opportunity for this individual to practice interacting with others at a limited level. None of the other options provides the opportunity to develop interpersonal skills. See reference: Early: Work, homemaking and childcare.

151. (D) Present only a few blocks at a time.
Similar to other children with this diagnosis, this

child most likely has poor impulse control and experiences great difficulty completing a task. By presenting a few blocks at a time (answer D), the COTA can help the child focus on a few relevant stimuli and make it possible to complete a short-term task successfully. This experience will then help the child increase attention span. Soft foam blocks (answer A) are less likely to cause injury if thrown, but their use is not likely to help increase his attention span. Providing blocks of only one color (answer B) may reduce visual stimulation somewhat, and using interlocking blocks (answer C) may make manipulation of the pieces easier, but the overwhelming stimulus caused by presenting all the blocks at once would make these strategies irrelevant. See reference: Case-Smith (ed): Cronin, AS: Psychosocial and emotional domains.

152. (D) in the upper cabinet to the left side.
This pattern of movement promotes the greatest degree of weight shift to the affected side. Putting groceries on the counter directly in front of the person (answer A), or in the upper cabinet to the right side (answer C), would not cause enough weight to be shifted to the affected side, and would even shift weight away from that side. When placing groceries on the counter to the left side (answer B), minimal weight shift occurs. See reference: Pedretti and Early (eds): Pope-Davis, SA: Proprioceptive neuromuscular facilitation approach.

153. (B) offer even-tempered acceptance, reflecting back what is heard without agreeing that the situation is hopeless. Answer B is the most helpful approach. In contrast, a cheerful approach (answer A) can be perceived as denying the importance of the person's feelings. Silence (answer C) may also be perceived as unaccepting. Answer D is incorrect because the COTA needs to provide the structure because initiating and maintaining discussions is often difficult for depressed individuals. See reference: Early: Responding to symptoms and behaviors.

154. (C) Following directions about objects located in front, in back, and to the side. Answer C is correct because a deficit in "position in space" refers to difficulty in perceiving the relationship of an object to the self. Answer A, identifying letters on a distracting page, is not correct because it refers to a problem of recognizing size and shape (form) constancy. Answer D, making judgments about moving through space, is incorrect because it refers to a problem in perceiving spatial relationships. See reference: Case-Smith (ed): Schneck, CM: Visual perception.

155. (C) increase swimming time to 25 minutes or to tolerance. This individual's goal is to maximize strength and endurance. Although ALS is a progressive degenerative disease, improvements in strength and endurance are possible if the individual was not previously functioning at maximum capacity. This individual's performance indicates potential for further improvement. The program should therefore be upgraded, not downgraded (answer B). Methods for improving endurance include increasing the frequency, intensity, or duration of the activity. The correct answer (answer C) increases the duration of the activity while recognizing the importance of avoiding fatigue. Answer A continues the program at a maintenance level. Using adaptive equipment (answer D), such as a flotation belt, is an energy saving strategy that would be appropriate if the individual were experiencing fatigue during swimming. See reference: Dutton: Biomechanical postulates regarding intervention.

156. (A) begin instruction in anger management strategies, such as relaxation. Beginning instruction in anger management techniques such as relaxation, conflict resolution and empathizing would be the next step in a plan to address anger management because the client has accomplished the first step of identifying key stressors leading to his anger and of defining his typical response to such stressors. Answer B, modifying treatment to focus on self-assertiveness, would not be an appropriate emphasis, and making such a change without collaboration with the OTR would be not appropriate. Answer C, providing activities as outlets for anger, may have the effect of "actually increasing anger" (p. 468). Though the client has made some progress towards goals, he has not achieved competence in anger management skills, therefore answer D, recommending discontinuation of services, is also incorrect. See reference: Early: Responding to symptoms and behaviors.

157. (A) Practice regular skin inspection. Children with lower extremity paralysis resulting from myelomeningocele usually experience impaired lower extremity sensation, placing them at risk for developing decubitus ulcers or burns due to contact with hot water or objects. Generally, children with myelomeningocele do not have oral motor or eating problems (answer B) or apnea episodes (answer C), unless Arnold-Chiari deformity is present. Tactile defensive behaviors and other sensory integrative disorders (answer D) can be present in children with spina bifida and myelomeningocele, but the issue of skin breakdown is more important at this time. See reference: Neistadt and Crepeau (eds): Erhardt, RP and Merrill, SC: Neurological dysfunction in children.

158. (A) Client will purchase 10 items at the supermarket with supervision. Short-term goals must relate to the long-term goal being addressed. Because the long-term goal being addressed is independence in grocery shopping, the short-term goal must relate to grocery shopping. Answers B and C do not relate to grocery shopping. "Goals need to be written to show what the patient will accomplish, not what the therapist will do" (p. 94). Answer D is an appropriate treatment intervention, but is written in a way that describes what the OT, not the client, will do. Answers B and C describe activities related to the task of shopping, but not the shopping itself. See reference: AOTA: Effective documentation for occupational therapy: Writing goals.

159. (A) Instruct the individual to wear clothes for 2 days and to then launder those items. Teaching the individual to recognize and judge when clothing needs to be laundered has been unsuccessful, indicating that the individual may not have the capacity to learn this skill. If the OT practitioner determines that the individual can usually wear clothes for 2 days before they need to be laundered, then providing a rigid schedule based on this average removes the need for judgment, and provides a schedule that will result in the individual wearing clean clothes most of the time, if not always. Assessment of the individual's clothing management capabilities (answer B), would have been performed before the implementation of the initial intervention. Taking the clothes to the dry cleaner (answer C), would be cost prohibitive and would still require judgment to determine when they needed to be cleaned. Turning the responsibility over to the staff (answer D), would not promote independence in clothing management. See reference: Bruce and Borg: Cognitive disability frame of reference.

160. (C) Provide a screen to reduce peripheral visual stimuli. Although all the answers given describe techniques that could assist the student, the use of a screen is most appropriate in a mainstream classroom, because the other methods or adaptations (answers A, B, and D) could have a negative impact on the other childrens' ability to learn. See reference: Case-Smith (ed): Schneck, CM: Visual perception.

161. (C) marking the end of each step with high-contrast tape. Difficulty in seeing contrast and color are two forms of decreased visual acuity that cannot be addressed by corrective lenses. Two effective environmental adaptations to these deficits are increasing background contrast and illumination. Using tape or paint to make the edge of each step contrast sharply with the rest of the step is an inexpensive way to adapt the environment. Installing a stair glide or handrails (answers A and B) are more costly adaptations that do not address the problems of decreased visual acuity. Instructing the patient to take only one step at a time (answer D) may cause the individual to be unnecessarily slow, and does not address the problems of decreased visual acuity. See reference: Pedretti and Early (eds): Warren, M: Evaluation and treatment of visual deficits.

162. (B) self-help group. Self-help groups are supportive and educational, and focus on personal growth around a single major life disrupting problem. Support groups (answer C) focus on assisting

members who are in crisis, until the crisis is past. Advocacy groups (answer A) focus on changing others or changing the system, rather than changing one's self. Psychotherapy groups (answer D) focus on understanding the influence of past experiences on present conflicts. See reference: Posthuma: Self-help groups.

163. (C) School newspaper. Anxiety disorder is characterized by extreme self-consciousness and anxiety about competence. Public exposure and pressure for on-the-spot performance heighten the anxiety. By becoming involved in the school newspaper preparation, the student will have an opportunity to develop a sense of competence without the pressure of a face-to-face audience or judged competition, as represented by activities described in answers A, B, and D. See reference: Case-Smith (ed): Cronin, AF: Psychosocial and emotional domains.

164. (B) Raise the toilet. The minimum doorway width that allows a standard wheelchair to pass through easily is 32 inches. A standard toilet is 15 inches, which is 3 inches lower than the standard wheelchair seat. Raising the toilet to 18 inches would make transfers easier for this individual. See reference: Neistadt and Crepeau (eds): Holm, MB, Rogers, JC, and Stone, RG: Person-task-environment intervention: A decision-making guide.

165. (A) Give frequently repeated one- or two-step instructions. The best method to use with an individual with Alzheimer's disease is short instructions of one to two steps, keeping them to the point and repeating them frequently. Demonstration with multiple-step instructions (answer B) can be confusing because it provides too much stimulation. Multiple-step written instructions (answer C) are unlikely to be retained in the individual's short-term memory after reading, or remembered in sequence. Also, written instructions could be lost if the individual puts them down. Verbally repeating directions over and over (answer D), or rehearsal, does not enable a person with Alzheimer's disease to retain information in the memory, and he or she may not repeat the instructions properly. See reference: Neistadt and Crepeau (eds): Holm, M, Rogers, J, and Birge-James, A: Treatment of occupational performance.

166. (D) doll house and dress-up clothes. To encourage symbolic play, the child should be exposed to toys offering imaginative, open-ended play opportunities, encouraging formulation of ideas and feelings. Answers A, B, and C are not only representative of the younger (answer A) or older child (answers B and C), but they also encourage more defined, closed-ended play with predictable results. See reference: Case-Smith (ed): Morrison, CD and Metzger, P: Play.

167. (A) wrist cock-up splint. Carpal tunnel syndrome is a condition that results from compression of the median nerve at the wrist. A wrist cock-up splint positions the wrist in 10 to 20 degrees of extension to alleviate symptoms and prevent further damage. Answer B refers to splints made out of thermoplastic materials, and does not indicate a splint type specific to carpal tunnel syndrome. Resting hand splints (answer C) are typically used to prevent deformity development in individuals with arthritis or quadriplegia. Dynamic MP flexion splints (answer D) are used to assist flexion at the MP joints when this motion is weak or absent. See reference: Trombly (ed): Trombly, CA and Linden, CA: Orthoses: Kinds and purposes

168. (B) calendars. An external memory device uses environmental adaptations or structure to assist an individual in remembering specific information. Examples include setting an alarm clock to wake up in the morning, labeling drawers according to contents, and using a log or calendar to keep track of events and activities. An internal memory device would be the use of internalized memory techniques to structure information. Visual imagery techniques (answer A), mnemonics (answer C), and repetition or rehearsal (answer D), are all examples of internal memory devices. See reference: Zoltan: Executive functions.

169. (C) ease the child to a lying position, remove or pad nearby objects, and loosen clothing. The most important action to take is to protect the child during the seizure by preventing injuries that can occur from falling or hitting objects during movements. Other protective measures include loosening clothing that is restrictive, and placing a blanket or cushion underneath the child if possible. Answer A is incorrect because checking breathing would not be done until the seizure has stopped. Answer B is incorrect because any attempt to restrain the child could result in injury. While it is important to let the seizure end without any interference, Answer D, taking no action except observation, would not help to protect the child from environmental hazards. See reference: Case-Smith (ed): Rogers, SL, Gordon, CY, Schanzenbacher, KE, and Case-Smith, J: Common diagnosis in pediatric occupational therapy practice.

170. (D) The individual asks for more beverages during meals, but appears surprised when the therapist indicates beverages in closed containers are on the meal tray. The subjective portion of the SOAP note should contain information that is gained through a chart review, or communication with the patient, his or her family, or staff. This information is not measurable, and therefore, is considered subjective. Answer A would be in the program plan. Answers B and C would be in the objective portion, because they are either measurable or based on specific observations. See reference: Trombly (ed): Trombly, CA: Planning, guiding, and documenting therapy.

171. (D) managing stigma. More stigma is attached to issues surrounding mental health than physical health, and individuals with mental illness frequently experience prejudice. It is important for individuals re-entering the community to be prepared for this with strategies that will enable them to cope with stigmatization. Self-esteem, assertiveness, and anger management (answers A, B, and C) are skills, which together, enable the individual with mental illness to effectively manage stigma. See reference: Cottrell (ed): Van Leit, B: Managed mental health care: reflections in a time of turmoil.

172. (A) The time he spends at the computer. Because computer work requires very little active movement, and lower extremities, trunk, and neck are generally held in a static position, it is essential to assess how much time the child spends in this position. The COTA must instruct the child to take regular breaks and maintain proper positioning while at the computer to avoid further strain. Answers B, C, and D address other relevant factors in computer use but none that would directly affect the symptoms described. See reference: Case-Smith (ed): Swinth, Y: Assistive technology: Computers and augmentive communication

173. (B) Patient reinstalled a door without reinjury. Answer B suggests that the patient used proper body mechanics. Using proper body mechanics would enable the individual with a back injury to lift heavy objects and perform activities in variety of potentially stressful positions, without increasing pain or chance of reinjury. The ability to work a full day without becoming fatigued (answer A) would more likely reflect the outcome of participating in a work-hardening program or using energy conservation techniques. Answer C would more likely result from instruction in joint protection techniques to reduce joint stress and pain. The ability to use a hammer for a sustained period of time (answer D) would reflect the result of participation in a strengthening or conditioning program. See reference: Pedretti and Early (eds): Smithline, J and Dunlop, LE: Low back pain.

174. (A) Subjective section. The subjective portion of a SOAP note (answer A) includes what the patient reports or comments about the treatment. The objective portion of the SOAP note (answer B) focuses on measurable and or observable data obtained by the OT practitioner through specific evaluations, observations or the use of the therapeutic activities. The assessment part of the SOAP note (answer C) addresses the effectiveness of treatment and any changes needed, the status of the goals, and justification of continuing occupational therapy treatment. The plan section of a SOAP note (answer D) includes statements related to continuing treatment, the frequency and duration of the treatment, suggestions for additional activities or treatment techniques, the need for further evaluation, and the recommendations for new goals as needed. See reference: Early: Medical records and documentation.

175. (B) self-monitor signs of illness and seek help if signs occur. Teaching a client to recognize the signs and symptoms of his or her particular condition provides the person with a specific tool to use for preventing relapse episodes. This strategy also provides an awareness of behaviors that alert the person to take the action of contacting or seeking support from a physician, case manager, peer or family member. Answer A, get adequate exercise, and answer C, maintain personal hygiene, are important for maintaining daily living skills, but do not specifically relate to relapse prevention. Making a life change (answer D) reflects the type of event that may trigger a relapse and knowledge of such triggers would be part of a relapse prevention education, not a recommended strategy for prevention of relapse. See reference: Early: Activities of daily living.

176. (C) assess the patient's ability to hold the toothbrush with a built-up handle. Progress is demonstrated by the ability to successfully perform an activity that was previously unsuccessful. A patient who was initially unable to hold a built-up handle may need to use a universal cuff (answer D). However, assessing the patient's ability to use a universal cuff is not an appropriate method for determining if she has achieved progress in this area. Evaluation using tools such as a goniometer and pinch meter (answers A and B) are formal, not functional, methods of evaluation. In addition, an individual using tenodesis may not have the strength to register a reading on these tools. See reference: Trombly (ed): Hollar, LD: Spinal cord injury.

177. (D) providing a variety of physical, creative, productive, and educational activities. A COTA is well qualified to serve as an activities director in nursing homes. The goals of an activities program in a nursing home are to promote the physical, social, and mental well-being of the residents through participation in activities. While the occupational performance (answers A and C) of individuals may be addressed by a COTA as part of an activities program to a degree, the primary emphasis is to provide a range of physical, creative, productive, leisure, spiritual, community, and educational activities to the nursing home population. Residents who are also receiving occupational therapy services will benefit when the OT practitioner and activities director coordinate their efforts to meet mutual goals. Medicare has established requirements for activities programming in nursing homes, however, it is not a billable service (answer B). See reference: Sladyk, K and Ryan, SE (eds): Ryan, SE: The role of the OTA as an activities director.

178. (C) Introduce and discuss concepts of community living, and give clients an opportunity to voice their concerns. Clients who have not left the hospital in many years are likely to be anxious about moving into a new environment. Introducing and discussing concepts of community living (answer C), allows the staff to provide information and allows the client to voice concerns and ask questions. Visiting future community settings and developing goals (answers A and B) are important, but would follow later. Because the patients have been receiving OT in the hospital for many years, evaluation (answer D) should already have occurred. See reference: Cottrell (ed): Baxley, S: Options for community practice: The Springfield Hospital model.

179. (A) Activities that promote mother-child communication and foster attachment. When working with the mother of infants, it is most important to develop the bond between mother and baby. Many of the mothers in this type of program engage in high-risk behaviors, including unprotected sex and substance abuse. They often have poor leisure skills, limited or no knowledge of child development, and do not know how to play appropriately with their children. Low frustration tolerance and limited awareness can result in inappropriate responses to problems with their children. Modeling and discussing appropriate disciplinary techniques (answer B) is an effective way of developing this skill for parents of toddlers and young children. Answers C and D also include important concepts for these teenage mothers and their children, who are at risk for cognitive, psychosocial and emotional deficits; however, in infancy, the mother-child bond is paramount. See reference: Cottrell (ed): Zeitz, MA: The mothers' project: A clinical case management system.

180. (B) fall prevention. All of the answers are important to the quality of life and independence for individuals living in an ALF. Falls, however, are the leading cause of death due to accident in people over 65 and are a major reason for nursing home placement. See reference: Bonder and Wagner (eds): Tideiksaar, R: Falls.

181. (C) environmental modification. Environmental modification is the area of intervention that can best assist in maintaining safety and supporting function at home by providing the physical and sensory environments to compensate for deficits. Strength and endurance activities (answer A) will have no direct effect on safety in the home. Cognitive rehabilitation techniques (answer B) are not indicated for conditions with progressive cognitive deterioration. Use of assertiveness skills (answer D) would be inappropriate for dealing with the kinds of communication problems encountered with persons who have Alzheimer's disease. See reference: Pedretti and Early (eds): Glogoski, C: Alzheimer's disease.

182. (C) recommend activities to develop fine coordination that teachers can incorporate into classroom programming. Recommending classroom activities that will develop the performance component of fine motor coordination would be the best population-based intervention because it involves addressing the occupational performance needs of many students. Answers A, B, and D focus OT efforts on individual intervention approaches. See reference: AOTA: Guide To Occupational Therapy Practice:

183. (B) providing staff education, recommendations, and support for restraint alternatives. Providing education on the effects of restraints, and recommendations, and program support for alternatives to the use of restraints, such as activities, distraction techniques, and environmental adaptations would be the most appropriate functions for the OT practitioner to provide. Answers A, C, and D would be elements of a facility's restraint reduction efforts, but would not be likely to be performed by the OT practitioner. See reference: Hellen: Physical wellness: Mobility and exercise.

184. (C) Preparing and consuming nutritional and normal-size portions of food. Individuals with eating disorders are generally well versed in weight-loss techniques (answer A), as well as in making food look appealing for others to eat (answer D). "They have extensive knowledge of the caloric content of foods (answer B), but little knowledge of other aspects of food content, such as vitamin and nutritive value. . .A cooking group would support the experience of preparing and consuming normal-size portions of food" (p. 143). See reference: Early: Understanding psychiatric diagnosis: The DSM-IV.

185. (A) Stocking the shelves at a local grocery. OT interventions for the transition from school to adult life should focus on real-life functional activities in actual work settings. Working in a natural setting affords students opportunities to develop skills necessary for success in community jobs. Working in a sheltered workshop or in their own school environment does not provide real-life settings for job training. Reading help wanted ads and role playing interviews (answer D) are not considered vocational training. See reference: Case-Smith (ed): Spencer, K: Transition services: From school to adult life.

186. (C) Program evaluation. Program evaluation is the compilation of the intervention results for a population of individuals. Final evaluations of clients involved in the program and client satisfaction surveys (answers A and B) may both be components of the program evaluation. Utilization review (answer D) evaluates the care that is provided to ensure that services were appropriate and not overutilized or underutilized. Utilization review also analyzes the services to ensure that the interventions were provided in an economical manner. See reference: Neistadt and Crepeau (eds): Perinchief, JM: Management of occupational therapy services.

187. (A) Daily, direct contact at the site of work. According to the AOTA document *Guide for Supervision of Occupational Therapy Personnel in the Delivery of Occupational Therapy Services*, an entry-level COTA must receive "close supervision" regardless of the working environment. Answers B, C, and D are appropriate for individuals requiring less than close supervision. See reference: AOTA: Guide for supervision of occupational therapy personnel in the delivery of occupational therapy services.

188. (A) Use disposable cotton swabs and have clients bring their own cosmetics. Universal precautions help prevent the spread of infection. Using disposable cotton swabs and having clients use their own cosmetics would be effective in reducing the risk of infection. Combing someone's hair (answer B) does not usually involve risks related to blood or bodily fluids. Washing equipment (answer C) that is used near eyes and mouths by several individuals is inadequate. Avoiding glass containers (answer D) is a safety precaution that is related to self-harm and not universal precautions. See reference: Early: Safety techniques.

189. (A) When the COTA consistently obtains the same results as the OTR. The term "service competency" indicates an interrater reliability between two OT professionals. Service competency is determined by skill level, not by years of experience (answer D). Passing the NBCOT examination (answer B) establishes entry-level competence, not service competence in a particular area. OT practitioners have a professional responsibility to maintain competence, and continuing education (answer C) is one method for maintaining competence and promoting lifelong learning. See reference: Neistadt and Crepeau (eds): Sands, M: Practitioners' perspectives on the occupational therapist and occupational therapy assistant partnership.

190. (D) Program evaluation. Program evaluation is a systematic collection and reporting of outcome data to document program effectiveness and cost-efficiency. Quality assurance (answer A) identifies problems and implements corrective actions. Peer review (answer B) is the system of other service providers assessing the provision of care to ensure appropriate interventions and documentation practices. Answer C, utilization review, is the process of analyzing the provision of services to promote the most economical delivery of service. See reference: Neistadt and Crepeau (eds): Perinchief, JM: Management of occupational therapy services.

191. (D) Discuss the observations with an OTR who is present. Although the COTA's own supervisor is absent, an OTR present would become the acting supervisor for the day. The COTA should always discuss concerns with the supervisor first. Going to the administrator (answer C) would not only disregard the chain of command, but could escalate a problem that should be handled internally. Training in ADLs is a skilled service beyond the scope of the service of an aide. The COTA should not allow the aide to finish the treatment session (answer A). It may not be feasible for the COTA to complete the session (answer B), but it would also be inappropriate to terminate the aide when simple review of procedures and role delineations would be indicated in this case. See reference: Early: Supervision.

192. (C) Supervision of noncertified personnel. Under the supervision of an OTR, COTAs often participate in orienting, training, and evaluating the performance of unlicensed or noncertified personnel. Quality assurance programs (answer A) should be established by team members, not independently. COTAs may supervise other COTAs (under the supervision of an OTR), but supervision of OTRs must be carried out by OTRs (answer B). Management responsibilities such as marketing (answer D) are also within the scope of practice of the OTR. See reference: AOTA: Occupational therapy roles.

193. (A) Read the facility's infection control plan. An infection control plan most likely incluldes appropriate techniques and procedures for storing and handling foods within the OT department. Such plans specify the shelf lives of certain foods, standards for storage of food, use of hair nets, and cooking temperatures and times. A risk management plan (answer C) addresses the issue of liability in reference to negligence and malpractice issues. The dietary department (answer B) would not be likely to have information regarding the handling and storage of food. Cooking with only canned foods (answer D) would still require the COTA to apply the principles of infection control. See reference: Sladyk, K and Ryan, SE (eds): Leary, CJ: Management issues and models.

194. (D) call 911. The OT practitioner should be knowledgeable about situations that may be potentially dangerous for patients. This question requires that the practitioner be knowledgeable about the appropriate ranges for heart rate and blood pressure. Both of the measures are above safe ranges and indicate that the patient is medically unstable. Therefore, immediate medical services would be necessary. Answers A, B, and C do not recognize the seriousness of the situation and could delay the necessary medical attention. See reference: Neistadt and Crepeau (eds): Ferraro, R: Cardiopulmonary dysfunction in adults.

195. (B) document services provided, and date the note as a late entry. It is the responsibility of the OT practitioner to document services provided. After an error is found, the OT practitioner should document the services as recalled. Answers C and D are incorrect because they do not provide for documentation of services. Answer A is unethical in that it is not appropriate for the therapist to document the note and backdate it. See reference: AOTA: Effective documentation for occupational therapy.

196. (D) Demonstrate service competency in the use of paraffin. "Physical agent modalities may be used by occupational therapy practitioners when used as an adjunct to or in preparation for purposeful activity by a practitioner who has demonstrated service competency" (p. 1075). Service competency in this area includes, but is not limited to, possessing the theoretical background and technical skills (answer A) for the safe and effective use of the modality. Although study and practice (answer B) are necessary to establish service competency, an OTR must determine that the COTA is competent before he or she can use physical agent modalities. Having an experienced OTR on-site (answer C) is not adequate if service competency has not been established. See reference: AOTA: Registered occupational therapists and certified occupational therapy assistants and modalities.

197. (D) use brochures, posters, videotapes, and films available from the AOTA to enhance the presentation. The emphasis of this question is that it is every OT practitioner's responsibility to promote the profession. Simple, daily public relations activities occur each time an OT practitioner (whether it is a COTA or an OTR) describes the services to be provided to patients and families. More complex public relations may include developing a plan to promote community awareness regarding the profession. A public relations program is designed to increase public awareness about the role and importance of OT services. See reference: Sladyk, K (ed): Bowler, DF: OT and political action.

198. (A) Contact administration to let them know of the unforeseen change in service delivery and make appropriate adjustments to billing. Occupational therapy practitioners are ethically bound to charge fairly and accurately for services. Billing is a form of documentation and should reflect skilled services that are actually provided. While patient education can and should be considered an appropriate skilled intervention under the right circumstances, time spent coaxing a client to participate (answer C) does not fall under this activity. Answers B and D both involve fraud and are unethical. See reference: AOTA: Occupational therapy code of ethics.

199. (C) collaborate with the OTR to determine discharge options and actions. COTAs may recommend discontinuation of OT services to the supervising OTR. The OTR is responsible for making the final determination regarding discharge and future recommendations (answer A). It would be unethical to continue seeing the client after OT goals have been achieved (answer B). See reference: AOTA: Standards of practice for occupational therapy.

200. (B) Based on his refusal, do not treat the individual and document the interaction in the chart. As stated in principle 3 of the *Code of Ethics*, "Occupational therapy personnel shall respect the individual's right to refuse professional services or involvement in research or educational activities" (p. 614–615). Answers A and C are incorrect because the therapist proceeded to treat the patient against his wishes. Answer D is incorrect because it does not meet with principle 5 of the *Code of Ethics*, "Occupational therapy practitioners shall record and report in an accurate and timely manner all information related to professional activities" (p. 615). See reference: AOTA: Occupational therapy code of ethics.

SIMULATION EXAMINATION 2

> **Directions:** Circle the correct answer to the following questions. When you have completed this examination, check your answers against the answer key that follows. As you will see, an explanation is given for each answer along with a reference for further study. The book author is listed as well as the chapter author. See the bibliography for complete references. Study the areas in which your comprehension was low, then test yourself again by taking Simulation Examination 3.

Evaluation

1. **An individual with depression refuses to participate in an initial evaluation process. He sits away from the other clients, does not make eye contact with anyone, and states he just doesn't "feel like doing anything right now." Which of the following actions is the MOST appropriate for the COTA to take?**
   A. Leave the client alone until he begins to make eye contact, indicating his readiness to participate.
   B. Approach the client briefly several times throughout the session without making any demands on him.
   C. Inform the client that his doctor will need to be notified of his refusal to participate.
   D. Explain to the client that once he lets you evaluate him, you'll be able to help him more effectively.

2. **While observing a newly referred child in the playground, the COTA suspects that the child has dyspraxia. The MOST relevant assessment to determine the child's level of performance will be one which determines the child's ability to:**
   A. print or write.
   B. read.
   C. calculate mathematics.
   D. plan new motor tasks.

3. **The BEST way for the OT practitioner to evaluate the presence of unilateral neglect is by using which of the following evaluations?**
   A. Six-block assembly
   B. Line bisection
   C. Proverb interpretation
   D. Identification of the square in four overlapping figures

4. **An OT practitioner wishes to identify how a patient spends his leisure time, which leisure activities he especially enjoys, and which others he has participated in that he would be interested in renewing. The MOST appropriate tool for this purpose is a(n):**
   A. evaluation of living skills.
   B. interest checklist.
   C. activity configuration.
   D. self-care evaluation.

5. **A young child with a diagnosis of spina bifida has been referred for an assessment. When collecting the initial data by interviewing the child's mother, the OT practitioner should focus PRIMARILY on:**
   A. the mother's concerns and goals for her child.
   B. medical management.
   C. equipment needs.
   D. the physical layout of the home.

6. **An OT practitioner is performing a home management evaluation of an ambulatory individual with cerebral palsy who is cognitively intact, but exhibits an ataxic gait pattern. The PRIMARY focus of the evaluation should be:**
   A. safety and stability.

B. the individual's ability to reach and bend.

C. whether the individual has adequate strength to perform homemaking tasks.

D. fatigue and endurance levels.

7. **An individual who has recently undergone a knee replacement is working on homemaking skills in the ADL suite. The PT has indicated the patient can ambulate with close supervision using a cane. While the individual has arrived for therapy on time for the past 3 days, she has consistently left her cane back in her room. When the COTA asks where her cane is, the individual replies, "Oh, that cane, it's just so ugly." Which of the following actions is MOST appropriate for the COTA to take?**

A. Discuss issues related to self-concept with the individual.

B. Evaluate the individual's short-term memory.

C. Evaluate the individual's long-term memory.

D. Devise strategies to address time management.

8. **While working with an 8-month-old child, the COTA observes him assume a quadruped position and then begin to rock back and forth. This behavior MOST likely indicates:**

A. perseverative tendencies.

B. normal development.

C. low muscle tone.

D. limitation in movement repertoire.

9. **When administering an evaluation of upper extremity function to a newly admitted patient with Guillain-Barré syndrome, it is MOST important to:**

A. test proximal muscle strength first.

B. perform the evaluation over several sessions.

C. include sensory testing.

D. evaluate range of motion.

10. **A COTA working in a long-term care facility frequently evaluates cognitive performance. Which of the following methods is BEST for evaluating remote memory?**

A. Name three items, and ask the individual to list the items 5 minutes later.

B. Ask the individual about the grade school he or she attended.

C. Have the individual state the place, date, and time.

D. Ask the individual what he or she had for breakfast that day.

11. **While observing a child for the first time, the COTA notes that the child responds to a loud noise by abducting and extending the arms. The reflex, or reaction, observed in this child is documented by the COTA as a:**

A. rooting reflex.

B. Moro reflex.

C. flexor withdrawal reflex.

D. neck righting reaction.

12. **An OT practitioner who is a member of an assistive technology team evaluating an adult with severe motor limitations is MOST likely to:**

A. make recommendations for ways of operating the technology.

B. recommend communication strategies.

C. seek funding sources for the technology.

D. solve mechanical or software problems.

13. **An individual with schizophrenia is newly admitted to the hospital. He is asked to describe what brought him to the hospital for admission. The individual responds by saying, "I took a cab." In the report, the OT practitioner is MOST likely to identify this response as:**

A. delusional thinking.

B. a distractible response.

C. a concrete response.

D. an insightful response.

14. **An OT practitioner observes a child with a learning disability use an unusually tight grip when writing with a pencil. The child also frequently breaks the pencil point by applying too much pressure on the paper. This type of problem is MOST likely caused by inadequate sensory information from the:**

A. vestibular system.

B. auditory system.

C. somatosensory system.

D. visual system.

15. **Which of the following methods is BEST for evaluating a hook grasp?**

A. Direct the individual to hold a sewing needle while it is being threaded.

B. Observe the individual lift a tall glass half filled with water.

C. Have the individual hold a heavy handbag by the handles.

D. Hand the individual a key to place in a lock.

16. **Which of the following activities would MOST effectively evaluate group interaction skills during a 45-minute OT session?**

    A. The clients make individual collages, sharing a set of magazines to complete the activity.
    B. All group members construct one tower that incorporates all of the pieces provided in a set of constructional materials (e.g., Legos, Tinkertoys, or Erector set).
    C. All group members work together to make pizza and salad for their lunch that day.
    D. Each client selects a short-term craft activity from four available samples.

17. **Through the evaluation process, the OT practitioner may consider many possibilities for intervention, however, the specific plan for implementation of intervention is MOST often developed at which point in the OT process?**

    A. After observation or screening
    B. After the interview
    C. After the evaluation
    D. After the development of the goals and objectives

18. **While observing a client who has just been admitted to the rehabilitation unit after a right CVA with left hemiplegia, the OT practitioner notices that the patient's left arm lays limply by the patient's side. This MOST likely indicates:**

    A. normal upper extremity function.
    B. flaccidity.
    C. subluxation.
    D. spasticity.

19. **What should the OT practitioner do FIRST to obtain accurate information about a patient's family situation and about their occupational, cultural, and educational backgrounds?**

    A. Read the medical record.
    B. Interview the patient's family.
    C. Interview the patient.
    D. Read the social worker's report.

20. **A child with motor delays is being evaluated to determine how he performs self-care activities. Which evaluation procedure is MOST likely to provide relevant information about self-care function?**

    A. Standardized tests of motor development

B. Review of the medical record
C. Developmental screening test
D. Home observation and parent interview

21. **An OT practitioner is evaluating two-point discrimination in an individual with a median nerve injury. The MOST appropriate procedure is to:**

    A. apply the stimuli beginning at the little finger and progress toward the thumb.
    B. test the thumb area first, then progress toward the little finger.
    C. present test stimuli in an organized pattern to improve reliability during retesting.
    D. allow the individual unlimited time to respond.

22. **When a new patient is referred for psychiatric services, the COTA and OTR both review the chart. The OTR then completes performance measures, and the COTA performs an interview. The COTA/OTR team relies on the interview part of the assessment to address the individual's:**

    A. diagnosis.
    B. current medications.
    C. ability to concentrate and solve problems.
    D. view of the problem and an overall goal.

23. **A child running in the playground trips and falls forward, landing on outstretched arms. This behavior is BEST described as a(n):**

    A. primitive reflex.
    B. righting reaction.
    C. equilibrium reaction.
    D. protective extension response.

24. **An individual who recently experienced an MI is now medically stable and has been referred to OT. To determine the individual's current endurance level, the OT practitioner plans to monitor performance of self-care activities. The FIRST step is to:**

    A. take the individual's vital signs after performance of self-care activities.
    B. observe the individual for signs and symptoms during self-care activities.
    C. take the individual's vital signs at rest.
    D. take vital signs 5 minutes after the individual has completed self-care activities.

25. **An OT practitioner is working on morning activities of daily living with a young adult who recently sustained a traumat-**

ic brain injury. The client requires prompting to apply shaving cream to his face and to pick up his razor. After these cues, the client is then able to complete the shaving activity. This MOST likely indicates a deficit in which of the following performance components?

A. Impulsivity
B. Initiation
C. Memory
D. Attention

26. A 4-year-old child with spina bifida has a lesion at the lumbar level that causes her bladder to be flaccid. The parents are requesting a bladder training program. The MOST appropriate response would be to:

A. explain to the parents that toilet training is not a feasible option.
B. recommend waiting until the child is 5 years old.
C. begin a toilet training program.
D. assess the child's ability to remove lower extremity garments.

27. An OT practitioner is performing an environmental assessment to determine accessibility for a client who will be returning home. The FIRST step in this process is to:

A. identify the barriers to movement and function in the home environment.
B. identify and analyze the tasks and occupations that the client will be performing in the home.
C. identify the aspects of the environment that support movement and function in the home.
D. determine the social environment of the client.

28. A homemaker recently diagnosed with early-stage Alzheimer's disease lives with her husband who is a high school teacher. Which of the following is MOST important to address in the initial evaluation?

A. Ability to chew and swallow
B. Kitchen safety
C. Anger management
D. Recognition of family members

29. During an initial interview, parents describe their child as having severe difficulty in communicating and interacting with others. The COTA also observes

that the child exhibits many repetitive and ritualistic behaviors. The behaviors described are MOST likely to be associated with:

A. attention deficit hyperactivity disorder.
B. childhood conduct disorder.
C. obsessive-compulsive disorder.
D. pervasive developmental disorder of childhood.

30. The MOST appropriate assessment instrument for the OT practitioner to use for measuring range of motion of the hand is a(n):

A. goniometer.
B. dynamometer.
C. pinch meter.
D. aesthesiometer.

31. A COTA working in a geropsychiatric day program runs a craft group after lunch. Many of the clients doze off during the group, which prevents them from benefiting from the activity. The COTA should recognize this as a problem with:

A. motivation.
B. interest.
C. level of arousal.
D. attention span.

32. An 11-month-old infant who was born 3 months prematurely demonstrates the ability to creep, pull to a standing position, put objects into containers, and respond to the word "no." She does not understand object permanence, cruise, or demonstrate a pincer grasp. Adjusted for prematurity, this child's developmental level should be considered to be:

A. 1 month delayed.
B. 2 months delayed.
C. 3 months delayed.
D. age appropriate.

33. An individual has been referred to OT following an upper extremity injury resulting in partial paralysis. Which of the following assessments would be MOST important for an OT practitioner guided by a biomechanical frame of reference?

A. Adaptive equipment needs
B. Tone, reflex development, automatic reactions
C. Strength, range of motion, coordination
D. Habits, values, roles

Treatment Planning

34. **Staff members in a group home report to the COTA that several of the men repeatedly try to touch the female clients and staff, and that they often make sexual gestures and comments. Which of the following environmental modifications would be MOST likely to reduce this behavior?**

    A. Provide a relatively active and stimulating environment with opportunities for these individuals to engage in real-life activities.

    B. Stand to the side of these individuals instead of face to face during interactions with them.

    C. Avoid having these individuals in close proximity to others to reduce opportunities for physical contact.

    D. Advise these individuals in a calm, nonjudgmental manner about the behavior you expect.

35. **To develop the MOST relevant goals and objectives for a child's OT program, the COTA should focus goals on:**

    A. the child's priorities.

    B. the priorities of the parents or caregivers.

    C. the therapist's priorities for solution of problems identified in the OT evaluation.

    D. child, caregiver, and therapist priorities.

36. **A COTA provides a leather-working activity to an individual with C7 quadriplegia in order to increase grip strength. Which component of this activity would be MOST effective in promoting this goal?**

    A. Holding the hammer

    B. Holding the stamping tools

    C. Squeezing the sponge to wet the leather

    D. Lacing with the needle

37. **A COTA is beginning training meal preparation with a homemaker after a TBI. The activity that should be introduced FIRST is:**

    A. making a peanut-butter-and-jelly sandwich.

    B. preparing a hot cup of tea with sugar.

    C. pouring a glass of orange juice.

    D. cooking a grilled ham-and-cheese sandwich.

38. **A child's long-term goal is to increase fine motor skills. The assessment has revealed a deficit in tactile discrimination,** specifically stereognosis. The MOST relevant short-term goal would be that the:

    A. child will correctly identify five out of five fingers touched when given tactile stimulus.

    B. child will correctly identify five out of five shapes drawn on the dorsum of her hand.

    C. child will correctly identify five out of five matching textures.

    D. child will correctly identify, by feel only, five out of five common objects.

39. **In establishing long-term goals for an individual with T4 paraplegia in a rehabilitation setting, the COTA would MOST likely predict that the patient will attain what level of independence with bathing, dressing, and transfers?**

    A. Complete independence with self-care and transfers

    B. Independence with self-care and minimal assistance with transfers

    C. Minimal assistance with self-care and moderate assistance with transfers

    D. Dependence with both self-care and transfers

40. **After administering an interest checklist, the COTA documents that an individual has identified a few solitary leisure interests, but no interests involving social interaction. Based on this information, what is the BEST activity to use in the next session of a leisure counseling group?**

    A. A leisure inventory assessment

    B. An activity exploring leisure opportunities and problems

    C. A magazine picture collage

    D. A calendar of community leisure activities for the first week after discharge

41. **Poor impulse control has been identified as the primary deficit in a 12-year-old boy with conduct disorder. Which of the following is the MOST effectively written functional OT goal?**

    A. Within 6 months, the client will participate in classroom activities for 1 hour without disruptive outbursts twice a day.

    B. Within 6 months, the client will attend to an activity for 30 minutes, demonstrating improved impulse control.

    C. The client will show a 50% reduction in the frequency of disruptive outbursts within 6 months.

    D. When presented with a new activity, the

client will follow directions without protest, four out of five times, within 6 months.

42. **A flight attendant with a back injury is participating in a work-hardening program. The client can successfully simulate distributing magazines to all passengers in a plane using proper body mechanics. To upgrade the program gradually, the COTA should NEXT request that the client simulate:**
    A. putting blankets in the overhead compartments.
    B. distributing full meal trays to the passengers.
    C. distributing magazines to half of the passengers in the plane.
    D. putting luggage in the overhead compartments.

43. **A college student has been referred to a day treatment program following hospitalization for an acute schizophrenic episode. The individual is uncomfortable in social settings, has difficulty sustaining conversations, is unable to make eye contact, and responds to others with bizarre comments. Which of the following would be the MOST effective treatment approach?**
    A. Vestibular stimulation and gross-motor exercises
    B. Modification of the environment
    C. Pleasurable activities that don't require conscious attention to movement
    D. Social skills training

44. **A child displays poor postural stability because of low muscle tone. To promote beginning antigravity control, the FIRST activity that should be performed is:**
    A. pull-to-sit, leaning back against a therapy ball.
    B. prone scooter obstacle course.
    C. hippity-hop races.
    D. batting a balloon while the child is suspended in net.

45. **A COTA is simulating cylindrical grasping activities with a client who desires to work on the skills necessary to be a carpenter. Which of the following activities would MOST likely address these needs?**
    A. Positioning a nail on a piece of wood
    B. Hammering a nail into a piece of wood
    C. Carrying a pail of bolts
    D. Unscrewing a lunchbox thermos

46. **The COTA is using a sensory integration approach with a group of regressed patients with limited attention spans. Most group members can tolerate a group situation for no more than a half hour. The BEST activity to begin the session with is:**
    A. ask each patient to introduce themself.
    B. pass around a scent box and ask each patient to smell the contents.
    C. ask each patient to read a favorite poem.
    D. discuss the menu for lunch.

47. **A 5-year-old child with autism needs a preparatory vestibular activity to decrease his level of arousal so that he will be able to concentrate on simple activities in school. The BEST activity would be:**
    A. bouncing while sitting on a large therapy ball.
    B. rocking in prone on a therapy ball, with feet touching the floor.
    C. spinning in supine while on a hammock swing.
    D. rolling down a large wedge.

48. **An individual has sustained a large, full-thickness burn to both upper extremities during a fireworks display. The client is in the acute care phase of treatment. Which of the following BEST represents an acute care rehabilitation goal?**
    A. Prevent loss of joint and skin mobility.
    B. Provide adaptive equipment.
    C. Provide compression and vascular support garments.
    D. Prevent scar hypertrophy through scar management techniques.

49. **Which aspects of psychosocial performance are MOST important to emphasize in developing a client's work potential in a prevocational program?**
    A. Punctuality, accepting directions from a supervisor, and interacting with coworkers
    B. Memory, sequencing of work tasks, attending to work tasks, and making decisions
    C. Standing tolerance, eye–hand coordination, and endurance
    D. Maintaining personal cleanliness and adhering to safety precautions

50. **When developing play activities for a child with acute juvenile rheumatoid**

arthritis, which of the following precautions should the COTA follow?

A. Avoid light touch.
B. Avoid rapid vestibular stimulation.
C. Avoid resistive materials.
D. Avoid elevated temperatures.

51. **After evaluation, a short-term goal for an individual who had a total hip replacement was to dress with minimal assistance, using adaptive equipment and verbal cues to follow hip precautions. After 1 week of treatment, the individual is able to dress with standby assistance, using adaptive equipment and verbal cues to follow hip precautions. What skills does this person need to demonstrate before changing the goal?**

A. Less time needed to perform dressing
B. Improved concentration
C. Ability to consistently follow hip precautions
D. Ability to use adaptive devices appropriately

52. **When planning treatment for individuals diagnosed with eating disorders, the COTA's initial OT treatment goals would MOST likely address:**

A. increasing self-awareness through expressive activities.
B. increasing awareness of nutritional issues.
C. improving school performance skills.
D. making recommendations or referrals for family therapy.

53. **A COTA/OTR team receives a consult for an infant in the NICU whose mother has a history of drug abuse during pregnancy. Using a sensory integrative approach, what is the FIRST action the COTA/OT team should take?**

A. Determine the mother's current medical status, parental involvement, and support systems.
B. Recommend a social work referral to address social concerns, provide emotional support and community program information, and make a referral to the Department of Human Services.
C. Modify the environment to protect the infant from excessive and/or inappropriate sensory stimulation prior to direct intervention.
D. Assess motor and behavioral skills to identify areas of developmental delay in order to educate family and medical staff of necessary positional and environmental strategies for skill acquisition.

54. **An individual demonstrates a left visual field cut as a result of a TBI, and demonstrates difficulty crossing the midline during many self-care activities. Which of the following activities would MOST effectively promote this individual's ability to cross the midline?**

A. Making a coil pot out of clay
B. Making a macramé planter
C. Stringing a bead necklace
D. Weaving on a frame loom

55. **The occupational therapist is a member of the interdisciplinary team providing transition services for a 17-year-old male with moderate learning disabilities. The goal is to help the student engage in part-time work at a local stationery store. Which of the following interventions is MOST appropriate?**

A. Have the student practice work tasks in the classroom with peers.
B. Observe performance at the job site and make recommendations to increase productivity.
C. Teach math and money management skills to help the student handle his pay check.
D. Teach the student interviewing skills to increase the likelihood of eventually obtaining full-time employment.

56. **A COTA is collaborating with a new teacher to plan classroom activities for a 6-year-old child with developmental dyspraxia. Which would be the MOST accurate description for the COTA to provide to the teacher to explain this problem?**

A. A problem with learning new motor skills
B. A sensory integration problem
C. A lack of development of higher order reflex reactions
D. A problem of poor balance

57. **A COTA working with a patient who has an above-the-knee amputation has planned an activity that requires the patient to retrieve food items (cans, boxes, etc.) from a bag of groceries on the floor and place them on cabinet shelves at various heights, from chest level to several feet above his head. The COTA has selected this activity PRIMARILY because it addresses the performance component of:**

A. postural control.
B. muscle strength.

C. functional mobility.
D. soft tissue integrity.

58. **A COTA is working with three individuals in a cooking group. The individuals demonstrate difficulty attending to tasks, frequently ask to leave the room, and do not interact with each other. Based on the developmental group concept, which of the following is the MOST appropriate goal for this group?**
   A. Each member will take a leadership role within the session.
   B. Members will share materials with at least one other group member.
   C. Each member will express two positive feelings about themselves within the group session.
   D. Each member will remain in the group without disrupting the work of others for 15 minutes.

59. **When planning a therapeutic program for a child who has deficits in visual discrimination, the FIRST step is to provide matching activities that require:**
   A. discrimination among the colors of objects.
   B. discrimination among the shapes of objects.
   C. discrimination among the positions of objects.
   D. the ability to recognize objects.

60. **The assessment results for an individual who is diagnosed with a CVA indicate that the patient exhibits a flaccid left upper extremity, impaired sensation throughout the arm, and marked pitting edema of the affected hand. Based on prioritization of this person's needs, the COTA's initial interventions would include:**
   A. positioning, compression glove, and edema massage, followed by passive range-of-motion exercises.
   B. splinting, elevation of the arm, and active range-of-motion exercises.
   C. no action until the edema subsides.
   D. having the individual attempt to squeeze a ball.

61. **A COTA is working with a man diagnosed with schizophrenia. He states that his main goal is to have a girlfriend. Which of the following statements would then be the MOST appropriate short-term OT goal?**

A. The client will develop a friendship with a female within 6 months.
B. After each group session, the client will identify the ways in which his disability has interfered with his thinking processes.
C. The client will initiate appropriate, casual greetings when beginning casual conversations with female staff.
D. During conversations with female group members, the client will make eye contact for 8 to 10 seconds, twice in each half-hour group.

62. **An adolescent with mental retardation is planning to enter a supported employment program in the community after leaving school. Which area of intervention would the COTA be MOST likely to focus on?**
   A. Developing the student's leisure interests and skills
   B. Developing the student's vocational interests, social skills, and community mobility skills
   C. Facilitating development of the student's gross motor skills
   D. Facilitating development of the student's fine motor skills

63. **Which type of splint would be MOST appropriate for an individual who has a diagnosis of ulnar nerve injury?**
   A. A wrist cock-up splint
   B. An anticlaw splint
   C. A resting hand splint
   D. A cone

Treatment Implementation

64. **A COTA is planning a group session in which the group members will be encouraged to participate in a game of chance. Which of the following would the COTA MOST likely introduce to the group?**
   A. Collecting baseball cards
   B. Bingo
   C. Charades
   D. Balloon volleyball

65. **A 16-year-old boy with juvenile rheumatoid arthritis is ready to begin shaving, but has difficulty as a result of limited range of motion in his shoulders and elbows. Which of the following is the BEST adaptation for him to use?**
   A. Electric razor attached to universal cuff

B. Safety razor with built-up handle
C. Safety razor with extended handle
D. Safety razor attached to universal cuff

66. **An individual with amyotrophic lateral sclerosis has asked a COTA how to maintain strength in weak (fair plus) wrist extensors. Which is the MOST appropriate intervention for the COTA to recommend?**
    A. A cock-up wrist support
    B. Playing Velcro checkers to tolerance
    C. Active range of motion of the wrist daily without resistance
    D. Wrist extension exercises several times a day against maximal resistance

67. **During hospitalization, an individual has made significant progress in the facility's return to work program, and is now being discharged to a group home. He has expressed fears regarding "working in the real world," but has demonstrated the interest and skills needed to return to some type of work in the community. Which of the following approaches would be MOST effective at this point?**
    A. Have the individual work around the group home.
    B. Assist the individual in identifying volunteer opportunities in the community.
    C. Have the individual schedule interviews for paid employment.
    D. Advise the individual not to think about work opportunities at the present time.

68. **When adapting a toilet for use by a child with poor postural control, the COTA should pay PRIMARY attention to which of the following issues?**
    A. Can the toilet paper be reached without a major weight shift?
    B. Is the flush handle easy to manipulate?
    C. Can the child's feet reach the floor?
    D. Is a nonskid mat placed on the floor to prevent slipping?

69. **A COTA student needs to design an adaptation and decides to focus on gardening for a client with a back injury. The MOST appropriate adaptation would be:**
    A. ergonomically correct hand tools.
    B. a wheelbarrow with elongated handles.
    C. a 12-inch high seat with tool holders.
    D. a raised-bed garden.

70. **A COTA is instructing a patient with left hemiplegia and unilateral neglect to put on a tee shirt. The MOST effective sequence to teach the patient would be to:**
    A. (1) place left hand into sleeve and pull up sleeve past elbow; (2) place right hand into sleeve and pull up sleeve; (3) pull shirt up over head; (4) pull shirt down over trunk.
    B. (1) position shirt on lap; (2) place left hand into sleeve and pull up sleeve past elbow; (3) place right hand into sleeve and pull up sleeve; (4) pull shirt up over head.
    C. (1) position shirt on lap; (2) place right hand into sleeve and pull up sleeve past elbow; (3) place left hand into sleeve and pull up sleeve; (4) pull shirt up over head.
    D. (1) pull shirt up over head; (2) place left arm into sleeve; (3) place right arm into sleeve; (4) pull down shirt over trunk.

71. **When instructing the parents of a toddler in the use and care of a hand splint, the COTA should put MOST emphasis on:**
    A. checking for irritation and pressure problems.
    B. avoiding excessive heat exposure.
    C. cleansing the splint regularly.
    D. adhering strictly to the wearing schedule.

72. **During a home visit, a client with rheumatoid arthritis informs the COTA that her joints have recently become very painful and inflamed. She reports she has been performing her activity program despite the pain, and demonstrates a series of briskly executed active range of motion movements. The COTA should instruct the client to:**
    A. continue performing her program as she has been.
    B. perform gentle active range of motion with weights as tolerated.
    C. eliminate all range-of-motion exercises for a week.
    D. perform only gentle active range of motion.

73. **An individual with mental illness wants to travel to the library independently, but keeps getting lost. Which of the following actions should the COTA take FIRST?**
    A. Take the individual to the library and obtain a library card.
    B. Assess the individual's ability to read.
    C. Identify the bus that goes to the library and obtain a bus schedule.

D. Assess the individual's topographical orientation skills.

74. Upon arrival to an infant's therapy session in the neonatal intensive care unit, the COTA finds the infant's parents present. Of the following, which is the OPTIMAL intervention to pursue?

A. Review the chart to complete birth history information and speak to the infant's primary nurse.

B. Introduce yourself as their child's OT practitioner, explain your role in their child's developmental care, and excuse yourself from the situation secondary to limited availability for intervention.

C. Issue written positioning and state regulation and readiness information for the parents to review.

D. Review appropriate behavioral and developmental positioning techniques with parental observation and interaction.

75. A COTA is fabricating a splint for a client with swan-neck deformities. The COTA should fabricate a splint that will prevent further:

A. hyperextension of the PIP and DIP joints.

B. hyperextension of the PIP joint and flexion of the DIP joint.

C. flexion of the PIP joint and hyperextension of the DIP joint.

D. hyperextension of the MP joint and flexion of the PIP joint.

76. A COTA is preparing to do a parachute activity as part of a sensory integration program and several of the patients in the group are taking antipsychotic medications. The COTA should be alert for which possible side effect that could occur as a result of this activity?

A. Postural hypotension

B. Photosensitivity

C. Excessive thirst

D. Blurred vision

77. The benefits that a correct sitting position has in relation to hand function is explained to the parents of a child with CP. The child currently uses compensatory movements because of the inability to sit independently. Which aspect of therapeutic positioning should the COTA stress?

A. Stabilizing the trunk

B. Placing weight on the arms

C. Stabilizing the pelvis, hips, and legs

D. Stabilizing the head and neck

78. A COTA is working on self-care activities with a client who recently had a total hip arthroplasty. Which of the following would the COTA MOST likely recommend the client use at home after discharge from rehab?

A. A wire basket attached to a walker

B. A padded foam toilet seat 1 inch in height

C. A short-handled bath sponge

D. A long-handled bath sponge

79. A COTA working in a sheltered workshop with adult clients with developmental disabilities is preparing for a group of clients functioning at Allen's Cognitive Level 4. Which of the following is the BEST method for introducing an assembly activity?

A. Provide repetitive, one-step activities.

B. Demonstrate a three-step assembly process.

C. Provide project samples for clients to duplicate.

D. Provide written directions for the individuals to follow.

80. A first-grade child has difficulty with finger isolation and handwriting. The MOST appropriate activity for the COTA to recommend to the child's teacher is:

A. crayon drawing on sandpaper.

B. copying shapes from the blackboard.

C. rolling out "Play Doh" with a rolling pin.

D. picking up raisins with pair of tweezers.

81. A COTA is working with a patient who demonstrates unilateral neglect. Of the following, which would be the MOST effective strategy for increasing attention to the left?

A. Encouraging participation in bilateral activities

B. Encouraging any available hemiplegic limb movements before or during a task

C. Participation in tasks that do not cross the midline

D. Participation in tasks placed on the uninvolved side

82. A client is being seen by the COTA to promote independence in meal preparation and clean-up activities. Which method of structured activity practice would BEST

promote retention of learning and transfer of skills?

A. Practice preparing a variety of foods using different cooking methods and recipes.
B. Practice cooking one meal from beginning to end in the same kitchen setting several times.
C. Practice making a sandwich until that is mastered, then practice preparing another part of a meal until the person has mastered that skill, and so on.
D. Practice performing each step of the food preparation process, such as cutting vegetables.

83. A child is having difficulty with reading skills as a result of a deficit in visual memory. Which is the BEST game to play with a child for the purpose of improving visual memory?

A. Dominoes
B. Concentration
C. Pick-up sticks
D. Checkers

84. An individual in the late stages of AIDS is bedridden, and flexion contractures have begun to develop in his right hand. Which of the following would the COTA MOST likely fabricate for this individual?

A. Dorsal wrist splint
B. Functional-position resting splint
C. Volar wrist cock-up splint
D. Dynamic finger-extension splint

85. A COTA is running a living skills group. Before the active involvement of the participants, the practitioner needs to review lecture materials for 30 minutes. The group composition that is MOST likely to result in an increased focus on the group leader, and decreased interaction among the group members is a:

A. group size of fewer than five members.
B. group made up of members of differing ages.
C. group size between seven and ten members.
D. group with members who have similar goals and abilities.

86. A young child has a diagnosis of spastic quadriplegia. The COTA is teaching the child's parents how to effectively position the child in sitting so that participation in family games can be facilitated.

What is the MOST important point the COTA can make?

A. Make sure the child's head is upright.
B. Make sure the child's arms are on the armrests.
C. Make sure the child's back is straight.
D. Make sure the child's hips are secured against the back of the seat.

87. A woman who had a CVA exhibits random movements in all four extremities. What is the MOST appropriate switch to use on the controls of her wheelchair?

A. Infrared switch
B. Sip and puff switch
C. Piezoelectric switch
D. Rocking lever switch

88. A physician has informed a COTA that her client's headache problem at work is primarily caused by the increased neck and shoulder tension that the individual experiences while typing on a computer. The BEST stress management approach for the COTA to suggest in this situation is:

A. assertiveness training focusing on increasing the individual's assertiveness with his or her supervisor.
B. progressive relaxation exercises and autogenic training.
C. training in cognitive reappraisal to decrease the frequency of the individual's tendency to generalize and exaggerate the negative side of work events.
D. teaching the individual more effective problem-solving strategies.

89. A sixth grade student has a diagnosis of juvenile rheumatoid arthritis. Which of the following leisure activities would BEST suit this child for helping him maintain range of motion?

A. Swimming
B. Basketball
C. Soccer
D. Aerobics

90. An individual confides to the COTA that he is concerned that lower extremity flaccidity may cause problems during sexual activity. The BEST strategy for the COTA to recommend is to:

A. use a sidelying position.
B. use pillows to prop up body parts into the desired position.
C. incorporate slow rocking into movements.

D. avoid movements that elicit a quick stretch.

91. **A COTA uses a remediation of functional performance deficits approach in addressing individuals treated in a psychosocial setting. The activity that is MOST consistent with this approach is:**
    A. an expressive group magazine collage.
    B. a class about job-seeking strategies.
    C. the modification of the environment to provide familiar visual cues.
    D. a review of the individual's balance of time among ADL, work, and leisure activities.

92. **A 17-year-old client who wears a hip brace is being measured for a wheelchair. The correct seat dimension for the COTA to recommend would be:**
    A. 2 inches wider than the widest point across the child's hips with the brace on.
    B. 2 inches wider than the widest point across the child's hips.
    C. 2 inches more than the distance from the back of the bent knee to the buttocks.
    D. the same as the distance from the back of the bent knee to the buttocks.

93. **An artist recently diagnosed with MS is interested in pursuing a leisure activity that will promote physical fitness. Because the individual's symptoms are limited to mild UE numbness and slight weakness in the dominant hand at this point, the BEST activity to recommend is:**
    A. volleyball.
    B. painting with the dominant hand.
    C. swimming in a cool water pool.
    D. jogging on a track or treadmill.

94. **A COTA is treating a patient who has difficulty maintaining attention to a task but is aware of the problem. The BEST example of a strategy that the COTA can teach the patient to control effects of attention deficits would be:**
    A. simplifying the instructions given to accomplish the task so only one step is presented at a time.
    B. learning the self-monitoring technique of asking oneself if any part of the task has been missed.
    C. providing practice in shape and number cancellation worksheets.
    D. removing unnecessary objects from around the task area to decrease distractions.

95. **A COTA is working with a preschooler with spina bifida who is about to transition to a fully inclusive kindergarten. Lower extremity weakness and postural control are primary concerns, as well as bilateral and fine motor coordination. Knowing there will be significant emphasis on writing activities, which of the following should the COTA/OTR team recommend?**
    A. Send the child to the OT room for fine motor activities when the class is working on writing skills.
    B. Arrange for the child to work in an area of the classroom where distractions can be minimized.
    C. Arrange for the child to have a flat desk to work on, in either standing or sitting positions.
    D. Provide a vertical work surface where writing and other hand skills can be practiced.

96. **An individual with Guillain-Barré syndrome complains of pain during passive range of motion to the shoulder. Which is the MOST important technique for the COTA to use while performing PROM with this individual?**
    A. Work proximal to distal.
    B. Proceed only to the point of pain.
    C. Limit the number of repetitions to 10.
    D. Gently encourage the individual to work through pain.

97. **In a long-term care facility, an elderly resident with dementia repeatedly asks for her mother and becomes increasingly upset. The MOST therapeutic strategy for responding to this resident is to:**
    A. use reality orientation by explaining that her mother has been dead for a long time.
    B. set limits by firmly telling the her to stop asking for her mother.
    C. use therapeutic "fibbing" by telling the resident that her mother will be coming shortly.
    D. respond to the emotional tone expressed by the words and provide extra attention and reassurance.

98. **A child with a learning disability has significant problems with visual memory. A COTA may use which of the following to better enhance visual memory?**
    A. Provide memory tasks that are of low interest to the child.
    B. Decrease visual attention before doing memory tasks.

C. Combine task with additional sensory input (tactile, proprioceptive, and auditory).

D. Repeat the visual memory task once.

99. A homemaker who sustained a CVA with subsequent left hemiparesis is returning home to live with her husband and children. To enable the individual to carry out her prior responsibility of meal preparation, which item would MOST likely be recommended for stabilization when cutting a potato?

A. A piece of nonskid backing under the cutting board

B. A plate guard around the edge of the board

C. A rocker knife

D. A cutting board with two nails in it

100. An individual in an OT group has a history of monopolizing the group without giving others an opportunity to participate in the group process. What is the most effective approach for working on the individual's social conduct and group skills during a gardening activity?

A. Give the individual a specific task such as filling up the water containers.

B. Have the individual assign tasks to various group members.

C. Have the individual observe the group.

D. Pair the individual with another group member for a specific task.

101. Which of the following BEST describes how a COTA would document a normally developing infant's first steps?

A. The infant uses a narrow base of support and low arm-guard position and takes big steps.

B. The infant uses a wide base of support and is independent in stopping and turning.

C. The infant uses a narrow base of support and low arm-guard position.

D. The infant uses a wide base of support and high arm-guard position and takes short steps.

102. A COTA is teaching several elderly clients with COPD energy conservation techniques in home management skills. Following learning principles for older adults, the MOST effective way to present the information would be for the COTA to:

A. present all the important principles to be covered together in a single presentation.

B. keep the presentation loosely structured, rather than highly organized.

C. attempt to persuade clients about the importance of those points on which the clients don't seem to agree.

D. present important principles in small units that are spaced at a slower than normal pace.

103. A COTA is working with a client who has severe cognitive deficits. Using a functional skill training approach, the MOST appropriate method to teach the client to brush his or her teeth is based on:

A. rote repetition of the task substeps with gradually fading cues.

B. practice of fine-motor activities that incorporate motions needed in tooth brushing.

C. teaching a caregiver how to set up the task and guide the client's performance.

D. use of instructional cards, which the client will learn to use as a reminder of how to perform the task.

104. A third-grade student receives direct OT services provided through the public school system. Which of the following activities should the COTA recommend to the gym teacher to BEST consolidate the child's skills in spatial organization and motor planning?

A. Relay races

B. Obstacle courses

C. Balance beam activities

D. Freeze tag

105. An individual uses a mouthstick when working with a computer. Which of the following devices will prevent the mouthstick from accidentally striking other keys?

A. A moisture guard

B. A key guard

C. An auto-repeat defeat

D. One-finger-access software

106. A resident of a long-term care facility is being seen by the COTA in the mornings to help the resident reestablish dressing routines after a period of illness. The client is in a weakened condition and has mild cognitive deficits. The BEST way to structure the task is to:

A. have the resident select the clothing they prefer, then have the COTA dress the client.

B. have the resident dress in bed with garments that are stretchy and one size larger than usual, and then preview each step of the process with the resident.

C. have the resident walk to retrieve clothing garments and encourage independent performance.

D. place clothing within close reach of the resident, encourage the resident to proceed dressing as you provide distant supervision.

107. A COTA has been working in a medical setting with a 6-year-old child who has had a traumatic brain injury. At what point should the COTA recommend discharge to the supervising OTR?

A. When the child refuses to attend OT

B. When the child is ready to make the transition to first grade

C. When the child has achieved a maintenance level of functioning

D. When the child is considered to be completely recovered

108. An individual with emphysema reports recently "having an accident" when unable to "make it to the bathroom in time." When the home health OT practitioner recommends a bedside commode, the idea is immediately rejected. Which of the following actions should the OT practitioner take FIRST?

A. Identify options and the consequences of each option.

B. Document the individual's reasons for rejecting the bedside commode.

C. Practice with a "demo" bedside commode.

D. Allow time for the individual to think about the bedside commode.

109. A patient in an OT group suddenly becomes assaultive toward another group member. What is the FIRST step the COTA should take in this situation?

A. Call for other staff.

B. Try to calm the patient.

C. Try to physically restrain the patient.

D. Remove the other patients from the area.

110. During an infant's OT session, the mother reports she has observed that her baby has difficulty with swallowing and frequently chokes. The COTA can position the infant to MOST effectively reduce the risk of aspiration and facilitate swallowing by keeping the head:

A. in a neutral position.

B. slightly flexed.

C. slightly extended.

D. rotated toward the feeder.

111. A COTA is working with a homemaker who sustained a partial thickness burn 6 months ago. Which scar management technique is MOST appropriate for the COTA to introduce during the rehabilitative phase of treatment?

A. Preventing scar development through static splinting

B. Controlling edema to prevent loss of range of motion

C. Minimizing scar hypertrophy through compression garments and proper skin care

D. Promoting self-care skills in order to resume the role of homemaker

112. A client with cognitive deficits has difficulty swallowing pills and refuses to take his medication. Which of the following solutions is BEST?

A. Check with the pharmacist to see which medications can be crushed and mixed in with applesauce.

B. Sort medications into a medication organizer that is labeled with days and times of the day.

C. Teach the client to use an alarm that signals the medication schedule.

D. Work with the individual on swallowing smaller pills and progress to larger pills when possible.

113. A 2-year-old child has hypotonia, extremely poor head control, and inability to maintain a sitting position. The BEST method for the COTA to use during the FIRST pre-sitting activity is to provide stability for the child as needed and then move the child:

A. forward and backward on a ball with the child in a prone position.

B. forward and side-to-side with the child sitting on the therapist's lap.

C. to a sitting position by pulling the child up from a supine position on a mat.

D. forward and side-to-side on a tilting board with the child in a quadruped position.

114. A COTA is treating a client who has refused to wear his splint over the past three sessions. The client now arrives to the clinic stating that he misplaced his splint. Prior to fabricating a new splint the COTA should FIRST:

A. give the client one last chance and refabricate the splint.

B. talk to the client to determine if there are any motivational or cultural issues interfering with splint-wear compliance.

C. ask the client to find the splint and demand that he begin wearing it or you will call his physician.

D. discharge the client because he has no interest in regaining function.

115. A client in a day program frequently does not make it to the bathroom on time. When asked if he needs to use the toilet, he usually replies that he does not. Which of the following approaches is MOST likely to succeed?

A. Ask him if he needs to use the toilet at least once an hour.

B. Place a timer at his seat and set it to go off once an hour.

C. Determine how frequently he needs toileting and take him without asking.

D. Move his seat closer to the bathroom.

116. Which of the following would be the BEST cup for the COTA to recommend using when working with a child who tends to drink too quickly?

A. A vacuum feeding cup

B. A "nosey cup" (cut out for the nose)

C. A mug with two handles

D. A cup with a large drinking spout

117. The supervising OTR of a hand clinic requests that the COTA treat a client with an edematous hand following a healed Colles' fracture. Which of the following is the COTA MOST likely to use to decrease the client's edema?

A. Contrast baths and retrograde massage

B. Hot pack applications

C. Paraffin treatments

D. Sensory re-education and pendulum exercises

118. A client who has MS is standing at a table folding laundry when she complains of fatigue. In response to the client's comment the COTA adapts the activity by:

A. suggesting the client complete the activity in a seated position.

B. recommending the client upgrade the activity by ironing all of the shirts prior to folding.

C. stopping the activity and breaking the task

into pieces to determine where the activity went wrong.

D. suggesting that the client stop the activity so a more effective task can be introduced.

119. A COTA is working with a student who experiences tremors while writing. She instructs the student to stabilize his forearm on the table when writing. The COTA recommends this position because the student is MOST likely demonstrating:

A. decreased vision.

B. poor endurance.

C. limited fine movement.

D. incoordination.

120. An OTR and COTA, together with the assistive technology team, has made specific recommendations for electronic assistive technology for an adult with muscular dystrophy. After the devices are ordered and modified as necessary, the NEXT step in the process of implementation is for the OT practitioners to:

A. evaluate how well the whole system works.

B. evaluate if the assistive technology devices match the needs of the client.

C. train the client in the operation of the AT system and in strategies for its use.

D. determine if funding is available for the recommended assistive technology.

121. A COTA is discussing skills that can help a client with substance abuse problems to develop an alcohol-free lifestyle. The area that the COTA is MOST likely to address first with the client is:

A. work or job performance.

B. self-care skills.

C. time management and use of leisure time.

D. medication management.

122. A child with a diagnosis of mental retardation is currently learning to independently tie her shoes. To facilitate generalization of this skill, the COTA should:

A. fit the child's shoes with Velcro closures.

B. have the child practice tying her shoes at home and in school.

C. use a backwards-chaining technique.

D. provide brightly colored shoelaces.

123. A COTA is working with an elderly client who has diabetes, poor vision, and peripheral neuropathies. The client has difficulty discriminating between med-

ications. The **BEST** adaptation for the **COTA** to provide is:

A. Braille labels.
B. labels with white print on a black background.
C. a pill organizer box.
D. brightly colored pills with each type of medication a different color.

124. **A patient in an acute care facility with severe depression is withdrawn and exhibiting a low energy level. Of the following, which would be the MOST appropriate type of intervention activities for the COTA to present in the initial stages of treatment for this patient?**

A. Selecting a leisure activity of interest and identifying materials needed
B. Performing a clerical task such as sorting papers
C. Practicing meditation
D. Writing suggestions for coping with daily life stresses

125. **A COTA is instructing the parent's of a newborn infant regarding the facilitation of the suck-swallow reflex. Prior to feeding the infant a bottle the COTA encourages the parent's to perform which of the following?**

A. Stroke the infant's cheek before feeding her a bottle.
B. Gently touch the infant's lips to encourage her to open her mouth and begin sucking motions.
C. Softly stimulate the infant's gums before bottle feeding.
D. Gently rub the infant's gums and cheek simultaneously before feeding the baby her bottle.

126. **Each morning, a COTA performs ADL training with a teenage client who has quadriplegia. On the first day, the practitioner works with arranging the shirt on the client's lap. When the client masters that particular skill, they work on sliding both arms into the sleeves and pushing the shirt up past the elbows. When this skill is mastered, they will work on gathering the shirt up at the collar and pulling it on over the client's head. The COTA is MOST likely using which of the following techniques?**

A. Repetition
B. Cueing
C. Rehearsal

D. Chaining

127. **An individual with severe cognitive limitations frequently chokes while drinking liquids. Which of the following is the MOST appropriate course of action?**

A. Use a straw for drinking liquids.
B. Use a "sippy cup" for drinking liquids.
C. Monitor fluid intake.
D. Add a thickening agent to liquids.

128. **The COTA is working with a child with low muscle tone who has difficulty engaging in activities against gravity. The COTA also wants to encourage the child to play. To best address these issues, the COTA would MOST likely position the child:**

A. long sitting along a wall.
B. side-lying on a mat.
C. supine on a large wedge.
D. prone over a bolster.

129. **A patient diagnosed with Parkinson's disease is being seen by a COTA to develop a routine for performing self-care activities. The COTA is MOST likely to begin this process by instructing the patient that self-care activities:**

A. are more easily performed if coordinated with consistent timing of medications.
B. should be performed before medications are taken.
C. should be attempted only with the assistance of others.
D. should be performed at intervals throughout the day until completed.

130. **A COTA is putting together an inpatient group for individuals with schizophrenia. Which of the following would the COTA MOST likely attempt to facilitate among group members?**

A. Self-disclosure
B. Development of insight regarding a person's feelings
C. Appropriate social and life skills
D. Strategies used for dealing with anger

131. **A COTA is treating a child with autism. To maximize the child's benefit from therapy, the COTA would present activities in a therapeutic environment that:**

A. is lively and colorful, facilitating active involvement.
B. provides many options, encouraging decision making.

C. involves many toys and activities, promoting exploratory learning.

D. is highly structured, facilitating step by step learning.

132. **A 60-year-old automobile mechanic with diabetes has been referred to OT following an above-knee amputation. The patient has impaired sensation in the remaining lower extremity and will be using a wheelchair for the foreseeable future. The FIRST patient education subject the COTA should cover is:**

A. skin inspection.

B. grooming techniques (shaving, trimming toenails, etc.).

C. retirement planning.

D. returning to work.

133. **An individual with mental retardation insists on wearing the same outfit day after day, regardless of whether it is clean or dirty. What is the BEST approach for the COTA to use?**

A. Force alternate clothing choices by limiting outfits available in the closet.

B. Encourage the caregiver to wash the outfit each night.

C. Tell the client the outfit is in the laundry and she will need to wear a different one.

D. Provide the client with several outfits similar to the preferred one.

134. **A COTA is working on prewriting skills with an 11-month-old child. Which of the following activities would be MOST appropriate for the COTA to instruct the child to perform?**

A. Scribble on a piece of paper.

B. Copy a triangle.

C. Copy a horizontal line on a chalkboard.

D. Copy numerals on a sheet of paper.

135. **The goal for an elderly client with lower extremity weakness is to be independent with bathing, but this requires the tub to be more accessible to the client who uses a walker. Which environmental adaptation would the COTA MOST likely recommend to achieve this?**

A. Place the light switch outside the door so the bathroom is lit before entering.

B. Provide long-handled adaptive devices to facilitate lower extremity dressing.

C. Provide a transfer tub bench and install grab bars.

D. Place nonskid decals in the tub and mats on the floor to prevent slipping on the wet floor.

136. **A COTA is ready to introduce decision-making opportunities to an individual in a craft group. Which choice should the COTA begin with?**

A. Which type of project is the client interested in: leather, wood, macramé or weaving?

B. Does the client want to paint the project blue or white?

C. Would the client like to give the finished project to a friend or relative?

D. Would the client like to work alone or in a group?

137. **A 5-year-old child has sustained burns to his bilateral upper extremities, hands, and trunk. The child is reluctant to perform any active range of motion despite encouragement from the OTR. The OTR has requested that the COTA attempt to engage the child in therapy because they seemed to have developed a good rapport together. Which of the following activities should the COTA attempt FIRST?**

A. Inform the child that if he does not participate in therapy he may have terrible scarring and limited range of motion.

B. Introduce active range of motion exercises through gentle swaying/dancing with the child's favorite music.

C. Introduce passive range of motion exercises while the child watches his favorite cartoon.

D. Attempt to position the child over a prone bolster while encouraging the child to reach for toys.

138. **While performing endurance training activities, an individual on a cardiac rehabilitation unit begins to slow down, using progressively smaller movements to perform the activity. Which of the following is the MOST appropriate action for the COTA to take?**

A. Stop the activity.

B. Upgrade the activity for the next session.

C. Modify the activity to make it less challenging.

D. Replace the activity with isometric exercises.

139. **A depressed client has completed a mosaic tray project. The end product that the client shows the COTA looks messy**

and poorly put together. Which type of feedback would be MOST appropriate?

A. "You did a fine job, this looks very good."
B. "This could be much better, let me show you how you could fix this."
C. "I see you've finished the project, is there anything else you'd like to do with it?"
D. "It's understandable that you did a poor job, don't worry about it."

140. Which of the following describes the BEST treatment activity for improving coordination?

A. Walking sideways on a balance beam
B. Crawling over and along a rope taped to the floor
C. Kicking a ball with alternating feet when sitting on a T-stool
D. Tossing a balloon with alternating hands

141. A COTA enters the room of a patient who recently had an RCVA with flaccidity to the left upper extremity. The COTA begins to perform upper extremity passive range of motion to the left arm when marked pitting edema of the left hand is noted. Which of the following should the COTA do FIRST?

A. Continue to perform PROM and then position and elevate the affected extremity.
B. Fabricate a resting splint for the affected extremity.
C. Take no action and wait for the edema to subside.
D. Have the individual attempt to squeeze a ball.

142. A lead guitar player in a band has been admitted to an inpatient psychiatric facility following a suicide attempt. At present, he is withdrawn and rarely participates during group activities. What would be the MOST effective method to use for increasing the individual's engagement in group activities?

A. Give him a guitar to play during break under the supervision of the COTA.
B. Give him a guitar to practice with in his room.
C. Have him compose music for the group.
D. Allow him to play the guitar in a separate room during group.

143. A COTA is treating a child with a standard above-elbow amputation who is experiencing hypersensitivity of the residual limb. The COTA would MOST likely

perform which of the following interventions in the preprosthetic phase of treatment?

A. Play activities to strengthen the residual limb
B. Activities to increase the range of motion of the residual limb
C. Play activities that incorporate tapping, application of textures, and weight bearing to the residual limb
D. Dressing activities for practicing putting on and taking off the UE prosthesis

144. Which of the following devices is required for an individual with C7-C8 quadriplegia when performing oral hygiene activities?

A. Mobile arm support with utensil holder
B. Universal cuff
C. Toothbrush with built-up handle
D. Wrist support with utensil holder

145. During a time management group, an individual with severe anxiety begins to provide a description of the physical symptoms she experienced while on a community outing the previous day. The COTA should:

A. report this to the individual's supervising OTR.
B. report this to the individual's physician.
C. encourage the individual to elaborate on her concerns.
D. redirect the individual to a more neutral topic.

146. A COTA is working with a group of 4- to 5-year-old children who have mild cerebral palsy. The goal of the group is to encourage the children to participate in some form of physical or "rough and tumble" play. Which of the following is the COTA MOST likely to recommend?

A. Drawing and puzzle activities
B. Constructing towers and buildings with blocks
C. Role playing with stories the children make up
D. Playing "Simon Says"

147. An individual with C4 quadriplegia is able to independently use a mouth stick to strike keys on a computer keyboard for 15 minutes. To upgrade this activity, the COTA should:

A. provide a heavier mouth stick.

B. have the individual work at the keyboard for 30 minutes.

C. progress the individual to a typing device that inserts into a wrist support.

D. teach the individual how to correctly instruct a caregiver in use of the keyboard.

148. **A COTA is working with a client who had a TBI and demonstrates deficits in sequencing and problem solving. The client has successfully prepared a cold meal in today's treatment session. The next meal preparation activity the COTA should have the client prepare is:**

A. brownies.

B. a cheese sandwich.

C. a casserole.

D. a spaghetti dinner with salad and garlic bread.

149. **A COTA is explaining to a teacher the kind of high technology aid that can be used to help a multiple handicapped student who has speech and writing deficits function in the classroom. The COTA would MOST likely recommend which of the following for a child with speech and writing limitations?**

A. Environmental control unit

B. Wanchik writer

C. Head pointer

D. Electronic augmentative communication device

150. **An elderly client, who has had several falls at home and ambulates with a cane, is preparing for discharge to the home of an adult child who is renovating some rooms for the parent. The COTA has been asked to recommend flooring for the client's rooms. The BEST recommendation for the COTA to make is:**

A. carpeting with low or looped pile.

B. wood floor.

C. area rugs.

D. carpeting with deep pile and padding.

151. **A group goal is to increase interpersonal skills. What is the BEST approach for a COTA to use during the first week of the group?**

A. Provide a variety of scenarios and incorporate role-playing activities.

B. Have the group members write and act out a play.

C. Watch a video and ask group members to critique the characters.

D. Have each group member complete a worksheet defining communication and his/her individual style.

152. **A young patient with neurological deficits has been unable to carry over skills learned previously in therapy, and has exhibited the inability to learn new information. The MOST appropriate strategy the COTA can suggest to the patient's mother to improve ADL functioning would be to recommend:**

A. repetitive practice of simple ADL under the COTA's guidance.

B. environmental adaptations and assistance for ADL.

C. ADL training in the familiar home environment.

D. forward or backward chaining techniques.

153. **A COTA is working with a client who complains of hypersensitive fingers. The client sustained a crush injury to the hand 10 weeks ago. Which of the following methods should the COTA introduce to achieve sensory desensitization?**

A. Textured material, rubbing, tapping, and prolonged contact

B. Massage, facilitory electrical stimulation, and a progressive desensitization program

C. Pressure, percussion, vibration, icing, and edema massage

D. Visual compensation and functional use of the extremity

Effectiveness of Treatment and Discharge Planning

154. **While preparing a client with an anxiety disorder for discharge from OT, the COTA is reviewing the client's plans for healthful activities. The BEST recommendation for activities to reduce the physical symptoms of muscle tension associated with anxiety disorder would be:**

A. sewing and handcrafts.

B. aerobic exercise.

C. line dancing.

D. woodworking projects.

155. **A preschooler has trouble with manipulation of small objects because of higher than normal muscle tone. He has just achieved his goal of independently releasing inch cubes into a cup, however, he uses full extension of his arm and a**

tenodesis pattern to effect the release. The COTA recommends to the OTR that the child's goal be updated to reflect the next level of achievement. The new goal should read: "Within 3 months the child will demonstrate increased manipulation skills by releasing:

A. foam balls into a basket placed 3 feet away from his standing position."
B. inch cubes into a cup placed on a tabletop at a distance of 8 inches."
C. raisins into a bottle placed on a tabletop at a distance of 1 foot away."
D. beanbags onto a target placed on the floor at his feet."

156. **A COTA is preparing an individual with burns to perform a home program of positioning and splinting. The MOST appropriate recommendation to prevent deformity would be to:**
A. discontinue the positioning and splinting program upon returning home.
B. continue the same positioning and splinting program that was indicated before discharge.
C. continue with the positioning and splinting program only during the day.
D. continuing with the positioning and splinting program only during the night.

157. **Several clients are about to be discharged from an inpatient psychiatric unit to a variety of community programs. Which of the following areas is MOST important to address in a discharge planning group?**
A. Developing ADL routines
B. Self-awareness
C. Relapse prevention
D. Social skills

158. **When preparing to discharge a child with juvenile rheumatoid arthritis, what is the MOST important information to share with the child's school teacher?**
A. A summary of the child's cognitive and visual perceptual skills
B. Methods of accommodation in the classroom
C. Information on the child's range of motion status
D. A summary of the child's progress in OT

159. **A long-term goal for a 60-year-old client with back pain is to be able to return to work as an illustrator. The client has**

achieved the short-term goal of sitting at a work table for 20 minutes. Which of the following is the BEST example of a revised short-term goal for this client?
A. Client will draw sitting at a work table.
B. Client will draw for 1 hour, taking stretch breaks every 20 minutes.
C. Instruct client in stretching techniques to be performed every 20 minutes.
D. Instruct client in the use of proper body mechanics that apply to prolonged sitting.

160. **An individual who is being discharged in 1 week is functioning at Allen's Cognitive Level 4, and needs to take two different psychotropic medications twice daily. Which of the following is the MOST appropriate discharge recommendation?**
A. Instruct the client to take medication at 9 A.M. and 9 P.M..
B. Instruct the client to take "one white and one blue pill" with the morning and evening meals.
C. Instruct the caregiver to remind the client to take medication twice daily.
D. Instruct the caregiver to place pills into client's hands at the designated times.

161. **A child with active juvenile rheumatoid arthritis has been fitted with hand splints. The COTA is explaining the purpose of the splints to the child's parents. Which is the MOST accurate description of how splinting will benefit the child?**
A. The splints will inhibit hypertonus.
B. The splints will increase range of motion.
C. The splints will prevent deformity.
D. The splints will correct deformity.

162. **An individual has been instructed to place towels, one at a time, on a high shelf in order to increase shoulder flexion. The individual is able to easily place 10 towels. Which of the following modifications would MOST effectively improve endurance in the shoulder flexors?**
A. Place the towels on a higher shelf.
B. Increase the number of towels from 10 to 20.
C. Place the towels on a lower shelf.
D. Add a 1 pound weight to each arm.

163. **An elderly patient has Alzheimer's disease and is about to be discharged to home where she lives with her husband. She does not always recognize her chil-**

dren, shows a tendency to wander, and has frequent episodes of incontinence. Which of the following is the MOST important item to include in the family discharge planning conference?

A. Strategies the patient can use for handling incontinence
B. Strategies the husband can use to prevent the patient from wandering
C. Strategies the patient can use to prevent wandering
D. Reality orientation techniques to increase recognition of the patient's children

164. A child with a swallowing dysfunction is being discharged with a home feeding program that includes eliminating foods with consistencies that are difficult to swallow. Which of the following food textures would the COTA MOST likely recommend that the child avoid?

A. Smooth semisolids (pureed bananas)
B. Lumpy semisolids (cottage cheese)
C. Liquids and solids combined (minestrone soup)
D. Thickened liquids (malted milk)

165. In preparing a patient with a unilateral below-knee amputation for discharge from a rehabilitation facility, the MOST important adaptive equipment for the COTA to recommend is:

A. lightweight cooking utensils.
B. a tub bench and toilet rails.
C. long-handled dressing devices.
D. a reacher.

166. An individual was unable to achieve the goal "the client will initiate two requests to other group members for sharing materials within a 1-week period." The BEST revised goal is:

A. the client will initiate two requests to other group members for sharing group materials within a 2-week period.
B. the client will initiate one request to one other group member for sharing group materials within a 1-week period.
C. the client will initiate two requests to each of the five group members for sharing one group tool within 2 weeks.
D. the client will say "hello" to the group leader at the start of each group session.

167. In reviewing a client's progress, a COTA would MOST likely recommend changing treatment activities when the activities:

A. continue to provide some degree of challenge.
B. reflect the client's priorities.
C. help to achieve the client's goals.
D. are easily accomplished by the client.

168. An individual with carpal tunnel syndrome has been fitted with a splint. Her long-term goal is to return to work as a secretary. The COTA would document that the person has attained the MOST relevant short-term goal when the person demonstrates:

A. understanding of work simplification techniques.
B. ability to put on and remove the splint correctly.
C. ability to type for 10 minutes with wrists in 10 degrees of flexion.
D. use of lightweight cookware for meal preparation.

169. The COTA is working with a patient who needs to be independent in medication management prior to discharge. The MOST effective technique for the COTA to teach the patient to remember whether he has taken his medications is to:

A. establish a routine of taking medications the same time every day.
B. keep the medications in a special, labeled location.
C. use a diary to record each dosage after it is taken.
D. arrange for a caregiver to remind the patient when medications should be taken.

170. A COTA has recommendations concerning adaptations for a child's artificial limb. This would require that the COTA consult the:

A. physiatrist.
B. orthotist.
C. prosthetist.
D. physical therapist.

171. A family would like to place grab bars around the toilets in the house for easy access during transfers by the mother, who uses a wheelchair and is of average height. The grab bars should be placed at a height range of:

A. 28 to 32 inches.
B. 33 to 36 inches.
C. 38 to 41 inches.
D. 43 to 46 inches.

172. **A mother of two children is about to be discharged to home following a brief hospitalization for substance abuse. Her husband asks the COTA what he "should do with her" for her first weekend at home. Which of the following suggestions is MOST appropriate?**

A. Throw a party for some close friends.

B. Take her to see her favorite band.

C. Take her and the kids on a mini-vacation.

D. Attend an AA meeting.

173. **A COTA is preparing the family for discharge of 5-year-old child diagnosed with developmental delay. The child has just achieved independence in self-feeding with a spoon. The BEST suggestion for the parents to help the child maintain her skill level at home is to:**

A. use hand-over-hand technique to reinforce correct technique.

B. consistently point out incorrect hand placement and/or movement patterns.

C. let the child's older sister feed her occasionally as a reinforcement.

D. praise her for what she does well to reinforce her independence.

174. **A patient is being discharged after hospitalization for a cerebrovascular accident and a 2-week inpatient rehabilitation program. He requires minimal assistance in advanced ADL, but is independent in most basic ADL, and his RUE function is improving. He plans on eventually returning to work as a cashier. Recommendations for continued OT services would MOST likely include:**

A. home health OT.

B. outpatient OT.

C. a work-hardening program.

D. discontinuation of OT services.

175. **An OTR and COTA are collaborating on a discharge summary. Which of the following is the MOST appropriate contribution for the COTA to make?**

A. Describe the treatment received.

B. Make the referral for community-based services.

C. Compare the initial and final status.

D. Formulate the OT follow-up plans.

176. **A COTA is helping a family plan a wheelchair ramp to the front door of their home. The minimum amount of space** needed in front of the door to allow easy wheelchair access is:

A. 3 feet by 5 feet.

B. 4 feet by 4 feet.

C. 4.5 feet by 3 feet.

D. 5 feet by 5 feet.

Occupational Therapy for Populations

177. **A COTA recently began a group at a mental health day program for those participants who have physical disabilities in addition to mental illness. After a few sessions, group members began expressing anger about the lack of accessibility in the building where the day program is housed. Which of the following offers the BEST action to take?**

A. Employ an OTR to assess the facility for ADA compliance.

B. Incorporate advocacy skill training into the group format.

C. Bring a lawsuit against the facility for violating the ADA.

D. Involve the clients in a stress management group.

178. **An 8-week stress management program can benefit a wide variety of populations. The MOST important activity to include in the first session is:**

A. a physical activity such as yoga or tai chi.

B. diaphragmatic breathing or progressive relaxation techniques.

C. providing information on the definition and physiological signs of stress.

D. role playing stressful situations.

179. **The goal of a work program for homeless youths is to develop job skills that will improve housing status. Which of the following must occur FIRST?**

A. Help clients feel safe and supported, and explore the meaning of the worker role.

B. Develop work skills, habits, and appropriate interpersonal and work behaviors.

C. Emphasize quality and productivity and identify realistic work interests.

D. Evaluate participants' performance strengths and weaknesses.

180. **One of the functions of the OT in the long-term care facility is to recommend changes in the physical environment that will accommodate age-related sen-**

sory changes. Which of the following is the MOST appropriate environmental recommendation to reduce visual discomfort from too much glare?

A. Avoid highly polished or glossy surfaces on walls, floors, and furniture.
B. Recommend residents wear darkened glasses indoors when in high-glare areas.
C. Reduce illumination throughout the facility by making lights dimmer.
D. Use color contrast to differentiate areas and objects from backgrounds.

181. A COTA is working in a day program with older adults with severe mental illness who have been institutionalized for many years. The COTA is developing ideas for a work and productive activities program. However, because of their age and severely impaired performance, these individuals will never move into paid employment. Which of the following is the MOST important concept for the COTA to integrate?

A. Incorporate activities such as wiping the tables after lunch, which are concrete, consistent, and predictable.
B. Train clients to sort objects like nuts and bolts, to prepare them for piece-work employment.
C. Teach clients jobs they can then generalize to their home environments, such as dusting furniture.
D. When available, involve clients in stuffing envelopes for non-profit agencies, to develop a sense of community membership.

182. A day camp for children with special needs offers a variety of indoor and outdoor activities emphasizing development of interpersonal and social skills. Which of the following activities provides the most appropriate opportunity for campers to BEGIN experiencing responsibility for others?

A. Having a buddy during a field trip to an amusement park
B. Roasting marshmallows over a fire
C. Feeding the camp pets
D. Lifeguarding at the kiddie pool

183. A COTA is working as a consultant to assist a health care facility achieving compliance with the Americans with Disability Act, Title III. The PRIMARY focus of the COTA's efforts would be to make recommendations about:

A. improving accessibility in building access, building interiors, and restrooms.
B. modifying equipment, providing assistive aides, and training in adaptive methods so a disabled person can perform a particular job.
C. providing education to persons who hire personnel concerning nondiscriminatory behaviors and procedures regarding persons with disabilities.
D. assistive technology systems to facilitate job performance of disabled employees.

184. A COTA has been hired as a program manager to develop a community-based program for individuals with chronic mental illness. The FIRST step in the process which the COTA must complete is:

A. program planning.
B. program implementation.
C. needs assessment.
D. program evaluation.

185. An OT practitioner is developing transition activities for a group of 16-year-old students diagnosed as trainable mentally retarded. Which of the following activities would be BEST for addressing goals related to transition?

A. Role play ordering food in the classroom.
B. Go out for lunch at a fast-food restaurant.
C. Order a takeout lunch by phone.
D. Select lunch items from a picture menu in the classroom.

186. An OT practitioner functioning in the role of a consultant in an adult day care facility would be MOST likely to be providing which of the following services?

A. Evaluate clients to determine OT needs.
B. Implement recreational activity groups.
C. Serve as a personal advocate for the client and family liaison.
D. Provide OT expertise to run the program and solve problems.

Service Management

187. A COTA and OTR jointly decide to discharge an individual after the goal of independence in ADLs has been achieved. However, they are instructed by the facility administrator to continue treating, or at least billing, the individual for two sessions per day for the next week, because his insurance will allow it. What

is the most appropriate action for the OT practitioners to take?

A. Continue to work on activities the individual particularly enjoys twice a day whenever possible.

B. Discontinue treatment, but continue to bill as directed by the administrator.

C. Inform the administrator they are unable to provide services to individuals who can no longer benefit from OT.

D. Compromise with the administrator, and agree to drop in and check on the individual once a day and bill accordingly.

188. An OT practitioner is working in a psychiatric OT department that uses a variety of craft paints, stains, and sharp tools. In order to ensure patient safety, the practitioner MUST complete which of the following activities on a daily basis?

A. Label chemicals used within the department.

B. Complete a tool count of departmental sharps.

C. Obtain a locked storage cabinet for sharps.

D. Offer activities other than crafts to individuals who are suicidal.

189. Which of the following is the BEST method for demonstrating service competency in a standardized evaluation?

A. Observe performance of the standardized test by a competent OT practitioner.

B. Observe a competent OT practitioner, then practice, then teach another individual how to administer the test.

C. Follow procedures exactly as outlined in the test manuals.

D. Obtain the same results as another OT practitioner who has demonstrated service competency.

190. The position of program director of an adult day care facility is vacant and a COTA employed by the facility has been offered the job. To accept the position, the COTA must:

A. stop providing OT services.

B. identify an OTR to provide supervision.

C. accept a salary cut.

D. demonstrate service competence.

191. During a routine transfer, a patient's legs buckle, causing both the COTA and patient to fall to the floor. The most appropriate way for the COTA to document this accident is in a(n):

A. incident report.

B. daily progress note.

C. letter to the department head.

D. verbal report to the department head.

192. An OT is working with a patient on an acute care floor when the patient's IV equipment disengages, splashing the therapist in the eye with medication and IV "backwash" fluid. The therapist's FIRST response should be to:

A. rub the eye and continue treatment.

B. rinse the eye with an eye wash or water immediately.

C. write an incident report.

D. cover the eye with a bandage and contact the immediate supervisor.

193. A referral for a woman who had a hip replacement is received in the OT department on a day when the only OTR is on vacation. The COTA observes that the patient is scheduled to be discharged before the OTR's return. The ONLY acceptable action for the COTA to take is to:

A. obtain collaboration with supervision from an OTR to screen the individual before beginning treatment.

B. perform an ADL evaluation.

C. provide the individual with the adaptive equipment she will need.

D. begin instruction in hip precautions.

194. COTAs requiring general supervision should:

A. practice only in the line of sight of an OTR.

B. receive supervision from an OTR at least once daily.

C. receive supervision from an OTR at least once a month.

D. receive supervision from an advanced-level COTA at least weekly.

195. A COTA and OTR are each working with two patients in the OT gym when the OTR suddenly becomes ill and goes to the emergency room. Which of the following is the most appropriate way for the COTA to use an aide in this situation?

A. Instruct the aide to call for someone to transport the patients back to their rooms.

B. Show the aide how to do the activities with the OTR's patients so the session can be completed.

C. Have the aide take over working with the

COTA's patients so the COTA can finish working with the OTR's patients.

D. Instruct the aide to involve the patients who are least acute in a balloon toss.

196. A COTA provided information about adaptations that will assist in resuming sexual activity to a patient with a spinal cord injury. Afterward, the patient confides to the COTA that there are serious personal issues affecting his sexual relationship with his wife. What is the BEST action for the COTA to take?

A. Encourage the patient to explain further about the problems he is having with his wife.

B. Explain that this is normal, and that divorce rates are actually higher after serious injuries.

C. Direct the patient to speak with his physiatrist about his concerns.

D. Encourage the patient to speak with the rehabilitation psychologist to discuss his concerns.

Professional Practice

197. A hospital's public relations department plans to take some pictures of the OT staff working with patients. Before proceeding, which of the following MUST be obtained?

A. The correct spelling of the patients' names for the photograph caption

B. The patients' written consents to take the photographs and use them for publicity

C. The department head's written consent to take the photographs and use them for hospital purposes

D. The correct spelling of the patients' diagnoses and names for the photographs' captions

198. A COTA is offered a job upon completion of fieldwork and accepts the position even though she had not yet applied for her temporary license. What would be the BEST action for this COTA to take under the circumstances?

A. Schedule an immediate start date and send for a temporary license.

B. Confide in the OT director and follow her recommendation to start as scheduled.

C. Decline the current offer, ask if company can wait to hire, and apply for a temporary license.

D. Start the job knowing that no one with the company will ask to see her license.

199. The OT department receives a telephone call with orders to complete an evaluation to assist with discharge planning for a patient leaving the hospital later that evening. The OTR has already left for the day. What is the BEST way for the COTA to respond?

A. Refuse the referral.

B. Initiate and complete the ADL portion of the evaluation, and provide recommendations based on the findings.

C. Request that PT be consulted instead because of availability issues.

D. Explain the OT role delineation for evaluations to the referring physician, and attempt to contact the OTR for further consultation.

200. A COTA learns that a nursing home resident fell during the night and may have sustained a new fracture. The individual still wishes to engage in therapy. What is the BEST course of action for the COTA to take?

A. Provide treatment as originally planned, based on the wishes of the individual.

B. Withhold treatment, but gather information on the course of events for documentation and consultation with the supervising OTR.

C. Provide treatment by observing performance in self-feeding, an area not listed as an OT treatment goal, but an ADL activity that the individual continues to perform despite the possible fracture.

D. Withhold treatment and leave all information gathering and treatment decisions to the OTR, despite the fact that the OTR may not be in the facility until the following week.

ANSWERS FOR SIMULATION EXAMINATION 2

1. (B) Approach the client briefly several times throughout the session without making any demands on him. This approach indicates to the individual that you accept his feelings and that you will not neglect him regardless of his withdrawn behavior. After several visits, the client will be more likely to respond. In addition, the OT practitioner should match the client's pace, and be careful not to make more demands of the individual than he is ready to handle. Depressed individuals may try to avoid contact with staff, and the OT practitioner must be careful not to reinforce this behavior by ignoring the client (answer A). Answers C and D both have a threatening or manipulative tone to them, and are unlikely to help establish a therapeutic relationship. See reference: Early: Responding to symptoms and behaviors.

2. (D) plan new motor tasks. Dyspraxia refers to difficulty planning new motor tasks (answer D). Inability to print or write (answer A) is termed "dysgraphia." The term "dyslexia" (answer B) literally means dysfunction in reading. Inability to perform mathematics (answer C) is known as "dyscalcula." See reference: Case-Smith (ed): Rogers, SL, Gordon, CY, Schanzenbacher, KE, and Case-Smith, J: Common diagnoses in pediatric occupational therapy practice.

3. (B) Line bisection. Line bisection is used as a method of determining unilateral neglect. The block assembly (answer A) is used for evaluating constructional apraxia. Proverb interpretation (answer C) evaluates an individual's ability to think abstractly. The overlapping figures (answer D) test figure-ground discrimination. See reference: Unsworth (ed): Corben, L and Unsworth, C: Evaluation and intervention with unilateral neglect.

4. (B) interest checklist. An interest checklist is frequently used to initiate discussion of how a patient usually spends his leisure time and to identify areas of specific interest. Although the evaluations of living skills and self-care (answers A and D) address the use of leisure time, they are used primarily to assess skills in personal care, safety and health, money management, transportation, use of the telephone, and work. An activity configuration (answer C) is used to assess the patient's use of time and his feelings about all of the activities he performs in a typical day or week. See reference: Early: Data gathering and evaluation.

5. (A) the mother's concerns and goals for her child. The caregiver's concerns are essential in planning effective intervention within the context of the family. Medical management (answer B), equipment needs (answer C), and the physical layout of the home (answer D) are important issues as well, but can be addressed at a later time. See reference:

Case-Smith (ed): Stewart, KB: Occupational therapy evaluation in pediatrics.

6. (A) safety and stability. Incoordination, tremors, ataxia, and athetoid movements may result from conditions that affect the central nervous system, such as Parkinson's disease, CP, multiple sclerosis, and head injuries. "The major problems encountered in ADL performance [for people with incoordination] are safety and adequate stability of gait, body parts and objects to complete the tasks" (p. 148). Strength (answer C) was not identified as an area of concern for this individual. The ability to reach and bend (answer B) is of primary concern for those with limitations in range of motion. Endurance level (answer D) is a primary concern for individuals with MS, Guillain-Barré syndrome, ALS, and other neurological conditions that cause them to fatigue quickly. See reference: Pedretti and Early (eds): Foti, D: Activities of daily living.

7. (A) Discuss issues related to self-concept with the individual. This individual has demonstrated competence in using the cane, but does not seem to want to use it. Her response indicates her discomfort with the cane is related to how it looks, or more likely, how it makes her look. The image of a woman with a cane is not consistent with her self-concept. Discussion about how she feels about using the cane may enable the individual to integrate it more successfully into her self-concept. Memory and time management (answers B, C, and D) appear to be intact, as indicated by her ability, to arrive for therapy on time each day. See reference: Neistadt and Crepeau (eds): Seymour, SG: Evaluation of psychosocial skills and psychological components.

8. (B) normal development. Proximal movement on a fixed distal limb component—that is, on hands and knees—is an example of the development of mobility superimposed on stability. This stage is essential in the development of coordinated antigravity movement. The development of this type of movement in the quadruped position occurs between the ages of 7 and 12 months. This pattern is typical of normal development and does not indicate answers A, C, or D. See reference: Case-Smith (ed): Nichols, DS: Development of postural control.

9. (B) perform the evaluation over several sessions. Upper extremity evaluation is lengthy and can be fatiguing, and fatigue should be avoided with individuals with Guillain-Barré syndrome. In addition, results may be invalid if the individual is fatigued and not performing at the highest level possible. Strength, range of motion, and sensory testing (answers A, C, and D) are all important when evaluating an individual with Guillain-Barré syndrome, but must be administered using a method that will yield valid results. See reference: Pedretti and Early (eds): Lehman, RM and McCormack, G: Neurogenic and myopathic dysfunction.

10. (B) Ask the individual about the grade school he or she attended. The ability to recall events from one's distant past is remote memory. It is commonly assessed through verbal interviews and informal testing, such as a question about an individual's recall of childhood events. Retention is determined by giving the individual information and asking about the same information a few minutes later (answer A). Orientation is determined by asking about the current time and date (answer C). Recent memory is determined by asking about meals eaten that day (answer D). See reference: Neistadt and Crepeau (eds): Golisz, KM and Toglia, JP: Evaluation of perception and cognition.

11. (B) Moro reflex. The Moro reflex is characterized by abduction, extension, and external rotation of the arms. The rooting reflex (answer A) is the turning of the head toward tactile stimulation near the mouth. The flexor withdrawal reflex (answer C) is characterized by flexion of an extremity in response to a painful stimulus. The neck righting reaction (answer D) involves body alignment in rotation after turning of the head. Only the Moro reflex causes an extension movement. See reference: Neistadt and Crepeau (eds): Kohlmeyer, K: Evaluation of performance components.

12. (A) make recommendations for ways of operating the technology. The OT practitioner on the assistive technology team usually determines which part of the body has sufficient motor control for operating the technology and then recommends the type of input access device (switch, keyword, software, etc.) that will best meet the client's needs. Answer B, recommending communication strategies, is most often the job of the speech and language pathologist. A social worker or other specialist in funding is usually responsible for seeking funding sources (answer C). Answer D, solving mechanical and software problems, is usually the role of the rehabilitation engineer. See reference: Angelo and Lane (eds): Angelo, J: A guide for assistive technology therapists.

13. (C) a concrete response. Literal and concrete responses to general inquiries indicate the difficulty that people with schizophrenia have in understanding questions with several possible meanings. Delusional responses (answer A) would most likely be completely off topic. A distractible response (answer B) would change the topic or stop in the middle of responding. An insightful response (answer D) would include reasons that led up to being hospitalized. See reference: Hemphill (ed): Shaw, C: The interviewing process in occupational therapy.

14. (C) somatosensory system. Many children who use an excessively tight grip on the writing tool and press too hard with the pencil on their paper have poor proprioceptive awareness (somatosensory). Answer A, vestibular system, is not the correct answer because, although it is difficult to completely separate one sensory system from another, the vestibular system primarily affects balance and general motor coordination. Answer B, the auditory system, is not the correct answer because the auditory system interprets sound for use in language. Answer D, the visual system, is not correct because although the visual system can monitor motor control such as pencil grip and pressure, use of a pencil requires unconscious awareness of body position and pressure at times when the task is not monitored visually. See reference: Case-Smith (ed): Amundson, SJ and Weil, M: Prewriting and handwriting skills.

15. (C) Have the individual hold a heavy handbag by the handles. The hook grasp is strongly based on the use of digits two to five. The thumb is not always required for the hook grasp and can remain inactive. A needle would be held with a two-point pinch while being threaded (answer A). A glass would be held with a cylindrical grasp (answer B). Finally, a key being placed in a lock would be held by a lateral pinch (answer D). See reference: Smith, Weiss, and Lehmkuhl: Wrist and hand.

16. (B) All group members construct one tower that incorporates all the pieces provided in a set of constructional materials (e.g., Legos, Tinkertoys, or Erector set). Activities used in evaluation groups should require group collaboration that can be done in approximately 45 minutes and emphasize process rather than end product. The collage and crafts (answers A and D) are individual activities and do not demand group interaction. Making pizza for lunch (answer C) is an end product that serves the group as a whole and usually takes longer than 45 minutes. The pizza activity and format is typically not an evaluation group, but is better suited as a task-oriented group activity in which self-awareness and self-understanding are primary goals. See reference: Mosey: Evaluation.

17. (D) After the development of the goals and objectives. The initial evaluation may incorporate observation, screening, interviews, and evaluations (answers A, B, and C). Goals and objectives are developed following evaluation. "Once short- and long-term goals have been agreed upon, an implementation plan must be made regarding how to provide services to meet these goals most effectively" (p. 256). See reference: Case-Smith (ed): Richardson, PK and Schultz-Krohn, W: Planning and implementing services.

18. (B) flaccidity. Flaccidity, or hypotonicity, is often present immediately after a stroke and may later change to spasticity (answer D) or increased muscle tone. The flaccid extremity feels heavy and hangs limply at the individual's side. The weight of the arm may eventually pull the humerus out of the glenohumeral joint, resulting in subluxation (answer C). Neither flaccidity, spasticity, nor subluxation are normal (answer A). See reference: Pedretti and Early (eds): Preston, LA: Motor control.

19. (D) Read the social worker's report. The social worker's report includes details about the patient's family situation, occupational, educational, and cultural background, and expected environment. Referring to this document eliminates the need to duplicate this information. Interviews with the patient and family by OT practitioners (answers B and C) are designed to obtain information concerning role and task performance, and performance levels in work, self-care, and leisure. It would be a waste of time to review the entire medical record (answer A) just to obtain information about an individual's social status. See reference: Early: Data gathering and evaluation.

20. (D) Home observation and parent interview. "Observation of children in familiar settings and routines allows more characteristic views of their abilities and may be actually more reflective of how children can be expected to perform....." (p. 207). Parent interviews provide information about the child's abilities from the parent's point of view and can identify the priorities of the child's caregiver. Answers A, B, and C provide necessary information about performance components, development, and other parameters, but are not as effective in helping the evaluator learn about the child's self-care functioning. See reference: Case-Smith (ed): Stewart, KB: Purposes, processes, and methods of evaluation.

21. (A) apply the stimuli beginning at the little finger and progress toward the thumb. The general guidelines for sensation testing are that an individual's vision should be occluded, the stimuli should be randomly applied with intermingled false stimuli (opposite of answer C), a practice trial should be performed before the test, and the unaffected side or area should be tested before the affected side or area (opposite of answer B). With a median nerve injury, the ulnar side of the hand is the uninvolved side, and should be tested first. Also, the tested individual should be given a specified amount of time in which to respond, therefore, answer D is incorrect. See reference: Trombly (ed): Bentzel, K: Evaluation of sensation.

22. (D) view of the problem and an overall goal. The interview is generally the component of the assessment process in which the OT practitioner asks about the individual's goals for treatment, and gains an understanding of the problems from the person's perspective. Diagnoses and medications (answers A and B) are most often found in a review of the chart. Abilities (answer C) are determined through perfor-

mance measures. See reference: Early: Data collection and evaluation.

23. (D) protective extension response. "Protective extension responses are postural reactions that are used to stop a fall or to prevent injury when equilibrium reactions fail to do so" (p. 74). Equilibrium reactions (answer C) involve "automatic, compensatory movements...used to maintain the center of gravity over the base of support" (p. 74). Righting reactions (answer B) "bring the head and trunk back into an upright position" (p. 74). Primitive reflexes (answer A) are automatic movements that occur involuntarily and disappear as the infant matures. See reference: Solomon (ed): Lowman, DK: Development of occupational performance components.

24. (C) take the individual's vital signs at rest. First, vital signs should be taken at rest. The individual should then perform a self-care activity while being monitored by the OT practitioner for any signs or symptoms (answer B). The third step is to take vital signs again immediately after completion of the activity (answer A). The final step is to retake vital signs after the individual has rested for 5 minutes (answer D). This process provides the OT practitioner with baseline information about the individual's endurance level. See reference: Dutton: Introduction to biomechanical frame of reference.

25. (B) Initiation. The inability to perform the first step of an activity without prompting indicates that the individual has initiation problems. A problem with impulsiveness (answer A) during self-care would be evidenced by the individual's attempting to complete several steps of an activity rapidly, which would probably result in this individual cutting himself or doing a poor job of shaving. Memory or attention deficits (answers C and D) are demonstrated by the individual skipping steps of the activity, either because he does not remember the steps or is distracted by internal or external stimuli. Memory deficits could also be evidenced by the performance of task steps out of correct sequence. The individual with initiation problems may be able to plan or carry out activities, but would be unable to begin until prompted by someone else. An individual who has difficulty with impulsivity, memory, or attention would have no difficulty with beginning the activity but would have difficulty in completing the task successfully. See reference: Zoltan: Executive functions.

26. (A) explain to the parents that toilet training is not a feasible option. Answer A is correct because "when the lesion is in the lumbar region or below, the bladder is flaccid (lower motor neuron bladder)...the reflex arc is not intact, and the bladder has lost all tone...Children with a flaccid bladder cannot be trained because the bladder has no tone to empty" (p. 508). As toilet training is not appropriate (answer C), these children are commonly provided with some type of catheterization after medical testing is performed. Although nighttime bowel and bladder control may not be accomplished until the normally developing child is 4 or 5 years of age, waiting another year (answer B) would not change anything for this child. Independence in lower extremity dressing (answer D) is an appropriate goal for this child, but it is not relevant to the issue at hand. See reference: Case-Smith (ed): Shepherd, J: Self-care and adaptations for independent living.

27. (B) identify and analyze the tasks and occupations that the client will be performing in the home. The first step in the process is to analyze the tasks and occupations that the client will be performing at home because this forms the basis of the entire assessment and recommendations that will be offered. This will also provide a framework for determining how well the client can perform the tasks within the particular environment being surveyed. Answers A, C, and D are also important aspects of the process, but occur after the first step. See reference: Pedretti and Early (eds): Smith, P: Americans with Disabilities Act: Accommodating persons with disabilities.

28. (B) Kitchen safety. Short-term memory loss is one of the earliest symptoms of Alzheimer's disease. Because her husband is still working, this individual may want to continue preparing meals. Kitchen safety issues, such as remembering to turn off the stove, would be the most important of the options listed to evaluate. The awareness of declining abilities may be very frustrating for some individuals, leading to anger, social withdrawal, and depression. There may be a need for anger management strategies (answer C), but this issue is a secondary concern to safety. Difficulty with motor abilities develop as the disease progresses, and the ability to chew and swallow (answer A) may need to be evaluated in the later stages. Severe memory loss (answer D), inability to process information, and loss of communication skills may also develop in the later stages of the disease. See reference: Neistadt and Crepeau (eds): Ward, JD: Psychosocial dysfunction in adults.

29. (D) pervasive developmental disorder of childhood. This disorder "is characterized by severe and complex impairments in social interaction, communication and behavior" (p. 164). Children with ADHD (answer A) display behaviors of inattention, hyperactivity, and impulsivity. Children with childhood conduct disorder (answer B) display repetitive and persistent antisocial behavior. Obsessive-compulsive disorder (answer C) is characterized by obsessive thoughts and displayed in compulsive behaviors such as handwashing. See reference: Case-Smith (ed): Rogers, SL, Gordon, CY, Schanzenbacher, KE, and Case-Smith, J: Common diagnosis in pediatric occupational therapy practice.

30. (A) goniometer. A goniometer measures available joint movement. A pinch meter (answer C) is

used to measure available thumb-to-finger pinch strength in all available positions. A dynamometer (answer B) measures grip strength in the hand. An aesthesiometer (answer D) measures two-point discrimination. See reference: Trombly (ed): Trombly, CA: Evaluation of biomechanical and physiological aspects of motor performance.

31. (C) level of arousal. Timing of group activities is very important. Individuals, especially the elderly, often become sleepy after eating lunch. Activities that require the highest levels of arousal should be planned for earlier in the day. Nonparticipation may also be caused by lack of motivation or interest (answers A and B), and a poor attention span (answer D) may limit an individual's ability to participate, but the age of the group members and the timing of the group provide clues to the correct answer. See reference: Neistadt and Crepeau (eds): Crepeau, EB: Activity analysis: A way of thinking about occupational performance.

32. (D) age appropriate. "Chronological age of preterm infants is usually 'corrected for prematurity' to better correlate with developmental expectations and performance" (p. 640). Corrected age is calculated by subtracting the number of weeks of prematurity from the chronological age. This child's corrected age would be 8 months. The developmental skills indicated in the question are appropriate for an 8-month-old child. Therefore, this child's developmental level would be considered age appropriate (answer D), when corrected for prematurity. See reference: Case-Smith (ed): Hunter, JG: Neonatal intensive care unit.

33. (C) Strength, range of motion, coordination. The biomechanical approach is based on enhancing strength, range of motion, and endurance (answer C). The biomechanical approach is typically used when impairment does not affect the intact central nervous system. This approach is primarily used for individuals who have had a traumatic injury or illness that has affected the musculoskeletal system. The rehabilitative approach (answer A) emphasizes making an individual as independent as possible, compensates for limitations, and incorporates the use of adaptive equipment (answer A). The neurodevelopmental approach (answer B) is used for individuals who are born with a central nervous system dysfunction, have experienced an illness, or have had an injury to the neural system. The neurodevelopmental approach is based on using sensory input and developmental sequences to promote function. Evaluation focuses on tone, reflex development, and automatic reactions. The Model of Human Occupation recognizes that human performance is organized and directed by volition, habituation, and mind-brain-body subsystems. This model emphasizes the importance of habits, values, roles (answer D), interests, and personal causation. See reference: Trombly (ed): Trombly, CA: Theoretical foundations for practice.

34. (C) Avoid having these individuals in close proximity to others to reduce opportunities for physical contact. Avoiding close proximity situations is the recommended environmental modification for sexual acting-out behaviors. Advising the client of your expectations (answer D) is an appropriate use of self in such situations. Standing to the side (answer B) is a recommended environmental modification for highly aggressive and hostile behavior risks. Providing real-life activities in a stimulating environment (answer A) has been found to be helpful with reducing some delusions. See reference: Early: Safety techniques.

35. (D) child, caregiver, and therapist priorities. The problems established in the OT evaluation are not the only basis for writing OT goals and objectives. The child's priorities, as well as the caregiver's needs and concerns, must be addressed so that immediate needs are met and there is a commitment on everyone's part to the success of the program. See reference: Case-Smith (ed): Richardson, PK and Schultz-Krohn, W: Planning and implementing services.

36. (A) Holding the hammer. Holding the hammer (answer A) is the only activity listed that requires gripping with the entire hand. Holding the stamping tools and needle (answers B and D) requires pinch patterns. Squeezing the sponge (answer C) offers less resistance than holding the hammer, and would therefore be less effective for strengthening. See reference: Breines: Folkcraft.

37. (C) pouring a glass of orange juice. Meal preparation is graded from cold to hot foods or beverages, and from simple to multiple steps. An individual beginning meal preparation training should start with a cold item involving the least number of steps possible, such as pouring a glass of juice or other cold beverage. Cold sandwich preparation (answer A) adds another step, as each topping to the bread is added, and as the use of utensils is introduced. After preparation of cold items has been mastered, training in hot food or beverage preparation (answers B and D) may be initiated. See reference: Neistadt and Crepeau (eds): Neistadt, ME: Overview of treatment.

38. (D) child will correctly identify, by feel only, five out of five common objects. Identifying an object by touch is termed "stereognosis" or "identification of solids." Stereognosis is a tactile discrimination skill needed for the development of fine hand manipulation. Answer A demonstrates localization of tactile stimuli, answer B demonstrates graphesthesia, and answer C is an example of the tactile discrimination of textures. See reference: Case-Smith (ed): Exner, CE: Development of hand skills.

39. (A) Complete independence with self-care and transfers. An individual with T4 paraplegia will have sufficient trunk balance, upper extremity strength, and coordination to complete self-care and transfers independently. Individuals with high cervical injuries are likely to be dependent in self-care and transfers (answer D). Individuals with low cervical and high thoracic injuries require assistance with transfers and some self-care (answers B and C). See reference: Pedretti and Early (eds): Adler, C: Spinal cord injury.

40. (B) An activity exploring leisure opportunities and problems. In the process of making choices about activities, the first step is developing awareness and knowledge. OT practitioners "... assist the clients in developing awareness of options and limits" (p. 387). This individual's leisure interests are already known, so answer A would be a duplication of information. Magazine picture collages could be adapted to further examine interests and values (answer C), but this answer does not describe such an adaptation. Answer D is premature at this point because the individual has not identified any goals around which to plan future leisure activities. See reference: Neistadt and Crepeau (eds): Knox, SH: Treatment through play and leisure.

41. (A) Within 6 months, the client will participate in classroom activities for 1 hour without disruptive outbursts twice a day. A functional goal relates the skill to be developed to a child's environment or life tasks, therefore making it more meaningful to the child and the family. Answers B, C, and D are measurable, but not functional goals, because they do not address the context in which the skill is applied. See reference: Case-Smith (ed): Richardson, PK and Schultz-Krohn, W: Planning and implementing services.

42. (A) putting blankets in the overhead compartments. When distributing magazines, the flight attendant uses negligible reaching and bending. Upgrading the activity increases the degree of reaching and bending and adds more resistance than that provided by magazines. Putting blankets in the overhead copmartments (answer A) would be an appropriate gradual upgrade. Handling full meal trays (answer B), which are significantly heavier than magazines, extending them to passengers, especially those in window seats, is more than a gradual increase or upgrade. Putting luggage into the overhead compartments (answer D) would be the final step in the work-hardening process, because it involves the most weight and the riskiest back position. Distributing magazines to half of the passengers (answer C) would be downgrading the activity. See reference: Pedretti and Early (eds): Smithline, J and Dunlop, LE: Low back pain.

43. (D) Social skills training. Social skills training can be used to develop the ability to relate appropriately and effectively with others. The sensory integration treatment approach, which aims to improve the reception and processing of sensory information within the central nervous system, uses vestibular stimulation and gross-motor exercise (answer A). This approach involves the use of pleasurable activities that don't require conscious attention to movement (answer C), and is best suited to individuals with chronic schizophrenia who have proprioceptive deficits. Environmental modification (answer B) is most appropriate for individuals with cognitive disabilities. See reference: Early: Some practice models for occupational therapy in mental health.

44. (A) pull-to-sit, leaning back against a therapy ball. While all answers involve antigravity control, answer A addresses beginning control in neck and shoulders. Because control develops cephalocaudally, neck and shoulder control should be addressed first. By using an incline, the pull of gravity can be reduced, thus facilitating maximum control. See reference: Case-Smith (ed): Nichols, DS: The development of postural control.

45. (B) Hammering a nail into a piece of wood. Hammering a nail into a piece of wood requires the individual to stabilize the object against the palm and fingers, while the thumb is positioned to perform as an opposing force. Answer A is a form of prehension commonly referred to as tip prehension. Answer C, carrying a pail of bolts, requires a hook grasp. This requires the MCP joints to be placed in extension, the PIP and DIP joints to be flexed, and may not include the use of the thumb. Answer D is considered a spherical grasp pattern that requires the fourth and fifth digits to assume a more flexed position for enhanced cupping of the palm. See reference: Pedretti and Early (eds): Belkin, J and Yasada, L: Orthotics.

46. (B) pass around a scent box and ask each patient to smell the contents. The sensory integrative frame of reference holds that patients can learn by receiving, processing, and responding to sensory stimulation. Starting a group for regressed patients with sensory stimuli such as touch and smell helps to get the patient's attention and arouse their interest. Asking patients in this type of a group to introduce themselves (answer A) can be confusing and time consuming, especially when dealing with regressed individuals with limited attention spans. Reading favorite poems (answer C), and discussing lunch menus (answer D), are activities more suited to patients functioning on higher levels than those in the group described. See reference: Stein and Cutler: Theoretical models underlying the clinical practice of psychosocial occupational therapy.

47. (B) rocking in prone on a therapy ball, with feet touching the floor. Answer B is correct because it employs slow, regular vestibular input in a comfortable and safe position with feet in contact

with the floor, which is inhibitory. Answers A, C, and D are vestibular activities, but they involve fast or irregular movements that will increase the level of arousal. See reference: Solomon (ed): Graham, G, McCreddy, P, and Solomon, JW: Sensorimotor treatment approaches.

48. (A) Prevent loss of joint and skin mobility. During the acute stage, when burn wounds are partial or full thickness in nature, maintenance of joint range of motion and skin mobility is the primary goal of intervention. Providing adaptive equipment (answer B) is typically performed during the surgical or postoperative stage, and compression and vascular garments (answer C), and the prevention of scarring (answer D) are goals most commonly implemented during the rehabilitation phase. See reference: Pedretti and Early (eds): Reeves, SU: Burns and burn rehabilitation.

49. (A) Punctuality, accepting directions from a supervisor, and interacting with coworkers. Psychosocial components include time management, social conduct, interpersonal skills, and self-control. Punctuality and accepting feedback are examples of important prevocational skills within these psychosocial performance components. Memory, decision making, attention to tasks, and sequencing (answer B) are considered to be cognitive components. Standing tolerance, endurance, and eye–hand coordination (answer C) are categorized as sensorimotor components. Grooming and adhering to safety precautions (answer D) are work performance areas, not psychosocial performance components. See reference: AOTA: Uniform Terminology for Occupational Therapy, ed 3.

50. (C) Avoid resistive materials. For a child with acute juvenile rheumatoid arthritis, the OT practitioner should always use techniques for joint protection and energy conservation. Activities requiring the manipulation of highly resistive materials such as clay, leather, and copper sheets should be avoided; the pressure applied to the joints could exacerbate the condition. Avoiding light touch (answer A) is a precaution more relevant for the treatment of a child with tactile defensiveness. Rapid vestibular stimulation (answer B) is contraindicated for a child who is prone to seizures. The need to avoid above-normal body temperature (answer D) is more relevant to a client with multiple sclerosis, because high temperatures exacerbate the symptoms. See reference: Case-Smith (ed): Rogers, SL, Gordon, CY, Schanzenbacher, KE, and Case-Smith, J: Common diagnosis in pediatric occupational therapy.

51. (C) Ability to consistently follow hip precautions. Many factors are considered when a short-term goal is reset. These factors may include consistency of performance, cognitive or perceptual impairments, the amount of time required, and any change in attention or concentration. For the short-term goal to be changed, the individual in this case needs to be able to demonstrate consistent performance in the use of hip precautions, because improved performance in dressing has already been demonstrated. If the amount of time needed, or concentration had been a problem, these issues would have been addressed as part of the original goal. The ability to use the adaptive equipment appropriately has also been demonstrated. See reference: Trombly (ed): Planning, guiding, and documenting therapy.

52. (A) increasing self-awareness through expressive activities. Increasing self-awareness would be an initial goal area because people with eating disorders are often out-of-touch with their bodies as well as their psychological and social needs. Expressive activities address psychosocial needs to increase self-awareness by providing opportunities for emotional self-expression and self-assertion (answer A). Answer B is incorrect because preoccupation with "good" versus "bad" nutrition may be part of the eating disorder. Answer C is incorrect because school performance tends to be unaffected when individuals have eating disorders unless they are physically ill. Family therapy referrals are typically performed by other disciplines on the team at the time of discharge, so answer D is also incorrect. See reference: Neistadt and Crepeau (eds): Ward, JD: Psychosocial dysfunction in adults.

53. (C) Modify the environment to protect the infant from excessive and/or inappropriate sensory stimulation prior to direct intervention. Preterm infants with histories of maternal drug abuse have multiple sensory needs often resulting in poor self-regulation and behavioral organization. Answers C and D both incorporate sensory integration approaches. However, answer C best demonstrates an initial intervention to promote the neurobehavioral organization required to tolerate direct handling. Answers A and B are important in determining appropriate treatment plans for the infant and family. However, a social work referral should be made after initial assessments are completed to make the most appropriate recommendations for social service involvement, if needed. Although identifying maternal medical status and treatment compliance issues are of great importance to best determine eventual educational and disposition recommendations, it is not the primary sensory intervention focus of the OT team. See reference: Case-Smith (ed): Hunter, JG: Neonatal intensive care unit.

54. (D) Weaving on a frame loom. Use of, and attention to the entire loom area, is essential for weaving on a frame loom. The shuttle must slide across the entire width of the loom, which involves crossing the midline. It is possible to build a coil pot (answer A), to make macramé objects (answer B), and string beads for a necklace (answer C) without crossing the midline. See reference: Breines: Folkcraft.

55. (B) Observe performance at the job site and make recommendations to increase productivity. One of the roles of the OT in transition services includes consulting with employers on adaptation to job activities to accommodate individuals with disabilities. The other members of the educational team can provide classroom-based instruction as in answers A, C, and D. See reference: Case-Smith (ed): Spencer, K: Transition services: From school to adult life.

56. (A) A problem with learning new motor skills. Answer A is correct because it describes the central problem of dyspraxia—difficulty in performing skills not previously mastered where motor planning is required. Answer B is not correct because, although developmental dyspraxia is considered a sensory integration problem, it does not explain what problems the child faces, which are praxic in nature. Answers C and D are incorrect because, although reflex integration and balance problems may be present with developmental dyspraxia, they are not problems of praxis or motor planning. Answers C and D are automatic motor activities, and dyspraxia is a problem of mastering motor activities that must be learned. See reference: Case-Smith (ed): Parham, LD and Mailloux, Z: Sensory integration.

57. (A) postural control. This activity requires the patient to reach in several directions and at various levels, which is useful for helping to improve balance by requiring postural adjustments to regain equilibrium. Postural control is particularly important to address with patients who have had lower extremity amputations, because this performance component will impact the ability to safely perform LE self-care and other daily activities. Answer B is incorrect because it is unclear how much resistance is involved in the activity. Answer C is incorrect because the patient is not moving through space. Answer D is incorrect because this activity would not have a direct affect on promoting soft-tissue integrity. See reference: Pedretti and Early (eds): Morris, PA: Lower extremity amputations.

58. (D) Each member will remain in the group without disrupting the work of others for 15 minutes. Parallel groups are most appropriate for people who do not have the ability to interact successfully with other group members. Participants in parallel groups are involved in individual tasks that require minimal, if any, interaction. Therefore, appropriate expectations for parallel groups focus on remaining in the group and working alongside others. Taking leadership roles (answer A) is a goal consistent with egocentric-cooperative groups. Sharing materials with another group member (answer B) is a project group goal. Expressing feelings within a group (answer C) is consistent with a cooperative group. See reference: Cole: Appendix B.

59. (D) the ability to recognize objects. Answer D is correct because a child must be able to recognize an object before they can discriminate among its specific visual attributes. Answers A, B, and C are not correct because the ability to discriminate among colors, shapes, and positions is a skill that develops later. See reference: Kramer and Hinojosa (eds): Todd, VR: Visual information analysis: Frame of reference for visual perception.

60. (A) positioning, compression glove, and edema massage, followed by passive range-of-motion exercises. The four measures given in answer A can be effective in the reduction of edema and prevention of further edema. The goal is to promote the movement of fluid back into normal circulation, rather than allowing it to collect in one area or body part. Gentle, passive range of motion is necessary to help maintain joint structure and provide nutrients to the joint. The actual movement of the extremity may serve as a "pump" to assist in moving excess fluid back into the body. These techniques are contraindicated for individuals who have deep vein thrombosis. Answers B and D are incorrect because both require some degree of active motion. Taking no action (answer C) would result in a prolonged period of edema and immobility of the upper extremity. See reference: Trombly (ed): Woodson, AM: Stroke.

61. (D) During conversations with female group members, the client will make eye contact for 8 to 10 seconds, twice in each half-hour group. The short-term goal that describes appropriate verbal and nonverbal interactions with female peers (answer D) is the best answer. A goal set for 6 months (answer A) is a long-term goal. Awareness of thought processes (answer B) is more appropriate to a goal related to self-awareness. Attempting to develop skills with staff (answer C) can pose some confusing boundary and ethical questions in a long-term goal related to developing future personal relationships. See reference: Early: Understanding psychiatric diagnosis: The DSM-IV.

62. (B) Developing the student's vocational interests, social skills, and community mobility skills. Answer B is correct because these skills are essential for functioning in the environment after school. Leisure interests and skills (answer A) are important in the student's life, but will not help preparation for employment. Answer C is not correct because, although it describes the student's motor control function, which may influence the type of job the adolescent performs, adaptation can be made in this area of need. Although developing fine motor skills (answer D) is a traditional OT role in school settings, it would not be an appropriate focus for this example of transition planning intervention. See reference: Case-Smith (ed): Rogers, SL, Gordon, CY, Schanzenbacher, KE, and Case-Smith, J: Common diagnosis in pediatric occupational therapy practice.

63. (B) An anticlaw splint. An ulnar nerve injury influences the flexion of the ring and small fingers that occurs during grasp, as well as wrist flexion and ulnar deviation. This injury may cause hyperextension of the metacarpophalangeal joint, resulting in a claw hand. An anticlaw splint (answer B) would therefore be the most appropriate splint for this type of injury. See reference: Pedretti and Early (eds): Kasch, MC and Nickerson, E: Hand and upper extremity injuries.

64. (B) Bingo. Luck is the key element in a game of chance. Bingo is a game where the outcome depends on the calling out of random numbers. Collecting baseball cards (answer A) is a hobby. Charades and balloon volleyball (answers C and D) are games based on strategy and skill. See reference: Early: Leisure skills.

65. (C) Safety razor with extended handle. The extended handle is the appropriate component that allows this individual to overcome limited shoulder and elbow range of motion in order to reach his face. Attaching a safety razor or electric razor to a universal cuff (answers A and D) would benefit an individual who is unable to grasp a razor, but would not enable this individual to reach his face to shave. A safety razor with a built-up handle (answer B) would benefit an individual with limited finger flexion or strength, but it would also be ineffective in enabling this individual to reach his face. See reference: Neistadt and Crepeau (eds): Holm, MB, Rogers, JC and James, AB: Treatment of activities of daily living.

66. (B) Playing Velcro checkers to tolerance. Gentle, repetitive, resistive exercises help maintain strength and endurance in weakened muscles. A wrist support (answer A) compensates for loss of muscle strength, but does not help to maintain strength. Exercising without resistance once a day (answer C) will also not help maintain strength. Exercising against maximal resistance (answer D) is contraindicated for individuals with ALS. See reference: Dutton: Biomechanical postulates regarding intervention.

67. (B) Assist the individual in identifying volunteer opportunities in the community. Working as a volunteer would ease the transition from the hospital to the community, and would also increase the individual's comfort level regarding "working in the real world." Volunteer work provides for greater flexibility and lays a foundation for future paid employment. Scheduling a real job interview (answer C) is probably too challenging at this time. While working around the group home (answer A) would be useful, it would not be as effective in moving in the direction of paid employment in the community as answer B. Advising the individual against working (answer D) ignores the individual's employment potential and his progress made. See reference: Early: Work, homemaking, and child care.

68. (C) Can the child's feet reach the floor? A relaxed position during toilet use is essential to success in elimination training. The seat should be low enough so the child's feet can be used to help with postural stability. In addition, a seat design featuring a wide base, back support, and placement at a height that enables the child to place their feet firmly on the ground or on foot supports, will give the child a sense of comfort and security. Answers A, B, and D describe other useful considerations that should be addressed after the issue of support has been resolved. See reference: Case-Smith (ed): Shepherd, J: Self-care and adaptations for independent living.

69. (D) a raised-bed garden. The individual with back pain must avoid activities that stress the lumbar spine, such as prolonged bending/flexing of the spine. A raised-bed garden would allow gardening without bending. A wheelbarrow with elongated handles (answer B) would be harder to control while pushing than a wheelbarrow with normal handles and would, therefore, place undue stress on the low back. A 12-inch high seat with tool holders could benefit an individual with low endurance, but working on the ground from that position would be very difficult for an individual with back pain. See reference: Pedretti and Early (eds): Smithline, J and Dunlop, LE: Low back pain.

70. (B) (1) position shirt on lap; (2) place left hand into sleeve and pull up sleeve past elbow; (3) place right hand into sleeve and pull up sleeve; (4) pull shirt up over head. Answer B would be the best sequence because positioning the shirt first on the lap may provide cues for patients with unilateral neglect. Also, starting with the left side allows the unaffected right hand to perform the first part of the task successfully, and requires the eyes to then scan to the left to locate the left arm. Answers A, C, and D are all examples of sequences that are less likely to be successful. See reference: Pedretti and Early (eds): Foti, D: Activities of daily living.

71. (A) checking for irritation and pressure problems. Because a toddler cannot communicate discomfort effectively, skin irritation may go unnoticed. A young child, therefore, is at higher risk for developing skin and pressure problems than an older, more verbal one. Although answers B, C, and D describe important factors in splint care, primary emphasis for the young child should be placed on answer A. See reference: Case-Smith (ed): Exner, CE: Development of hand skills.

72. (D) perform only gentle active range of motion. Gentle active range of motion allows the individual to control the movement and avoid overstretching of inflamed joint tissues. Brisk active range of motion (answer A) and the addition of resistance (answer B) are likely to cause further damage to the joints by increasing stress, which results in in-

creased inflammation. The individual must be taught in therapy, the importance of joint protection during exercise. Eliminating all range of motion exercise (answer C) would result in further joint stiffness and loss of range of motion. See reference: Trombly (ed): Feinberg, JR and Trombly, CA: Arthritis.

73. (D) Assess the individual's topographical orientation skills. To plan an appropriate intervention, the individual's community mobility skills must first be assessed. Constantly getting lost is a strong indicator that the individual may be impaired in the area of topographical orientation. Learning to take the bus and obtaining a library card (answers A and C), are important steps toward independent library use, but should occur after evaluation has been completed. Individuals may enjoy using a library whether they can read or not, so the ability to read is not essential to this goal and does not need to be evaluated (answer B). See reference: Early: Activities of daily living.

74. (D) Review appropriate behavioral and developmental positioning techniques with parental observation and interaction. The NICU environment can often undermine the importance of the family. Therefore, implementing and integrating parental involvement with daily neonatal care becomes of primary importance for the carryover of learned techniques to best promote developmental acquisition. Answers B, C, and D are all family-centered strategies and are recommended for NICU intervention. However, answer D is clearly the optimal strategy for fostering parental observation and interpretation skills, building positional and handling skills, and responding to their infant's behaviors. Initial chart review and updating with nursing staff (answer A), are essential assessment steps made prior to initial contact with the infant and family, and are the least optimal intervention strategy to pursue with the family present. See reference: Case-Smith (ed): Hunter, JG: Neonatal Intensive Care Unit.

75. (B) hyperextension of the PIP joint and flexion of the DIP joint. Answer B is the only answer provided that describes a swan-neck deformity. The pattern of hyperextension of the PIP and DIP joints (answer A) may be seen in lower motor-neuron palsies. Flexion of the PIP joint and hyperextension of the DIP joint (answer C) is descriptive of a boutonniere deformity. An individual who has overstretched the volar plates at the PIP and DIP joints would have hyperextension of the MP joint and flexion of the DIP joint (answer D). See reference: Pedretti and Early (eds): Buckner, WS: Arthritis.

76. (A) Postural hypotension. A frequent side effect of neuroleptic drugs is a decrease in blood pressure in response to sudden movements, specifically up and down, resulting in faintness or loss of consciousness. The parachute activity involves significant up and down body movements and, therefore, warrants the COTA's full attention with this patient population. Answers B, C, and D are also potential side effects of antipsychotic medications, but would usually not be problematic with parachute activities. See reference: Early: Psychotropic medications and other biological treatments.

77. (C) Stabilizing the pelvis, hips, and legs. Answer C is correct, because when the pelvis, hips, and legs do not provide a good central base of support, the child resorts to compensatory movements. Stabilizing the trunk (answer A) is not correct because unless the pelvis is stabilized, arm movements may still be compromised. Answer B is not correct, because use of a lap board or chair arms for weight bearing of the upper extremities will compromise the use of the arms and hands to stabilize the body. Stabilizing the head and neck (answer D) is not correct because the pelvis continues to be unstable and, therefore, is not a good base for arm movements. See reference: Case-Smith (ed): Nichols, DS: Development of postural control.

78. (D) A long-handled bath sponge. A person with a total hip arthroplasty must avoid hip flexion of 80 degrees or greater, hip adduction, and internal rotation. A long-handled bath sponge (answer D) would allow the person to adhere to the precautions stated above by providing an extended reach during bathing of the lower extremities. A wire basket attached to the walker (answer A) would not allow the person to come close to a counter without having to step sideways, which causes hip adduction. A padded foam toilet seat 1 inch height (answer B), or a short-handled bath sponge (answer C), would be inadequate in that they would cause the person to flex the hip past 80 degrees while performing self-care tasks. See reference: Trombly (ed): Bear-Lehman, J: Orthopaedic conditions.

79. (C) Provide project samples for clients to duplicate. Individuals functioning at cognitive level 4 are able to copy demonstrated directions presented one step at a time. They find it easier to copy a sample than to follow directions or diagrams. Individuals functioning at cognitive level 3 are capable of using their hands for simple, repetitive tasks (answer A), but are unlikely to produce a consistent end product. Those functioning at cognitive level 5 can generally perform a task involving three familiar steps and one new one (answer B). Individuals functioning at cognitive level 6 can anticipate errors and plan ways to avoid them. These individuals would be capable of following written directions (answer D). See reference: Early: Some practice models for occupational therapy in mental health.

80. (D) picking up raisins with a pair of tweezers. While all answers describe methods to promote some aspect of handwriting skills, this activity is the only one that targets isolated finger use. Drawing on sandpaper (answer A) can be used to increase kinesthetic awareness and finger strength. Copying shapes (answer B) is primarily a perceptual motor task. Rolling out "Play Doh" (answer C) is an activity that can promote bilateral hand use and the development of palmar arches. See reference: Case-Smith (ed): Amundsen, SJ and Weil, M: Pre-writing and handwriting skills.

81. (B) Encouraging any available hemiplegic limb movements before or during a task. Any contralesional limb movement (even shoulder elevation) will activate additional motor units, which will then increase attention to the left. Bilateral activities (answer A) may reduce attention to the left by inhibiting function of the affected hemisphere. Activities that do not cross the midline (answer C), and activities that focus on the uninvolved side of the body (answer D) only reinforce neglect of the involved side of the body. See reference: Unsworth (ed): Evaluation and intervention with unilateral neglect.

82. (A) Practice preparing a variety of foods, using different cooking methods and recipes. Recent findings in motor learning suggest that practicing a variety of tasks in a nonsystematic, but repetitive way (variable practice), can enhance learning retention and transfer of skills, because the novelty introduced into the task engages more cognitive effort. The practice methods identified in answers B, C, and D focus more on systematic practice. This type of practice may result in better performance of different parts of the task, or of one task, but not in improved learning retention and skill transfer. See reference: Neistadt and Crepeau (eds): Neistadt, ME: Theories derived from learning perspectives.

83. (B) Concentration. Concentration is a game that requires the player to remember visual cues. Dominoes (answer A), pickup sticks (answer C), and checkers (answer D), do require visual skills, but not visual memory. See reference: Case-Smith (ed): Schneck, CM: Visual perception.

84. (B) Functional-position resting splint. Bedridden individuals are often provided with splints to prevent the development of flexion contractures in the hand that can lead to problems with maintaining hygiene. A functional-position resting hand splint is most appropriate, because it will prevent flexion contractures from developing and allow the caregiver access to his hand for cleaning. Neither the dorsal nor volar wrist splints (answers A and C) would keep the fingers in extension, which is necessary to prevent development of finger contractures. Dynamic finger-extension splints (answer D) are appropriate for individuals who have active finger flexion, but limited active finger extension. See reference: Neistadt and Crepeau (eds): Fess, EE and Kiel, JH: Neuromuscular treatment: Upper extremity splinting.

85. (A) group size of fewer than five members. Group size strongly influences how members relate to one another. In general, an ideal group size is seven to ten members (answer C) for the most interaction among members. However, groups with fewer than five members tend to increase the focus on the leader in their interactions (answer A). Group membership of similar goals (answer D) improves cohesiveness more than interactions. Differing ages (answer B) is not known to have an impact on interactions. See reference: Neistadt and Crepeau (eds): Schwartzberg, SL: Group process.

86. (D) Make sure the child's hips are secured against the back of the seat. The hips are one of the key points of control when positioning a child. Positioning the hips securely against the back of the seat with a seat belt or an abductor wedge (or both) in the correct angle serves to break up the extensor pattern and facilitates the positioning of the other body parts (answers A, B, and C), so that the child can participate in family games. See reference: Case-Smith (ed): Wright-Ott, C and Egilson, S: Mobility.

87. (B) Sip and puff switch. A sip and puff switch (answer B) is operated by breath control and is unaffected by random movements of the extremities. An infrared switch (answer A) sends an infrared beam from the switch to a surface that reflects the light back to the switch. When the beam is broken, the switch is activated. The switch may be activated by an eye blink or finger twitch. Random movements of the extremities may misalign the person's head or body, causing false activation. A P switch (answer C) is a piezoelectric sensor that is activated by tensing a muscle so that a signal is relayed to a switch. A rocking lever switch (answer D) activates a device when one side of the switch is pushed, and turns the device off when the other side of the switch is pushed. Infrared switches, P switches, and rocking lever switches could all be activated accidentally by random movements. See reference: Angelo and Lane (eds): Switches.

88. (B) progressive relaxation exercises and autogenic training. Progressive relaxation exercises (answer B), are the most relevant to the client's shoulder tension. This technique "involves tensing and relaxing muscle groups, one group at a time, from head to foot" (p. 462), while autogenic training utilizes the concept of mental imagery in order to "achieve muscle relaxation and vasodilation" (p. 462). Answer A is for individuals who are unable to distinguish between assertive and aggressive behaviors, and, therefore, do not respond assertively when necessary. Answer C is useful for individuals whose irrational beliefs and thought processes lead to maladaptive behaviors. Answer D applies to individuals who have difficulty selecting effective solutions or identifying the source of their problems. See reference: Neistadt and Crepeau (eds): Giles, GM and Neistadt, ME: Treatment for psychosocial components: Stress management.

89. (A) Swimming. Swimming provides active movement through wide ranges of motion with minimal impact on the joints. The sports in answers B, C, and D involve bouncing, jumping, and kicking, which place additional stress on the joints. Resistive activities such as these would be contraindicated. See reference: Neistadt and Crepeau (eds): Newman, EM, Echevarria, ME and Digman, G: Degenerative diseases.

90. (B) use pillows to prop up body parts into the desired position. An individual with low tone may benefit from supportive positioning devices such as pillows, towels, or bolsters that can help to prevent overstretching and fatigue. Slow rocking (answer C), and avoidance of quick stretch (answer D), are both methods for reducing tone and would not be beneficial to an individual having a problem with low tone. A sidelying position (answer A) would be a very difficult position for an individual with lower extremity flaccidity to maintain during sexual activity, but may be preferable for someone requiring energy conservation. See reference: Pedretti and Early (eds): Burton, GU: Sexuality and physical dysfunction.

91. (B) a class about job-seeking strategies. The COTA's remediation of identified deficits can be organized into three general approaches in psychosocial settings, that is, enhancing the individual's skills and performance, assisting the individual in adjusting his or her perspective on skills and performance, and altering the environment. Teaching and training methods predominate the skill and performance remediation approach. Answer A is more consistent with object relations approaches; answer C is consistent with cognitive disabilities; and answer D is consistent with occupational behavior and human occupation approaches. See reference: Zoltan: Executive functions.

92. (A) 2 inches wider than the widest point across the child's hips with the brace on. Measuring the child with the brace on and adding 2 inches (answer A), allows the child to easily get in and out of the chair, while preventing pressure to the child's sides. Answer B measures only the hips and would not allow enough room for the child to sit or move easily in the chair while wearing the brace. Answers C and D are both incorrect measurements for seat length, because both would have the seat too deep for the individual's leg length. The correct length of the seat should be 2 inches shorter than the distance from the back of the bent knee to the back of the buttocks. See reference: Pedretti and Early (eds): Adler, C and Tipton-Burton, M: Wheelchair assessment and transfers.

93. (C) swimming in a cool water pool. Swimming is an excellent activity for promoting physical fitness, and the cool water pool (temperature under 84°) will prevent the overheating that is contraindicated for individuals with MS. Jogging and volleyball (answers A and D) are both likely to result in overheating, and volleyball would probably also fatigue weak hand muscles. Painting (answer B) is a lightweight activity that would probably appeal to an artist, but would do very little to promote physical fitness. See reference: Pedretti and Early (eds): Schultz-Krohn, W, Foti, D, and Glogoski, C: Degenerative diseases of the central nervous system.

94. (B) learning the self-monitoring technique of asking oneself if any part of the task has been missed. Teaching the client to self-monitor is an example of a strategy to control the tendency to miss details involved in the task process. Answer A, simplifying instructions, is an example of a method of adapting the amount of information presented during the task. Answer C, practicing shape and number cancellation worksheets, is an example of a remedial skill training activity. Answer D, removing unnecessary objects from the task area to decrease distractions, is an example of adapting the environment to compensate for attention deficits. See reference: Neistadt and Crepeau (eds): Toglia, JP: Cognitive-perceptual retraining and rehabilitation.

95. (D) Provide a vertical work surface where writing and other hand skills can be practiced. A vertical work surface encourages an upright posture, upper body strengthening, and eye-hand coordination. A horizontal work surface (answer C) would result in a hunched posture during writing activities. A distraction-free environment (answer B) is helpful for children who are easily distracted, but there is no indication this child requires such an accommodation. Pulling out the child to an OT room (answer A) when adaptations can be made that allow the child to fully participate, would be counterproductive to the philosophy of an inclusive setting. See reference: Neistadt and Crepeau (eds): Erhardt, RP and Merrill, SC: Neurological dysfunction in children.

96. (B) Proceed only to the point of pain. Care must be taken to avoid fatigue and irritation of inflamed nerves when working with individuals with Guillain-Barré syndrome, so ranging only to the point of pain is the most important consideration here. While keeping that precaution in mind, the COTA could begin with proximal muscles and move in a distal direction (answer A). The number of repetitions is at the discretion of the COTA (answer C), the quality of the stretch being more important than the quantity. See reference: Pedretti and Early (eds): Lehman, RM and McCormack, GL: Neurogenic and myopathic dysfunction.

97. (D) respond to the emotional tone expressed by the words and provide extra attention and reassurance. Listening for the feelings behind the words will best help to identify and address the needs of the person who has lost the ability to use words effectively. The resident's searching for her

mother may reflect sense of loneliness. Explaining the factual truth (answer A) can have the effect of unnecessarily confronting the person with his or her deficits, and they may respond to the news as if hearing it for the first time. Telling the person to stop the behavior (answer B) will not address the need that is being expressed verbally. Answer C, telling a therapeutic fib, might work for a brief period of time, but may backfire if the person continues to question the story given, or if it causes sadness or anger. See reference: Hellen: Communication: Understanding and being understood.

98. (C) Combine task with additional sensory input (tactile, proprioceptive, and auditory). Answer C is correct because additional sensory input, when combined with a visual memory task, facilitates memory. Answer A is not correct because interest in the task should be high in order to enhance visual memory. Answer B is not correct because visual attention is a prerequisite to visual memory. Answer D is incorrect because serial or varied repetition enhances visual memory. See reference: Kramer and Hinojosa (eds): Todd, VR: Visual information analysis: Frame of reference for visual perception.

99. (D) A cutting board with two nails in it. The potato is placed on the nails to hold it in place while working. The "Dycem" (answer A) would only hold the cutting board in place, not the potato being cut. A plate guard (answer B) would not be secured tightly enough to the plate to withstand the force of cutting the potato. A rocker knife (answer C) would be unable to both stabilize the potato and be used for cutting. See reference: Trombly (ed): Stewart, C: Retraining housekeeping and child care skills.

100. (A) Give the individual a specific task such as filling up the water containers. Assigning a specific and concrete task allows the individual to focus on the task at hand, while sending the message that the individual is a valued member of the group. Giving the individual control over other group members (answer B), feeds into the individual's issues. Pairing the individual with another group member (Answer D) will give the other person little opportunity for involvement. Limiting participation to observation (answer C) will only increase the individual's frustration and lead to feelings of isolation. See reference: Early: Group concepts and techniques.

101. (D) The infant uses a wide base of support and high-arm guard position and takes short steps. Answer D is correct because according to Case-Smith, "the infant's first efforts toward unsupported movement through walking are often seen in short erratic steps, use of a wide based gait, and arms held in a high guard" (p. 80). Answers A, B, and C are not considered typical for a normally developing infant. See reference: Case-Smith (ed): Case-Smith, J: Development of childhood occupations.

102. (D) present important principles in small units that are spaced at a slower than normal pace. According to learning principles for older adults, learning will be more effective if the information is presented in small units at a slower pace. Answer A is incorrect because learning will be impeded if information is presented too quickly and in large chunks. Answer B is incorrect because presentations that are highly organized will enhance retention of information more than loosely structured presentations. Attempts to persuade clients on points that may not be in agreement of the older adult's preconceived ideas, values, or habits may also impede learning (answer C), whereas a more collaborative approach may result in better learning of concepts. See reference: Larson, Stevens-Ratchford, Pedretti, and Crabtree (eds): Stevens-Ratchford, RG: Occupational therapy services within the rehabilitation health care system.

103. (A) rote repetition of the task substeps with gradually fading cues. Functional skill training focuses on mastery of a specific task. It requires the client to repeatedly practice the substeps of a task with the number of cues given for each step gradually decreasing or fading. Answer B, fine-motor activities, is incorrect because the functional training approach does not emphasize underlying performance components. Answer C, caregiver training, and answer D, use of instructional cards, represent adaptation and compensation approaches, rather than actual skill training. See reference: Neistadt and Crepeau (eds): Toglia, JP: Cognitive-perceptual retraining and rehabilitation.

104. (B) Obstacle courses. This child should be exposed to situations that require problem solving by challenging the child to move his or her body in relation to objects in the environment. Although all of the answers involve motor planning in response to the environment to some degree, running obstacle courses more clearly emphasize the spatial element. Obstacles also consist of static items and therefore facilitate success in adjustment (motor planning) more easily than moving objects. See reference: Case-Smith (ed): Parham, LD and Mailloux, Z: Sensory integration.

105. (B) A key guard. A key guard is a device that covers computer keys and provides a guide for a finger or stick without punching extra keys. A moisture guard (answer A) is a flexible plastic cover that protects the keys from drool, moisture, or dirt. An auto-repeat defeat mechanism (answer C) stops repetition of letters or numbers caused by overlong or involuntary depression of keys. One-finger-access software (answer D) allows the user to lock out keys such as "shift" or "enter." This enables an individual who uses only one finger or a stick to type capital letters or perform other keyboard functions that require simultaneous depression of more than one

key. See reference: Angelo and Lane (eds): Angelo, J: Low technology interface devices.

106. (B) have the resident dress in bed with garments that are stretchy and one size larger than usual, and then preview each step of the process with the resident. The resident who is resuming the dressing activity has low endurance as well as cognitive deficits, so they would most likely benefit from an adapted, structured approach. Dressing in bed will require less energy initially, and the larger, stretchy garments will make dressing easier. Reviewing each step before it occurs will provide cognitive cues. Answer A, having the client only select clothing, does not provide enough participation to be therapeutic. Answers C and D are too demanding and do not provide the structure necessary to ensure safety and successful performance. See reference: Hellen: Daily living care activities.

107. (C) When the child has achieved a maintenance level of functioning. Because this child may never be considered completely recovered (answer D), or may refuse OT services because of his head injury (answer A), discharge should be discussed with the OTR when the child is no longer making significant progress. Transition to the first grade (answer B) is an educational consideration that is not directly relevant to the provision of services under a medical model. See reference: Case-Smith (ed): Case-Smith, J, Rogers, J and Johnson, JH: School-based occupational therapy.

108. (A) Identify options and the consequences of each option. Individuals are frequently resistive to changes that will affect the familiar home environment, such as moving furniture or adding medically necessary equipment. To accept change, the feelings and cultural attitudes and beliefs of the client must be recognized. Then the following steps can be implemented to encourage acceptance of change: (1) identify options and the consequences of each option; (2) allow time for reflection and consideration of options (answer D); (3) practice with a "demo" device (answer C); (4) reassess the decision; (5) if acceptable, order the equipment; and (6) if rejected, document the steps taken and the reasons for rejection (answer B). See reference: Bonder and Wagner (eds): Hunt, LA: Home health care.

109. (A) Call for other staff. Calling for more staff is the first step. Several staff members may be needed to calm or restrain the individual or assist the other patients. Once help is called for, removing the other patients (answer D) and trying to calm the patient (answer B) can be initiated. As a general rule, physically trying to restrain the patient (answer C) should not be attempted. See reference: Early: Safety techniques.

110. (B) slightly flexed. Postural alignment is important in promoting oral motor function. The spine and pelvis should be in a neutral position. Normally, the head should be in a position neutral or slightly flexed (answer A). When a child has difficulty swallowing, however, tucking the chin slightly can reduce the risk of aspiration and can facilitate swallowing. Positioning the infant with the head in extension (answer C) can increase the risk of choking. Rotating the head (answer D) does not facilitate swallowing. See reference: Case-Smith (ed): Case-Smith, J and Humphry, R: Feeding intervention.

111. (C) Minimizing scar hypertrophy through compression garments and proper skin care.
Minimizing scar hypertrophy through compression garments and proper skin care is imperative upon wound closure. Answer A, preventing scar formation via static splinting, is typically performed during the surgical or postoperative phase of treatment. Controlling edema (answer B), and promoting self-care skills (answer D), are not goals directly related to scar management and are more commonly initiated during acute care intervention. See reference: Pedretti and Early (eds): Utley-Reeves, S: Burns and burn rehabilitation.

112. (A) Check with the pharmacist to see which medications can be crushed and mixed in with applesauce. This is a good and immediate solution for people who have difficulty swallowing pills. An individual who has difficulty swallowing pills may do better with smaller ones (answer D), but not all medication is available in smaller sizes. In addition, it could take a long time to get the individual to the point where he could take his medication successfully. Answers B and C are both good compensatory methods for individuals who have trouble remembering when to take medication, but do not address the swallowing issue. See reference: Neistadt and Crepeau (eds): Holm, MB, Rogers, JC, and James, AB: Treatment of activities of daily living.

113. (B) forward and side-to-side with the child sitting on the therapist's lap. Answer B is correct because the position of the child requires the least resistance to gravity. By tilting the child in this position, the practitioner controls how much the child will work against gravitational pull and assures that the child is well supported. Answers A and D are incorrect because they would require the child to lift his or her head directly against gravity. Answer C is also incorrect because the child's head is positioned against gravity in the quadruped position and a child with extremely poor head control probably could not hold this position. See reference: Case-Smith (ed): Nichols, DS: Development of postural control.

114. (B) talk to the client to determine if there are any motivational or cultural issues interfering with splint-wear compliance. Prior to fabricating another splint, the COTA must determine if the individual is likely to comply with a new splinting program. Some individuals refuse to wear splints due to

cultural norms, while others are simply embarrassed to wear a splint in public. Some people demonstrate a low motivational level in regard to regaining function, while others may overdo their splinting program in the hopes that it will facilitate healing. In the given case, it would not be indicated to refabricate the splint, answer A, unless the client agrees to adhere to a splint wear program. Answer C, requesting that the client find the splint or you will threaten to call his physician, would not be the first step to take in the process. Contacting the physician regarding the client's non-compliance as well as providing accurate, concise documentation of client performance is indicated, but not something to be used to threaten the client. Answer D, discharging the client, would not be appropriate until the COTA discusses the case with the supervising OTR, physician, See reference: Pedretti and Early (eds): Belkin, J: Hand splinting: Principles, practice and decision making.

115. (C) Determine how frequently he needs toileting and take him without asking. This individual appears to lack the awareness and/or motivation to achieve reliability with toileting. He is unlikely to respond appropriately when asked (answer A) or to respond to a timer (answer B). Moving his seat closer to the bathroom (answer D) would benefit an individual who attempts to make it to the bathroom, but doesn't make it in time. See reference: Neistadt and Crepeau (eds): Holm, MB, Rogers, JC, and James, AB: Treatment activities of daily living.

116. (A) A vacuum feeding cup. Children with impulsive behavior or poor judgment often attempt to drink too quickly. The rate of intake can be limited by using a drinking spout with a small opening, pinching a straw, or using a vacuum feeding cup with a control button. A cup with a large drinking spout (answer D) would increase the rate of intake, which could result in choking or spills. A "nosey cup" (answer B) allows children with dysphagia to maintain a tucked-chin position while drinking, which is necessary for a good swallow. A mug with two handles (answer C) would benefit a child with limited grasp or coordination. See reference: Trombly (ed): Konosky, KA: Dysphagia.

117. (A) Contrast baths and retrograde massage. Contrast baths cause vasodilation and vasoconstriction, which facilitate a pumping out of the edema. Retrograde massage assists with the facilitation of blood and lymph movement. Answers B and C, hot packs and paraffin, can assist with soft tissue and joint mobility as well as pain, but are often contraindicated in cases where edema is present because the direct heat source increases blood flow to the area and, subsequently, increases edema. Answer D, sensory re-education, would address the client's limitations with sensation, not edema, and pendulum exercises are typically performed in a dependent position to increase shoulder ROM, thus potentially increasing edema in the hand. See reference: Pedretti and Early (eds): Kasch, MC and Nickerson, E: Hand and upper extremity injuries.

118. (A) suggesting the client complete the activity in a seated position. Answer A best represents the process of activity adaptation. The COTA effectively modified (adapted) the activity to address the client's needs. "Adaptation is a change that facilitates performance" (p. 481). Answer B, recommending the client work on ironing prior to folding, is an example of grading of an activity. However, in this case, the client is in need of downgrading, not upgrading. Answer C is an example of activity analysis. Activity analysis consists of breaking an activity apart in to smaller components, while examining each step of the task. Answer D is representative of clinical reasoning, the problem-solving process that a practitioner implements to reflect upon client treatment. See reference: Early: Analyzing, adapting, and grading activities.

119. (D) incoordination. A student with tremors or poor coordination can reduce instability by stabilizing the limb proximally before working distally. Stabilization adds a secure base of support from which to work. Reduced vision, poor endurance, and limited fine movement (answers A, B, and C) do not require stabilization when writing; the effects of these deficits can be reduced by the use of paper with high-contrast guiding lines, more frequent rests, or built-up writing tools. See reference: Trombly (ed): Retraining basic and instrumental activities of daily living.

120. (C) train the client in the operation of the AT system and in strategies for its use. Training activities in the use of the assistive devices are the next critical step after setup of the system, and are essential because the complex nature of assistive technologies can require many hours of practice to master. Evaluating how well the whole system works (answer A) usually occurs after training is completed during the follow-up phase. Evaluating the match between the client and the technology (answer B) is done earlier in the process to ensure maximum success and because expensive technological devices may only be ordered once. Funding sources (answer C) are also determined before ordering equipment. See reference: Pedretti and Early (eds): Anson, D: Assistive technology.

121. (C) time management and use of leisure time. One of the lifestyle characteristics of people with substance abuse problems is that most time and effort eventually becomes structured around obtaining and using of the abused substance. Time management and use of leisure time are very important areas for the OT practitioner to address with a newly sober client who has been counseled to avoid situations and people associated with drinking alcohol. Identifying leisure interests and establishing

plans for structuring large amounts of time without drinking can help support attempts to remain substance free. Answer A, work performance, would also be an area to explore, but would probably not be an area of skill development introduced early in the OT intervention process. Answer B, self-care skills, may need to be addressed as part of daily living skills performance, but would not impact as directly on avoiding substance abuse. Medication is not typically a feature of treatment for substance abuse, so answer D is also incorrect. See reference: Early: Understanding psychiatric diagnosis: The DSM-IV.

122. (B) have the child practice tying her shoes at home and in school. Children with mental retardation often have difficulty generalizing learning from one setting to another. For instance, they learn to tie their shoes in the OT clinic, but are unable to perform the same skill at home or at school. The ability to generalize is essential in making the new skill functional in this child's daily life. Answers A, C, and D are adaptations or teaching techniques that do not address generalization. See reference: Logigian and Ward (eds): Ward, JD: Mental retardation.

123. (B) labels with white print on a black background. White print on a black background is easier to see for individuals with poor vision. Using Braille labels (answer A) is not appropriate for individuals with peripheral neuropathy, because they have decreased tactile sensation in their fingertips. A pill organizer box (answer C) is useful for taking pills on schedule and is particularly helpful for individuals who have memory deficits or complex medication regimens. If the pills were presorted in the box, the client could safely take them without actually identifying them. Using the pill organizer, however, does not address the issue of medication identification. Brightly colored pills (answer D) would make it easier for identifying different medications, however, the therapist has no control over how pills are manufactured and what colors are used. See reference: Sladyk, K and Ryan, SE (eds): Jamison, PW: A retired librarian with sensory deficits.

124. (B) Performing a clerical task such as sorting papers. The most appropriate type of activities to begin treatment for a person with severe depression are repetitive, structured and simple enough to ensure success, such as "...housework, folding laundry, simple cooking, sanding, clerical tasks, and sewing" (p. 246). Engagement in leisure exploration (answer A), meditation (answer C), and stress management activities (answer D), would eventually be relevant intervention activities for a person with depression. However, in the early stages of depression, attention span, concentration, and energy level may to be too impaired to benefit from these types of activities. See reference: Early: Responding to symptoms and behaviors.

125. (B) Gently touch the infant's lips to encourage her to open her mouth and begin sucking motions. Answer B, gently touching the infant's lips would most likely facilitate the suck-swallow reflex. "When the infant's lips are touched, the infant's mouth opens and sucking movements begin" (p. 91). Answer A, touching the infants cheek before feeding, would most likely facilitate the rooting reflex. Answer C would most likely facilitate the phasic-bite reflex, while answer D, rubbing the infant's lips and cheeks simultaneously, would most likely frustrate the infant, because several different reflexes are being encourage at the same time (e.g., the rooting reflex and phasic-bite reflex). See reference: Solomon (ed): O'Brien, JC, Koontz Lowman, D, and Solomon, JW: Development of occupational performance areas.

126. (D) Chaining. Teaching a task one step at a time, gradually adding more steps as each are mastered, is called chaining. Chaining is frequently used when teaching a multistep task, because it is easier to learn one step at a time than it is to learn a complete activity. Repetition and rehearsal (answers A and C) involve repeating the whole activity repetitively until the activity is learned. Cueing (answer B) uses an external source to remind a person of the next step or part of that step. See reference: Zoltan: Executive functions.

127. (D) Add a thickening agent to liquids. Individuals with swallowing problems usually have more difficulty with thin liquids than with thicker ones. A straw (answer A) is useful for individuals who are unable to lift a cup or glass to their mouth. "Sippy cups" (answer B) benefit individuals who tend to spill when they are drinking. It may be important to monitor fluid intake (answer C) for individuals who drink too much or don't drink enough. See reference: Neistadt and Crepeau (eds): Holm, MB, Rogers, JC, and James, AB: Treatment activities of daily living.

128. (B) side-lying on a mat. "Side-lying is a good positioning choice for children whose muscle tone becomes too high or low in prone or supine positions. Side-lying positions also give children a stable, midline head position and keep their hands in their line of vision…hands remain free to reach for and manipulate objects without having to resist the pull of gravity" (p. 354). Answer A, long-sitting, answer C, supine positioning, and answer D, prone positioning, all require the child to work against gravity, and would most likely be too difficult for the child to maintain while engaging in play activities secondary to low tone. See reference: Solomon (ed): Wandel, JA: Positioning and handling.

129. (A) are more easily performed if coordinated with consistent timing of medications. A patient with Parkinson's disease needs to learn to use the period of reduced symptoms and improved mobility resulting from medication use, to best advantage for performing ADL. Medications taken regularly and consistently aid the establishment of routines for self-care. Performance of self-care activities before medications (answer B), and stretched out throughout the day (answer D), would not make best use of the medication's positive effects. Answer C is incorrect because it discourages attempts for independent functioning. See reference: Pedretti and Early (eds): Schultz-Krohn, W, Foti, D and Glogoski, C: Degenerative diseases of the central nervous system.

130. (C) Appropriate social and life skills. Answer C is correct because practicing life skills is essential for learning, and has been found to be helpful in improving functional performance. Answers A, B, and D reflect verbally focused, rather than activity focused group environments that include insight development, self-disclosure, confrontation, and the open expression of anger. Intense treatment milieus that focus on these group environments have been found to be contraindicated in the inpatient treatment of individuals with schizophrenia. Structured, supportive milieus with an emphasis on enhancing positive social and life skills have been found to be helpful. See reference: Bonder: Schizophrenia and other psychotic disorders.

131. (D) is highly structured, facilitating step by step learning. Therapeutic activities should be presented in an environment free from extraneous stimuli to help the child focus on a task. The activities should be carefully graded and presented in a sequence tailored to the sensory capacities and preferences of each child. Stimuli-laden therapeutic environments such as those described in answers A, B, and C can be more beneficial to the child who is better able to use imagination and self-direction than to the autistic child. See reference: Case-Smith (ed): Rogers, SL, Gordon, CY, Schanzenbacker, KE and Case-Smith, J: Common diagnosis in pediatric occupational therapy practice.

132. (A) skin inspection. Visual inspection of an insensate area is essential for preventing pressure sores, which may develop when there are no sensory cues to alert a person to skin breakdown. Nail trimming (answer B) is an important issue to address with individuals with diabetes, but is secondary to skin inspection in importance. Many individuals with diabetes have abnormalities in nail growth, and instead of trimming their own nails, they have them trimmed by a podiatrist. Moreover, the nursing staff may address this issue with the patient. Retirement planning (answer C), and returning to work (answer D), are issues that may be addressed when discussing discharge plans. See reference: Trombly (ed): Bentzel, K: Remediating sensory impairment.

133. (D) Provide the client with several outfits similar to the preferred one. This option meets the client's need to wear the outfit of her choice, while having enough clean outfits. Answers A and C limit the client's freedom of choice, and will result in an unhappy individual. Washing the outfit each night (answer B) is burdensome for the caregiver and will quickly wear out the outfit. See reference: Neistadt and Crepeau (eds): Holm, MB, Rogers, JC, and James, AB: Treatment activities of daily living.

134. (A) Scribble on a piece of paper. The Bayley scales on infant development suggest that a child will be able to scribble on a piece of paper (answer A) between the ages of 10 to 12 months. Copying a triangle (answer B) is a task that is not anticipated until the age of 5 to 6 years. Copying a horizontal line (answer C) is typically not seen until the age of 2, while copying numerals (answer D) is typically not observed until the age of 5 to 6 years old. It is important to appreciate that despite these age/developmental generalizations, each child's skill level can vary. See reference: Case-Smith (ed): Amundson, SJ: Prewriting and handwriting skills.

135. (C) Provide a transfer tub bench and install grab bars. The best adaptation to achieve access to the tub would be providing the client with a transfer tub bench, which is recommended for individuals who cannot step over the edge of the tub. Bathroom grab bars should also be installed to provide stability during the move into the tub. Answer A, repositioning the light switch, would help to enhance visual cues and safety. Providing long-handled adaptive devices (answer B) would enhance bathing performance if the individual had difficulty with reaching their legs and feet. Answer D, nonskid decals and mats are primarily safety measures to prevent slipping and falling. See reference: Pedretti and Early (eds): Smith, P: Americans with Disabilities Act: Accommodating persons with disabilities.

136. (B) Does the client want to paint the project blue or white? The COTA should provide an individual who is just beginning to make decisions with limited, simple choices. The client is not yet ready to choose from four broad categories of activities (answer A); it would be better to ask him if he would like to make a leather key ring or a wooden coaster. Projecting about what the client will want to do with the finished project (answer C) is premature. The decision to work alone or in a group (answer D) should be made by the COTA, not the client, depending on how the environment would be best structured to benefit the individual. See reference: Early: Analyzing, adapting and grading activities.

137. (B) Introduce active range of motion exercises through gentle swaying/dancing with the child's favorite music. By introducing gentle, non-threatening activities (such as dancing to his favorite music), the child will have time to develop trust with the COTA in addition to having some sense of power over the situation by choosing his own type of music. Informing the child that he will most likely scar if he

does not participate in therapy is not the first thing the COTA should do (answer A). This may make the child feel scared, and given his age, even more frightened to participate in therapy. Patient education, especially when done with children, is something that should be done slowly and in a non-threatening manner. Answer C, introducing passive range of motion, does not assist the child to move actively, a crucial component to resuming activities of daily living post burn injury. While positioning the child over a bolster (answer D) is a viable option, it would not be the first activity to select in this particular case, because the child is unlikely to allow the COTA to touch his body in order to appropriately position him until further trust is established. See reference: Richard and Staley (eds): Reeves, SU, Warden, G and Staley, MJ: Management of the pediatric burn patient.

138. (C) Modify the activity to make it less challenging. The COTA should recognize subtle signs of fatigue, such as frustration, slowing down, hurrying to finish, lessening range of motion, and use of substitution movements, which indicate the training level was too difficult and should be downgraded. Other signs include the individual's heart rate exceeding the target heart rate; increase of more than 20 bpm above resting pulse; failure to return to resting heart rate after a 5 minute rest; and systolic pressure that does not increase at all, or that increases more than 20 mm Hg from baseline. Stopping the activity (answer A) is necessary if the individual experiences symptoms such as dyspnea, chest pain, lightheadedness, or diaphoresis. The activity should be upgraded (answer B) only when the individual is able to perform the activity without signs of fatigue or cardiac symptoms. Isometric exercises (answer D), which interfere with bloodflow through the muscles and create a heightened demand on the cardiovascular system, should not be used in individuals with cardiac conditions. See reference: Dutton: Introduction to biomechanical frame of reference.

139. (C) "I see you've finished the project, is there anything else you'd like to do with it?" This comment is best because it acknowledges the patient's effort to engage in the activity, rather than the quality of the finished product. Craft projects completed by depressed patients may show inattention to detail, and minimal effort as a result of their low energy level. Answer A, provides false praise which the client would probably recognize as unrealistic and untrustworthy. Answer B would put pressure on the client to improve performance, which could reinforce feelings of low self-esteem. Answer D minimizes the effort that the client put forth in attempting and completing the activity. See reference: Early: Responding to symptoms and behaviors.

140. (B) Crawling over and along a rope taped to the floor. The crawling activity requires both sides of the body to work together in either reciprocal or bilateral movements. Weight bearing provides proprioceptive input, and having the rope between arms and legs develops awareness of body sidedness from a visual standpoint. The remaining choices do not provide reciprocal or bilateral movement, which would develop coordination of the body sides in rhythmic patterns. See reference: Case-Smith (ed): Parham, LD and Mailloux, Z: Sensory integration.

141. (A) Continue to perform PROM and then position and elevate the affected extremity. Positioning, the use of a compression glove, edema massage, and PROM exercises are all effective methods for reducing edema and preventing further edema. The goal is to promote the movement of fluid back into normal circulation, rather than allowing it to collect in one area or body part. Gentle PROM is necessary to help maintain joint structure and provide nutrients to the joint. The actual movement of the extremity may serve as a "pump" to assist in moving excess fluid back into the body. These techniques are contraindicated for individuals who have deep vein thrombosis. Edema is caused in part by the loss of movement in an extremity because there is no contraction of muscles, which helps to pump the fluid to the heart. Splinting (answer B) is effective in preventing deformity, but compression gloves are more effective in reducing edema. Taking no action (answer C) could result in permanent damage to the tissue of the involved extremity. Having the individual attempt to squeeze a ball (answer D) would be inappropriate because the left arm is flaccid. See reference: Trombly (ed): Woodson, AM: Stroke.

142. (A) Give him a guitar to play during break under the supervision of the COTA. Participation in meaningful activity will promote self-esteem and self-concept. This will also facilitate development of rapport with the COTA, while providing a safe environment for the individual. Activities such as answers B and D isolate the individual from the group process, and would be contraindicated for an individual who recently attempted suicide. The responsibility of composing music (answer C) would probably be too challenging at this time. See reference: Early: Leisure skills.

143. (C) Play activities that incorporate tapping, application of textures, and weight bearing to the residual limb. Massage, tapping, use of textures, and weight bearing on the distal end of a residual limb are techniques used to develop tolerance to touch and pressure in the hypersensitive limb. Answers A and B will not affect hypersensitivity, and answer D is incorrect because the child is in the pre-prosthetic phase and does not yet have access to the prosthesis. See reference: Trombly (ed): Celikol, F: Amputation and prosthetics.

144. (C) Toothbrush with built-up handle. An individual with C7-C8 quadriplegia has the hand strength to hold a toothbrush with a built-up handle. An alternate method can be to position the toothbrush be-

tween the fingers. An individual with a C5 injury may require a MAS for brushing teeth (answer A). Other individuals with injuries at the C5-C6 level may be able to use a universal cuff (answer B), or a wrist support with a utensil holder (answer D), to hold the toothbrush. See reference: Christiansen (ed): Garber, SL, Gregorio, TL, Pumphrey, N, and Lathem, P. Self-care strategies for persons with spinal cord injuries.

145. (D) redirect the individual to a more neutral topic. In depth discussion of physical symptoms is not helpful for individuals with anxiety disorders, and they should be redirected, not encouraged (answer C), to speak further about somatic symptoms. It is best to "focus on what clients are concerned about, listen to their fears, and then gradually turn their attention to a neutral topic or something more constructive" (p. 241). Because individuals with anxiety often fixate on their physical symptoms, and because the problems occurred the previous day, it is probably not necessary to report them to the OTR or physician (answers A and B). See reference: Early: Responding to symptoms and behaviors.

146. (D) Playing "Simon Says." Playing "Simon Says" is the most appropriate choice because it promotes a gross motor activity, a major component of the physical or "rough and tumble" form of play. "Children from 2 to 5 years of age are extremely active and almost always ready to engage in rough and tumble play...activities such as running, hopping, skipping and tumbling are performed without any typical goal" (p. 86). The game of "Simon Says" can be downgraded so children can play from a wheelchair, mat, or standing position. Drawing and putting together puzzles, and constructing towers out of blocks (answers A and B), are activities typically introduced to encourage constructive play (activities used to encourage creativity with construction). While answer C, role playing (telling stories within the group, playing dress up and imaginary play), is an activity utilized to support the concept of dramatic play, it is not necessarily physical in nature. See reference: Case-Smith (ed): Case-Smith, J: Development of childhood occupations.

147. (B) have the individual work at the keyboard for 30 minutes. Increasing the duration the individual is able to tolerate working on the computer is the most appropriate way to progress this individual. A heavier mouth stick (answer A) would make the task more difficult and yield no benefit. An individual with C4 quadriplegia would not have the potential to use a typing device that inserts into a wrist support (answer C). Teaching the individual how to correctly instruct a caregiver in use of the keyboard (answer D) would be downgrading the activity. See reference: Christiansen (ed): Garber, SL, Gregorio, TL Pumphrey, N, and Lathem, P: Self-care strategies for persons with spinal cord injuries.

148. (B) a cheese sandwich. The most basic level of meal preparation is accessing a prepared meal, which involves tasks such as opening a thermos and unwrapping a sandwich. When an individual becomes proficient at this level, he or she can, and should, progress to a higher level. More advanced meal preparation activities can be structured to increase in complexity in the following sequence: prepare a cold meal (answer B); prepare a hot one dish meal (answers A and C); and prepare a hot multidish meal (answer D). See reference: Neistadt and Crepeau (eds): Rogers, JC and Holm, MB: Evaluation of activities of daily living (ADL) and home management.

149. (D) Electronic augmentative communication device. An augmentative communication keyboard is a high-technology aid that can compensate for expressive deficits and assist a student with communication. Answer A is incorrect because an environmental control unit is a device that allows a person with severe disabilities to operate appliances or devices. It may be used to turn on a tape recorder for note taking, but it would not be used as the primary method for conversation and graphics in the classroom. Answers B and C are incorrect because both the Wanchik's writer and a head pointer are low-technology aids for communication, rather than high-technology devices. See reference: Angelo and Lane (eds): Angelo, J: Written and spoken augmentative communication.

150. (A) carpeting with low or looped pile. Carpeting with low pile (answer A) would be the best choice for an elderly person who may be prone to falls, because it provides the fewest tripping hazards and provides a sense of security during walking. Answer B, a wood floor, is a hard surface that can be slippery and hazardous for someone who may fall easily. Answer C, area rugs, would not be recommended because of the potential for tripping on the rug edges. Answer D, carpeting with deep pile and padding may be comfortable and provide cushioning if the person does fall, but can add resistance or "drag" when walking, presenting an additional tripping hazard. See reference: Larson, Stevens-Ratchford, Pedretti, and Crabtree (eds): Christenson, MA: Environmental design, modification and adaptation.

151. (D) Have each group member complete a worksheet defining communication and his/her individual style. Determining that each member understands the concept of communication and having them identify their own style is the best initial activity. Answers A, B, and C are effective methods to use later on in the group. See reference: Early: Psychosocial skills and psychological components.

152. (B) environmental adaptations and assistance for ADL. A patient who exhibits no capacity for new learning will be unable to benefit from therapy interventions that require the ability to transfer learning (answers A, C, and D). A compensatory approach of adapting the environment and recommending assistance for safe performance of daily activities is the most appropriate intervention. See reference: Neistadt and Crepeau (eds): Neistadt, ME: Theories derived from learning perspectives.

153. (A) Textured material, rubbing, tapping, and prolonged contact. Sensory desensitization helps the individual recalibrate altered sensory perceptions and improve sensibility. This type of program is initiated when light-touch sensation is intact. The modalities listed in answer A are used as graded tactile stimuli. Treatment is most successful when carried out and controlled by the individual. With a severe injury such as a burn, it is also necessary to train the individual in protective precautions. Answers B and C, techniques that provide an ungraded or nonspecific level of touch, would be tolerated with difficulty by a person with hypersensitivity, because much of the input is facilitory and would be interpreted as painful. Visual compensation and functional use of the extremity (answer D) are techniques used with individuals who have impaired sensation. See reference: Trombly (ed): Bentzel, K: Remediating sensory impairment.

154. (B) aerobic exercise. Gross motor activities, involving either aerobic exercise or stretching and relaxation, can help to reduce the physical symptoms associated with anxiety. Although line dancing (answer C) involves all of the elements of gross motor activities, it requires the individual to follow specific steps and movements, which could cause the patient to become more anxious. Sewing and handcrafts (answer A) and woodworking (answer D) would not be the best recommendation for reducing physical symptoms of muscle tension, because they are primarily fine motor activities that require sustained attention. See reference: Early: Responding to symptoms and behaviors.

155. (B) inch cubes into a cup placed on a tabletop at a distance of 1 foot." Releasing cubes into a cup a foot away will help the child to develop arm and hand control in the midranges, by releasing objects in a controlled way without using his full extension pattern. This is achieved by placing target containers closer to his body, requiring gradually increasing elbow flexion with wrist extension. Answers A and D involve larger, softer objects for release and require either throwing or gravity-assisted movement, both of which require less control. Answer C requires the manipulation of smaller objects and more precision, i.e., a more advanced skill than given in answer B. See reference: Case-Smith (ed): Exner, CE: Development of hand skills.

156. (B) continue the same positioning and splinting program that was indicated before discharge. It is necessary to continue positioning and splinting after discharge, because active scar development continues for many weeks, depending on the severity of the burn. The same positioning and splinting devices used at the hospital are used at home, with changes made as needed during follow-up visits. Individuals stay in the hospital until their conditions can be managed at home, with outpatient visits to maintain status. Individuals are not kept at hospital until they are completely healed, which would be the only situation in which a home program would not be necessary. If an individual follows the home program only as he or she deems appropriate during the day or night, instead of as scheduled by the therapist, the position time may not be sufficient to prevent deformity from occurring. See reference: Trombly (ed): Alvarado, MI: Burns.

157. (C) Relapse prevention. Relapse prevention, symptom identification and reduction, and medication management are the areas that are emphasized in discharge planning groups. Developing ADL routines, self-awareness, and social skills (answers A, B, and D) are all areas that would be addressed throughout hospitalization, and possibly after discharge as well. See reference: Early: Treatment settings.

158. (B) Methods of accommodation in the classroom. The most essential information for parents and teachers to receive from the OT is how to provide accommodations for the child in the classroom, along with information on juvenile rheumatoid arthritis, and how the various symptoms may affect the child's ability to participate in school activities. Information on the OT evaluation (answers A and C) and progress in OT (answer D) are of lesser importance, and may be unimportant in terms of the child's current functional problems. See reference: Case-Smith (ed): Rogers, SL, Gordon, CY, Schanzenbacher, KE, and Case-Smith, J: Common diagnoses in pediatric occupational therapy practice.

159. (B) Client will draw for 1 hour, taking stretch breaks every 20 minutes. Goals should be functional, measurable, and objective. This answer meets those criteria. Answer A is not measurable. "Goals need to be written to show what the patient will accomplish, not what the [OT practitioner] will do" (p. 94). Answers C and D describe what the OT practitioner will do. See reference: AOTA: Effective documentation for occupational therapy.

160. (B) Instruct the client to take "one white and one blue pill" with the morning and evening meals. Cognitive disabilities' levels of function distinguish the types of assistance an individual needs to safely complete everyday tasks. Cognitive level 4 functioning involves having a routine goal in mind. Linking medications with meals helps the goal become routine. Answer A is consistent with cognitive level 5, answer C is consistent with level 3, and answer D is consistent with level 2. See reference: Ear-

ly: Some practice models for occupational therapy in mental health.

161. (C) The splints will prevent deformity. A child with juvenile rheumatoid arthritis will need splinting to prevent deformity and maintain range of motion. Hypertonus (answer A) is not a characteristic of this condition. Due to the active nature of the child's condition, increasing range of motion (answer B) may be contraindicated. The correction of deformity (answer D) may also be contraindicated with this child due to the active nature of the disease. See reference: Case-Smith (ed): Rogers, SL, Gordon, CY, Schanzenbacher, KE, and Case-Smith, J: Common diagnoses in pediatric occupational therapy practice.

162. (B) Increase the number of towels from 10 to 20. Endurance is improved by increasing the number of repetitions so the muscle has to work over a longer period of time. Placing towels on a higher shelf (answer A) would help to increase range of motion. Placing towels on a lower shelf (answer C) decreases the difficulty of the activity, and does not lengthen the period of time needed to improve endurance by providing more repetitions. The arm could be strengthened by adding a 1 pound weight (answer D), but that would not increase the repetitions needed to improve endurance. See reference: Pedretti and Early (eds): Breines, EB: Therapeutic occupations and modalities.

163. (B) Strategies the husband can use to prevent the patient from wandering. Although wandering, incontinence, and failure to recognize family members (answers A, C, and D) are all important issues, wandering is the only potentially dangerous one. Because the patient's dementia is advanced, most of the discharge planning is directed toward her husband. Discussion with the patient will have no effect on her ability to manage her incontinence. At this point, environmental adaptation will be more effective than attempting to change the patient's behavior. See reference: Early: Understanding psychiatric diagnosis: The DSM-IV.

164. (C) Liquid and solids combined (minestrone soup). Answer C is correct because it combines two food consistencies. Liquids are very difficult for children with poor oral motor organization to manage in eating. When solids are added to liquid, the child will have difficulty managing two different forms of food. Answers A, B, and D, are easier to move and manage within the mouth, depending on the child's oral motor skills. See reference: Case-Smith (ed): Case-Smith, J and Humphry, R: Feeding intervention.

165. (B) a tub bench and toilet rails. A tub bench and toilet rails make bathroom transfers easier and safer, and allows the person with a unilateral LE amputation to transfer independently. Lightweight cooking utensils (answer A) are recommended for those individuals with weakness or joint involvement of the upper extremities. Answers C and D are incorrect because long-handled dressing devices and reachers are more likely to be recommended when compensation for hip or trunk flexion is needed, and use of these devices might discourage the normal bending activity in the person with LE amputation. See reference: Pedretti and Early (eds): Keenan, DD and Morris PA: Amputations and prosthetics.

166. (B) the client will initiate one request to one other group member for sharing group materials within a 1-week period. Reducing the number of requests and the variety or number of individuals the client is expected to interact with, is the best way to simplify the initial goal. Extending the amount of time to accomplish the goal (answer A) does not make the goal easier to achieve. Increasing the number of individuals (answer C), and subsequently the number of requests, also makes the goal more difficult to achieve. Changing interactions to the group leader (answer D) moves the goal away from the original problem area of peer social conversation to authority conversations. See reference: Early: Analyzing, adapting, and grading activities.

167. (D) are easily accomplished by the client. Answer D is correct because activities that are easily accomplished offer no challenge and, therefore, will not enhance learning of skills and development of competence. During the process of reassessment, such activities require changing through a grading process to make them somewhat more difficult. Activities which continue to provide some level of challenge (answer A), or reflect the client's priorities (answer B), or directly relate to the client's goals (answer C) will all continue to motivate the client to continue with therapy. See reference: Neistadt and Crepeau (eds): Neistadt, ME: Overview of treatment.

168. (B) ability to put on and remove the splint correctly. Knowing how to correctly put on and remove a splint it is crucial for anyone using one. Because the patient will wear the splint to prevent further trauma to the median nerve at work, demonstrating this ability would be most relevant for attaining the long-term goal of returning to work. Work simplification (answer A) is modifying task performance to conserve energy, which is important for individuals with limited endurance, such as those with arthritis or COPD. Typing with wrists in flexion (answer C) is contraindicated and would aggravate the individual's symptoms. Lightweight cookware is appropriate for this individual, but it is related to a homemaking goal, not her goal of returning to work as a secretary. See reference: Pedretti and Early (eds): Kasch, MC and Nickerson, E: Hand and upper extremity injuries.

169. (C) use a diary to record each dosage after it is taken. Using a diary to record each dosage would be most effective because it would provide the patient with a written record of when the medication was taken. Answer A, establishing a routine, and answer B, keeping the medications in a special location, could be helpful in reminding the patient to take the medication, but would not be as effective as a diary for remembering whether the medications were taken. Answer C, arranging to have a caregiver remind the patient, would not facilitate independence to medication management. See reference: Early: Activities of daily living.

170. (C) prosthetist. Prosthetists are professionals trained to make and fit artificial limbs. The physiatrist (answer A) is a physician with specialized training in physical medicine. The orthotist (answer B) specializes in fitting and fabricating permanent splints and braces. The physical therapist (answer D) is a rehabilitation professional trained to administer exercise and physical modalities to restore function and prevent disability. See reference: Case-Smith (ed): Rogers, L, Gordon, CY, Schanzenbacher, KE, and Case-Smith, J: Common diagnoses in pediatric occupational therapy practice.

171. (B) 33 to 36 inches. This is the proper height for grab bars to allow for the upper extremities to lift the body with enough clearance to transfer onto the toilet seat. A height of 28 to 32 inches (answer A) would be too low to allow the body to clear the toilet seat when the arms are straightened. A height of 38 to 41 inches or 43 to 46 inches (answers C and D) would be too high to effectively push down with the arms to lift the body onto the toilet seat. See reference: Rothstein, Roy, and Wolf: American's with disabilities act and accessibility issues.

172. (D) Attend an AA meeting. An individual who has recently been discharged from drug/alcohol rehabilitation is likely to need support (such as Alcoholics Anonymous) her first weekend at home. People in recovery should avoid situations, people, and places that lead to abuse of substances. Parties and clubs/concerts (answers A and B) are often closely associated with access to substances and should be avoided. A mini-vacation with the kids (answer C) would probably be too stressful for her first weekend at home. See reference: Early: Understanding psychiatric diagnosis: The DSM-IV.

173. (D) praise her for what she does well to reinforce her independence. Since the child has just achieved independence in spoon feeding, she may still need frequent reinforcement of the new skill. It is more effective to encourage her for what she does well, than to point out her mistakes (answer B). To provide assistance either by using a hand-over-hand technique (answer A), or by feeding her as a reward may be counterproductive, causing her to lose independence in this skill. See reference: Case-Smith (ed): Case-Smith, J and Humphrey, R: Feeding intervention.

174. (B) outpatient OT. "It is no longer expected that patients discharged to home will be totally independent. . .these patients are frequently capable of achieving further gains and could appropriately be followed. . .in an outpatient setting" (p. 682). A patient with such high levels of function is not an appropriate candidate for a home health referral (answer A). Work-hardening programs (answer C) are for individuals who are severely deconditioned as a result of disease or injury, or for those who have significant discrepancies between their symptoms and objective findings. If the patient has potential for further functional improvement, continuationrather than discontinuation (answer D) of services is indicated. See reference: Trombly (ed): Woodson, AM: Stroke.

175. (A) Describe the treatment received. According to the 1991 *Role Delineations for OTRs and COTAs*, COTAs can record factual information at the time of discharge. Making referrals to outside agencies, comparing initial and final status, and independently making follow-up plans (answers B, C, and D) are not within the entry-level COTA's responsibilities. See reference: Early: Medical records and documentation.

176. (D) 5 feet by 5 feet. An outward opening door needs a space of 5 feet by 5 feet to allow for a wheelchair to be maneuvered around the door. A standard wheelchair requires 5 feet of turning space for a 180 or 360 degree turn. An area that is 3 feet by 5 feet (answer A), 4 feet by 4 feet (answer B), or 4.5 feet by 3 feet (answer C), would not provide enough space to allow the wheelchair to be turned. See reference: Pedretti and Early (eds): Smith, P: Americans with disabilities act: Accommodating persons with disabilities.

177. (B) Incorporate advocacy skill training into the group format. It is essential for individuals with disabilities to have the skills to advocate for themselves. The sense of empowerment that comes with self-advocacy internalizes the locus of control. These same advantages would not be recognized through a stress management group (answer D). Assessing the site for ADA compliance (answer A) is a possible option, and if the COTA can perform the assessment, it would not be necessary to hire an OTR. Suing the facility for non-compliance (answer C) would be a last resort, after many other attempts to resolve the situation have been made. See reference: Cottrell (ed): McConchie, SD: Establishing support and advocacy groups.

178. (C) providing information on the definition and physiological signs of stress. It is important to have a basic understanding of stress to effectively develop stress management skills. Answers A, B, and D are all effective stress management techniques. Other techniques include healthy eating, assertiveness skills, changing attitudes, and balancing work, rest, and leisure. See reference: Cottrell (ed):

Mueller, S and Suto, M: Starting a stress management program.

179. (D) Evaluate participants' performance strengths and weaknesses. The first step in any intervention is almost always evaluation. The next step in this process, which is based on a developmental model because of the age and backgrounds of the clients, is developing trust and exploration (answer A). This is followed by skill development (answer B). Once basic skills are in place, greater emphasis is placed on work quantity and quality (answer C). See reference: Cottrell (ed): Kannenberg, K and Boyer, D: Occupational therapy evaluation and intervention in an employment program for homeless youths.

180. (A) Avoid highly polished or glossy surfaces on walls, floors, and furniture. Indirect glare results when light reflects off a shiny surface. Avoiding or changing highly polished surfaces can reduce uncomfortable levels of glare. Recommending residents wear darkened glasses indoors (answer B) might reduce glare, but would dim the visual field and decrease vision, possibly causing the individual to bump into objects; also it is not an environmental recommendation. Answer C, reducing illumination, is incorrect because older adults need increased illumination to accomplish visual tasks, and the appropriate type of increased illumination (low-glare, high-intensity lighting) enhances visual function. Use of color contrast (answer D) is an adaptation that facilitates perception and differentiation of objects in the environment but would not reduce indirect glare. See reference: Larson, Stevens-Ratchford, Pedretti, and Crabtree (eds): Christenson, MA: Environmental design, modification, and adaptation.

181. (A) Incorporate activities such as wiping the tables after lunch, which are concrete, consistent, and predictable. Many of these clients have never held a job. Those who have held jobs have most likely experienced failure when attempting to work. In addition to inadequate skills for job performance, bizarre behavior and appearance, resulting from poor social and self-care skills, have led to stigma and rejection in the past. Work activities for these individuals must be concrete, predictable, consistent, and meaningful. These individuals are usually unable to generalize learning from one environment or situation to another; therefore, answers B and C, which involve generalization of new learning, are impractical. In addition, sorting nuts and bolts is not a meaningful activity. Mail management activities (answer D) are a good choice for this population, but this answer is less than optimal because "when available" does not provide the necessary consistency. See reference: Cottrell (ed): Coviensky, M and Buckley, VC: Day activities programming: Serving the severely impaired chronic client.

182. (C) Feeding the camp pets. Camp can provide a normalizing environment for children with special needs who don't always have the opportunity to engage in normal children's activities. Taking care of pets, in particular, can provide these children with an opportunity to be responsible for the well-being of another, as well as the chance to be the caregiver rather than the care recipient. Amusement parks (answer A), which are highly stimulating environments, can challenge any child's sense of responsibility, and would not be appropriate for beginning level responsibility. Roasting marshmallow (answer B) involves responsibility for one's self near a fire. Lifeguarding (answer D) is an inappropriate activity for someone who is not qualified. See reference: Fazio: Intervention and support programming in day camps, sleep-away camps, and adventures.

183. (A) improving accessibility in building access, building interiors, and restrooms. Title III of the ADA addresses accessibility of facilities used by the public and focuses on removal of structural barriers to allow access to the premises and use of the facilities, including parking areas, walks, ramps, entrances, etc. Answers B, C, and D may be relevant areas for OT consultation, however, these relate to Title I of the ADA which addresses employment of persons with disabilities. See reference: Pedretti and Early (eds): Smith, P: Americans with Disabilities Act: Accommodating persons with disabilities.

184. (C) needs assessment. Needs assessment (answer C) is the necessary first step of gathering data about a population, treatment needs, and resources available. Program planning (answer A) involves establishing goals and objectives based on the results of the needs assessment. Program implementation (answer B) occurs following program planning and involves coordination, assessment, and intervention selection. Program evaluation (answer D) occurs after implementation, and involves systematic review and analysis of the program based on achievement of program goals. See reference: Cottrell (ed): Grossman, J and Bortone, J: Program development.

185. (B) Go out for lunch at fast-food restaurant. A key principle in intervention for effective transition includes using natural environments and cues, and increasing community-based instruction as the student gets older. Classroom-based activities (answers A, C, and D) are not as effective in promoting development of the community member role as activities that actually take place in the community. See reference: Case-Smith (ed): Spencer, K: Transition services: From school to adult life.

186. (D) Provide OT expertise to run the program and solve problems. An OT practitioner could perform all of the functions identified. The OT consultant in this setting typically offers information and skill knowledge to both OT and non-OT staff, and ad-

ministration to help plan programs that meet the needs of the clients. Answer A, evaluating clients, would be the function of the OT direct-care practitioner. Implementing activity groups (answer B) would be the role of the activity program director, which could be performed by an OT practitioner. Answer C is the function of the case manager, which is one of the newer roles that an OT practitioner may perform in this setting. See reference: Larson, Stevens-Ratchford, Pedretti, and Crabtree (eds): Conyers, KH: Adult day care.

187. (C) Inform the administrator they are unable to provide services to individuals who can no longer benefit from OT. Answers A, B, and D involve falsifying documentation, financial exploitation of insurance carriers, inaccurate recording of professional activities, and are violations of the *Code of Ethics*. It is unethical to bill for services not rendered or to provide services to individuals who can no longer benefit. In this case, the individual reached his full potential for independence in self-care and no longer requires OT services. See reference: AOTA: Occupational therapy code of ethics.

188. (B) Complete a tool count of departmental sharps. Although answers A and C are required and necessary, the only activity that would be done daily is a tool count. It is recommended that tool counts be completed before and after patient activities. This ensures that sharps are not removed by patients who may harm themselves or others. Strictly monitoring clients with suicidal ideations (answer D) must be mandatory, but denying these individuals the opportunity to participate in therapy is not an appropriate choice of treatment. See reference: Early: Safety techniques.

189. (D) Obtain the same results as another OT practitioner who has demonstrated service competency. To establish service competency, it is necessary to obtain the same results as a competent OT practitioner when performing a treatment technique or evaluative procedure. Demonstrating service competency often requires more than one trial in order to refine techniques to obtain the same results. Answers A, B, and C are methods for developing service competency, but do not provide the opportunity for the OT practitioners to compare and contrast their techniques and measurements in order to obtain the same results. See reference: Neistadt and Crepeau (eds): Sands, M: Practitioners' perspectives on the occupational therapist and occupational therapy assistant partnership.

190. (D) demonstrate service competence. COTAs are often well qualified to accept positions outside of OT service delivery. In these situations, "supervision by an OT is not required to oversee performance" (p. 593). However, when functioning outside of OT service delivery, services may not be referred to as "occupational therapy." There is no reason to believe a salary cut (answer C) would be necessary; in fact, a raise would probably be appropriate. Service competence (answer D) refers to the ability to consistently demonstrate skills related to the OT process and related areas. There is no mechanism for demonstrating service competency for a position such as program director. The administrator responsible for filling the program director position must determine whether the COTA is qualified for the position based on performance appraisals, a resume, educational background, and other relevant information. See reference: AOTA: Guide for supervision of occupational therapy personnel in the delivery of occupational therapy services.

191. (A) incident report. Facilities use incident reports to document incidents such as this. Although the incident may be referred to in a daily progress note (answer B), an incident report must also be filed. An incident report form includes a level of detail that may not be achieved in a letter (answer C), and a verbal report (answer D) is not a form of documentation. See reference: Pedretti and Early (eds): Buckner, WS: Infection control and safety issues in the clinic.

192. (B) rinse the eye with an eye wash or water immediately. It is necessary to immediately wash the eye because the "backwash" fluid in the IV is unidentifiable body fluid and universal precautions should be followed. It is recommended to flush an exposed area with warm water or normal saline immediately. Therefore, answers A, C, and D are incorrect. Following the cleansing of the eye, it is recommended to contact the immediate supervisor and report the exposure through the facility reporting system. See reference: Occupational Safety and Health Administration: Standard #1910.1030, 1 FR 5507, February 13, 1996.

193. (A) obtain collaboration with supervision from an OTR before beginning treatment. According to the *AOTA Statement of Occupational Therapy Referral*, a COTA may identify or screen individuals for potential referral, but may not accept or enter a case without the supervision or collaboration of an OTR. Answers B, C, and D are all actions the COTA would take after accepting the case. See reference: AOTA: Statement of occupational therapy referral.

194. (C) receive supervision from an OTR at least once a month. General supervision requires that a COTA receive a minimum of monthly direct contact with an OTR, with additional supervision as needed by phone or other forms of communication. Close supervision requires daily, direct contact (answer B) at the work location. Although advanced-level COTAs may contribute to the supervisory process of less-experienced COTAs (answer D), the minimum required supervision must be provided by an OTR. Some regulations require that students perform in

the line of sight of the supervisor (answer A), however, this is not a requirement for COTAs. States may vary in their supervisory requirements, and state law takes precedent over AOTA guidelines. See reference: AOTA: Guide for supervision of occupational therapy personnel in the delivery of occupational therapy services.

195. (A) Instruct the aide to call for someone to transport the patients back to their rooms. Aides are limited to performing non–client-related tasks, such as preparation of the work area and maintenance. Aides may perform specific client-related tasks when they have been trained, the outcome is predictable, no judgment is required, and they remain in sight of the OT practitioner. Answers B, C, and D are all spontaneous actions, and there is no indication the aide is trained to perform any of them. See reference: AOTA: Guidelines for the Use of Aides in OT practice.

196. (D) Encourage the patient to speak with the rehabilitation psychologist to discuss his concerns. OT practitioners often need to address functional issues related to sexuality when working with individuals who have been seriously injured or disabled, and should be well versed and comfortable with the topic. Rather than moving into an area requiring skills beyond the scope of the COTA (answer A), the COTA should refer the individual to the psychologist, whose role is to provide more extensive sexual or marital counseling, which appears to be what is required in this situation. The physiatrist (answer C), a physician specializing in rehabilitation, is responsible for attending to the medical needs of the individual and coordinating the rehabilitation process. Discussing the increased chances of divorce (answer B), while true, would not be helpful to this individual at this vulnerable time. See reference: Neistadt and Crepeau (eds): Cohn, ES: Interdisciplinary communication and supervision of personnel.

197. (B) The patients' written consents to take the photographs and use them for publicity. A photograph of a person who is being treated at a health care facility would release privileged information and would violate confidentiality just as much as releasing the individual's name or diagnosis (answers A and D). No information about a person may be released without a written consent. It is not necessary to obtain permission of the department head to use a photograph to promote a positive image for the facility (answer C). See reference: Bailey: Final preparation before implementing the research plan.

198. (C) Decline the current offer, ask if company can wait to hire, and apply for a temporary license. All OT practitioners must hold a current, updated state license if residing in a licensed state. Students completing fieldwork II placements should apply for a temporary license prior to beginning their job search. The *AOTA Code of Ethics* addresses this issue in Principle 4, section A, stating that "occupational therapy practitioners shall hold the appropriate national and state credentials for the services they provide" (p. 615). It is essential that all practitioners maintain a high level of professional standards. See reference: AOTA: Occupational therapy code of ethics.

199. (D) Explain the OT role delineation for evaluations to the referring physician, and attempt to contact the OTR for further consultation.
COTAs may contribute to the evaluation process under the supervision and knowledge of an OTR. It is the role of the OTR to analyze and summarize assessment data for both intervention and discharge planning purposes. COTAs may contribute to this process only under the supervision of the OTR, therefore answer B is incorrect. It would not be appropriate to direct the patient to PT for OT services

(answer C). And, while it may not be possible to see the patient (answer A), attempting to contact the OTR is the first step. See reference: AOTA: Standards of practice for occupational therapy.

200. (B) Withhold treatment, but gather information on the course of events for documentation and consultation with the supervising OTR.
The treatment plan may need to be revised as a result of the change in the individual's status. The OTR must modify the intervention process to reflect changes in status; therefore, answer C is incorrect, although COTAs may contribute to this re-evaluation process. Treatment cannot continue as originally planned (answer A), because of the change in status, until reviewed by the OTR. Waiting for the OTR to return and collect information about the change in status (answer D) could delay resumption of treatment. See reference: AOTA: Standards of practice for occupational therapy.

151 D.
152 B.
153 A.
154 B.
155 B.
156 B.
157 C.
158 B.
159 D. B
160 A B
161 C.
162 B
163 C. B
164 C.
165 B
166 B
167 D.
168 B
169 C.
170 C.
171 A. B.
172 C. D.
173 D.
174 C. B
175 A
176 A D.
177 B
178 B. C
179 B.
180 C A

181. A.
182. C.
183. A
184. D, C
185. B.
186. B D
187. C.
188. B
189. C. D.
190. D.
191. A
192. B
193. B A
194. B. C.
195. D. A
196. A. D
197. B.
198. C.
199. B. B
200. B.

Obama — 4 AM (1)
6 high/normal
-63   206 755-1682   68%

#2 Exam
-9   -10   -14   6   -8   44

1. d. b	31. C.	61. D	91. D. B	121. D. C
2. d.	32. D	62. B	92. A	122. B
3. b.	33. C.	63. A. B	93. D. C.	123. B.
4. b.	34. C.	64. C. B	94. B	124. A B
5. a.	35. D	65. B C	95. D	125. A B
6. a.	36. C. A	66. C. B	96. B	126. D.
7. a	37. C.	67. B.	97 D	127. D.
8. b.	38. D	68 C	98. B. C	128. B.
9. a. b	39. A	69. D.	99. D	129. D. A
10. b	40. C. B	70. B.	100. A.	130. C.
11. D.	41. B. A.	71. B. A	101. D.	131. D.
12. b. a	42. B. A.	72. D.	102. D	132. A
13. a. C	43. D	73. D.	103. A.	133. D.
14. C.	44. A.	74. B	104. B	134. A
15. B	45. B.	75. B	105. B.	135. C.
16. B.	46. B.	76. B. A	106. B.	136. B.
17. A. d.	47. A. B	77. A C	107. C.	137. b.
18. B.	48. D. A	78. D B	108. C. A	138. A. C
19. D.	49. A.	79. B C	109. A A	139. A. C
20. D.	50 C	80. D	110. B.	140. D. B
21. D. a	51. C.	81. D B	111. C.	141. A
22. D. b	52. B. A.	82. B. A	112. A	142. A
23. D.	53. C.	83. A C.	113. C B	143. C.
24. C.	54. D	84. B	114. B.	144. C.
25. B.	55. A B	85. A	115. B C	145. B. D
26. D. a.	56. A.	86. D	116. A.	146. D.
27. B.	57. A B	87. D B.	117. A	147. B.
28. B.	58. D.	88. B.	118. A	148. B.
29. C. d.	59. A D	89. D. A.	119. B. B	149. D
30. B	60. A	90. A B.	120. C.	150. A

SIMULATION EXAMINATION 3

Evaluation

1. **Which of the following is BEST to use when assessing three-jaw chuck strength?**
   A. An aesthesiometer
   B. A pinch meter
   C. A dynamometer
   D. A volumeter

2. **During a group activity, a COTA observes a client making frequent negative comments pertaining to the collage activity that the group is working on. These comments are MOST likely an indication of:**
   A. passivity.
   B. insecurity.
   C. hopelessness.
   D. indecision.

3. **While working with a child diagnosed with CP, the COTA observes that the child's movements appear writhing, purposeless, and uncontrollable. These movements would BEST be described as:**
   A. athetoid.
   B. hypertonic.
   C. spastic.
   D. hypotonic.

4. **Which is the MOST appropriate technique for assessing light touch sensation in a client who has just been admitted to the rehabilitation unit after a RCVA with left hemiplegia?**

   A. Test the affected extremity before testing the unaffected extremity.
   B. Demonstrate the procedure on the unaffected extremity, then occlude the client's vision while testing the affected extremity.
   C. Demonstrate the procedure on the affected extremity, then explain the evaluation process to the client.
   D. Interview the client and assess only the areas that the client reports as impaired.

5. **In evaluating an adolescent with psychosocial problems, an OTR would be MOST likely to begin the process by screening the adolescent's level of function in which areas?**
   A. Play and social behavior, overall development, and visual motor skills
   B. Socialization, task performance, daily living skills, and time management
   C. Interest in work, leisure, and self-care
   D. Motor skills, sensory processing, and cognition

6. **At a team meeting, a teacher reports that a child is having difficulty copying letters, doing mazes, and using scissors. This behavior MOST likely indicates a problem in which of the following areas?**
   A. Visual-motor integration
   B. Visual acuity
   C. Visual tracking
   D. Visual perception

7. **While assessing dressing skills with a patient who recently had a stroke, the**

OT practitioner notes that the individual is unable to see buttons on a printed fabric. This **MOST** likely indicates that the individual may be having difficulty with:

A. spatial relations.
B. figure-ground perception.
C. body image.
D. visual closure.

8. **The OT practitioner has just completed observation of a child eating lunch. Which of the following statements BEST describes an objective observation?**

A. The child did not appear to like the food presented.
B. The child demonstrated tongue thrust.
C. The child was uncooperative and kept pushing the food out of her mouth.
D. The child was obviously not hungry at the time.

9. **Which of the following performance components are MOST important to consider when analyzing activities for use with adults with psychosocial problems?**

A. Self-control demands, time management demands, self-expression opportunities, and interest in the activity
B. Age appropriateness, prehension patterns required, and the presence of small pieces that could be mistakenly swallowed
C. Tactile, kinesthetic, visual, and olfactory properties
D. Space requirements, equipment and supply needs, cost, and safety considerations

10. **An infant has begun to sit and is leaning forward onto his arms. The COTA notes that the infant is able to coactivate muscle groups around the shoulder and arm in order to bear weight on arms in sitting. This demonstrates that the infant has MOST likely developed which type of reactions?**

A. Protective
B. Equilibrium
C. Rotational righting
D. Support

11. **An individual who had a myocardial infarction has been transferred from the acute care unit to a rehabilitation unit. During the initial interview, he displays good memory of information processed before the MI, but poor recall of the period spent in the acute care facility. He is able to recall information since the**

transfer. The OT practitioner would **MOST** likely document these behaviors as:

A. orientation problems.
B. long-term memory deficits.
C. anterograde amnesia.
D. retrograde amnesia.

12. **A woman who had a stroke tries unsuccessfully to put on a blouse using a one-handed technique. She states, "I can do it, I'm just not trying hard enough." The COTA most accurately recognizes this as:**

A. denial.
B. projection.
C. rationalization.
D. regression.

13. **A COTA working with an infant observes the presence of the first stage of voluntary grasp. Which of the following would be the MOST appropriate statement for documenting this behavior?**

A. The infant is exhibiting radial palmar grasp.
B. The infant is exhibiting pincer grasp.
C. The infant is exhibiting ulnar palmar grasp.
D. The infant is exhibiting palmar grasp.

14. **During evaluation, the COTA asks a client with rheumatoid arthritis to flex her shoulder. The client's range of motion is limited to 90 degrees and she can tolerate moderate resistance in this position. The COTA further observes that passive range of motion is the same as active range of motion. The manual muscle test grade for shoulder flexion would MOST likely be documented as:**

A. normal (5).
B. good (4).
C. fair (3).
D. fair minus (3-).

15. **By using an interest checklist that includes a report of both interests and actual participation in activities, an OT practitioner will MOST likely collect information on a client's:**

A. use of time.
B. developmental level.
C. mood and affect.
D. communication skills.

16. **When working with a child who exhibits tactile defensiveness, which of the following areas should be evaluated FIRST?**

A. Reading skills
B. Dressing habits
C. Social skills
D. Leisure interests

17. **A client who recently started using a wheelchair will be returning to work. An OT practitioner is evaluating the client's workplace for accessibility according to ADA guidelines. The doorway to the client's office has a clear opening of 28 inches. Which of the following recommendations would be the MOST appropriate to facilitate clear passage of the wheelchair through the doorway?**

A. The doorway width needs to be expanded to have a minimum clear opening of 32 inches.
B. The client needs to obtain a wheelchair narrower than 28 inches.
C. The doorway width needs to be expanded to have a minimum clear opening of 45 inches.
D. The doorway width is satisfactory and needs no modification.

18. **Using the Model of Human Occupation as a frame of reference, evaluation of an individual should focus PRIMARILY on which of the following?**

A. Identification of problem behaviors that need to be extinguished
B. Clarification of thoughts, feelings, and experiences that influence behavior
C. Cognitive function, including assets and limitations
D. The effect of personal traits and the environment on role performance

19. **A preschooler with a diagnosis of developmental delay is very withdrawn and passive. While working on toileting skills, the child reaches out for a toothbrush and starts to brush her hair with it. The OT practitioner recognizes the PRIMARY importance of this behavior as:**

A. demonstrating attention-getting behavior.
B. a sign of cognitive limitation.
C. indicating initiative and beginning task-directed behavior.
D. demonstrating misinterpretation of cues because of a visual deficit.

20. **A patient who is asked to show the path she would take to get from her room to the therapy clinic at the other end of the** corridor becomes easily confused and makes several wrong turns. This behavior MOST likely indicates:

A. spatial relations disorders.
B. figure-ground discrimination deficits.
C. topographical disorientation.
D. form discrimination deficits.

21. **An adolescent with a history of shoplifting and gang violence has been hospitalized with a diagnosis of conduct disorder. During a craft group, the COTA should pay particular attention to the individual's:**

A. perceptual-motor performance.
B. leisure and vocational interests.
C. attention span and social interaction skills.
D. interest in, and ability to, perform multiple roles.

22. **A child avoids playground equipment that requires her feet to be off the ground. This behavior MOST likely indicates:**

A. tactile defensiveness.
B. developmental dyspraxia.
C. gravitational insecurity.
D. intolerance for motion.

23. **During a coloring activity, an OT practitioner observes a preschooler stabilizing a crayon between the thumb and first two fingers. The practitioner MOST accurately documents this grasp as:**

A. pincer grasp.
B. radial-digital grasp.
C. palmar grasp.
D. lateral pinch.

24. **An individual with an anxiety disorder has been placed on new antianxiety medication. The COTA has been asked to observe the individual closely for side effects during OT activities over the next few days. The COTA should be particularly observant for which of the following?**

A. Akathisia
B. Confusion
C. Extrapyramidal syndrome
D. Tardive dyskinesia

25. **A 6-month-old child, when pulled into sitting with several trials, demonstrates a head lag. This behavior MOST likely indicates that head control is:**

A. developing in a typical manner.
B. slightly delayed by 1 month.

C. significantly delayed by several months.

D. advanced.

26. **As part of an initial evaluation of an individual with carpal tunnel syndrome, the OTR evaluates light touch sensation using a cotton ball. After wearing a wrist splint for 2 weeks, the patient returns for a reevaluation, which the COTA performs. At this time, the MOST appropriate method for reevaluation of light touch is:**

A. a cotton ball.

B. an aesthesiometer.

C. Semmes-Weinstein monofilaments.

D. a pin or straightened paper clip.

27. **An individual who had a traumatic brain injury is beginning OT. The OT practitioner needs to assess whether this person can transfer learning from one activity to another in order to plan treatment appropriately. The MOST appropriate way to observe this patient's learning ability would be to:**

A. describe situations that might be unsafe and ask the individual how he would respond.

B. give the individual a simple jigsaw puzzle to solve.

C. have the individual perform a simple cooking task, then use a different food at the next session.

D. give the individual simple calculations to perform.

28. **A 4-month-old infant being seen for an OT assessment shows a strong preference for the left hand when reaching for a rattle at midline. Considering the development of dominance in normal children, the COTA should conclude that:**

A. further observation and evaluation of right-sided dysfunction is indicated.

B. development of hand dominance is proceeding in a typical manner.

C. hand dominance will not develop until the child is 1 year old.

D. unilaterality precedes bilaterality in typical development.

29. **An OT practitioner is assessing hand function in a man with arthritis by observing him as he makes a peanut butter sandwich. The individual is unable to remove the lid from a 28 ounce peanut butter jar, but is able stand at the counter,** spread peanut butter on the bread with a knife, and replace the lid when he has finished making the sandwich. These observations would **MOST** likely reflect a deficit in which of the following?

A. Range of motion

B. Coordination

C. Endurance

D. Strength

30. **An individual diagnosed with major depression and recently admitted to an acute inpatient psychiatric unit has arrived for her 9:00 AM OT evaluation late, hair uncombed, clothing disheveled, and smelling badly. Chart review indicates the individual has been reluctant to engage in conversation with staff and peers. Which of the following methods is MOST appropriate for assessing the individual's self-care skills?**

A. Have the individual demonstrate dressing, hygiene, and grooming skills to the OT practitioner.

B. Interview the individual using open-ended questions that encourage the client to describe how she is doing with things like personal hygiene, bathing, dressing, and grooming.

C. Briefly interview the individual using closed-ended questions, targeting the individual's premorbid and current self-care performance levels.

D. Based on observation of the individual's appearance, the OT practitioner can determine that the individual demonstrates significant self-care deficits.

31. **Working with a preschooler in the home, the COTA observes the child climb into a highchair and jump up and down on a toy trampoline. When presented with a new rocking horse as a birthday present, however, the child is unable to determine how to mount the horse. This MOST likely indicates a problem in the area of:**

A. fine motor skills.

B. gross motor skills.

C. reflex integration.

D. motor planning.

32. **While performing a hand reassessment, the COTA notices a deformity developing in the client's second digit. The client's PIP joint appears flexed, and the DIP ap-**

pears to be hyperextended. The COTA can BEST describe this condition as a:

A. mallet deformity.
B. boutonnière deformity.
C. subluxation deformity.
D. swan neck deformity.

33. **A COTA is interviewing an individual diagnosed with Alzheimer's disease to obtain information about his level of independence in ADLs and IADLs. Halfway through the interview, the COTA realizes the client is confabulating. Which of the following options is MOST appropriate?**

A. Complete the interview using closed-ended questions.
B. Stop the interview and complete it the next day.
C. Interview a reliable informant instead of the individual.
D. Administer a written questionnaire using a checklist format.

Treatment Planning

34. **A client is working on prehension skills in order to return to work as a mechanic. Which of the following BEST resembles a prehension activity?**

A. Loosening nuts and bolts
B. Removing an air filter
C. Cranking a car jack
D. Grasping a hammer

35. **An individual learning to use an augmentative communication system has mastered the task of understanding picture symbols and their use. The next step would be:**

A. sequencing of picture symbols.
B. recognizing letters of the alphabet.
C. recognizing whole words.
D. spelling letter by letter.

36. **A child has low muscle tone resulting in problems in the following printing and handwriting subskill areas: (1) postural stability, (2) shoulder stability, and (3) grasp of the pencil. If the COTA uses a proximal-to-distal approach to skill development, which of the following treatment sequences is BEST?**

A. Improve posture, then improve shoulder stability, then improve grasp.
B. Improve shoulder stability, then improve posture, then improve grasp.
C. Improve grasp, then improve posture, then improve shoulder stability.
D. Improve shoulder stability, then improve posture, then improve grasp.

37. **A COTA is planning to practice transfers using a transfer board with a patient who has bilateral lower extremity amputations. The COTA must have the patient use a wheelchair which has:**

A. detachable footrests.
B. detachable arms.
C. anti-tip bars.
D. brake handle extensions.

38. **A COTA has begun working with a client in a psychosocial treatment setting and is explaining the therapy process. Which of the following introductory statements would the COTA MOST likely use to describe the therapeutic relationship between the COTA and the individual within psychosocial frames of reference?**

A. The most important aspect of the therapy is the relationship that develops between the client and the therapist.
B. We will be working together to achieve your goals.
C. The process of therapy should be the beginning of a good friendship between us.
D. Your situation is unfortunate and I hope that our relationship can improve the situation.

39. **A treatment plan for a child with a visual discrimination problem would MOST likely include which of the following adaptations of visual materials?**

A. Low contrast and defined borders
B. High contrast and defined borders
C. High contrast and unclear borders
D. Low contrast and unclear borders

40. **Which of the following activities would BEST represent an expected outcome for an individual who completes an energy-conservation program?**

A. Getting dressed without becoming fatigued
B. Lifting heavy cookware without pain
C. Doing handicrafts without damaging his or her joints
D. Dusting and vacuuming more quickly

41. **A COTA has been assigned to develop an expressive activity group for women who have experienced emotional and physi-**

cal abuse. The **BEST** choice of activity would be:

A. mediation and yoga exercises.
B. writing a soap opera.
C. personal hygiene and grooming classes.
D. aerobics and fitness program.

42. **A COTA is planning activities for a child with CP. A short-term goal of the treatment plan is to inhibit flexor spasticity in the child's hand to improve the child's ability to manipulate objects during play. The activity that would be MOST appropriate in meeting this objective would be:**

A. building a block tower.
B. active release of blocks into a container.
C. traction on the finger flexors.
D. weight bearing over a small bolster in prone.

43. **A COTA is planning to discharge an individual who recently had a stroke. Plans are to discharge the client home to live independently. The practitioner has worked with other individuals in similar situations, and has developed a keen sense for many of the issues that may arise and need to be problem solved. The form of clinical reasoning that this practitioner is MOST likely to use based on past experience will be:**

A. procedural reasoning.
B. conditional reasoning.
C. interactive reasoning.
D. narrative reasoning.

44. **A COTA and an OTR confer with a client with a mood disorder to establish program goals. It is most improtant that the developed goals include:**

A. specific measurable statements with time frames.
B. time frames for what will be accomplished.
C. specific measurements of the individual's skill and performance.
D. activities to be completed that correspond with the goals and objectives.

45. **A young child has just learned to sit independently on the floor. Which of the following is the NEXT step toward refining her postural reactions in sitting?**

A. Sit straddling a bolster with both feet on the floor.
B. Maintain sitting balance on a scooter while being pulled.
C. Ride a "hippity-hop" without falling off.

D. Maintain floor-sitting position with the therapist providing pelvic support.

46. **An individual with a C6 spinal cord injury has been referred to OT 2 days post-injury. Immobilized with a halo brace, the individual demonstrates fair plus wrist extension and poor minus finger flexion. Which of the following interventions should be implemented FIRST?**

A. Volar resting pan splints to prevent flexion contractures
B. Wrist support with universal cuff to promote independence
C. Wrist splints to promote development of tenodesis
D. Instruction in bed mobility techniques to prevent decubiti

47. **Which of the following is the MOST appropriate goal to address when working with clients diagnosed with progressive cognitive disorders?**

A. Improve their social skills in relating to others.
B. Create new habits of time use.
C. Implement compensatory strategies to manage the environment.
D. Facilitate resumption of previous life roles.

48. **A COTA/OTR team is considering the use of classical sensory integration therapy for a child with a learning disability. Which of the following techniques would be MOST consistent with this approach?**

A. Include the child in a group of children using a program of sensory stimulation activities.
B. Encourage the child to participate in activities that are passive and do not require adaptive responses.
C. Design an individualized program directed at the underlying neurologic deficit.
D. Promote the development of specific motor skills, such as balance and coordination.

49. **Which of the following is MOST important to include in the initial intervention for an individual with complete paralysis as a result of Guillain-Barré syndrome?**

A. ADL training
B. Balance and stabilization activities
C. Passive ROM, positioning, and splinting
D. Resistive activities for the intrinsic hand muscles

50. **A COTA is planning a simple meal preparation activity that will result in success**

for a patient with cognitive deficits. The **SIMPLEST** activity would be preparing:

A. a can of soup.
B. a casserole.
C. brownies from a box mix.
D. a meal with two side dishes and an entrée.

51. **A COTA is working with a withdrawn child and their OT objectives include increasing the ability to express feelings and conflicts. Which of the following activities will MOST effectively promote this skill?**

A. Drawing a picture entitled "This is me"
B. Playing adapted soccer with a large ball
C. Playing a structured board game, such as "Monopoly"
D. Singing folk songs in a group

52. **A COTA is planning intervention for an individual who recently experienced a left CVA resulting in right-sided hemiplegia and motor apraxia. To BEST facilitate the individual's attempts to perform morning ADL the COTA should plan to:**

A. provide the individual with detailed, step-by-step commands for each task throughout the ADL process.
B. make the environment as simple and uncluttered as possible and use sharp contrast to make objects clearly stand out.
C. have the individual visualize the task first and then provide general statements such as "Let's get ready."
D. teach the individual to move slowly through the environment and encourage touching of objects during the task.

53. **A middle-aged client with a diagnosis of reactive depression is admitted to the hospital following an overdose of sleeping pills. The client was recently forced to retire from a job in public relations. His present goals are to increase his sense of competence and encourage development of enjoyable leisure activities. Based on the client's OT goals, what is an appropriate activity to recommend FIRST?**

A. Pouring and glazing chess pieces
B. Designing and building a doll house
C. Copper tooling using a template
D. Learning how to play bridge

54. **Results of an OT evaluation show that a young child has many tactile defensive behaviors. The MOST appropriate begin-**

ning activity for intervention to normalize sensory processing would require that:

A. the therapist has the child play "sandwich" between heavy mats.
B. the therapist applies a feather brush lightly to the child's arms and legs.
C. the child is blindfolded and must guess where he or she is touched on the body.
D. the therapist has the child play the "Duck, duck, goose" circle game.

55. **A COTA is fabricating a splint for a client who has rheumatoid arthritis. Which of the following splints is MOST appropriate for the purpose of resting the joints, decreasing pain, and preventing contractures?**

A. A protective MP joint splint
B. A wrist stabilization splint
C. An ulnar drift positioning splint
D. A volar pan splint for hand and wrist

56. **A COTA working in a partial hospitalization program needs to select a game that allows group members equal opportunities to win and can be played by individuals functioning at various levels. The game type that BEST suits this purpose is:**

A. games of strategy.
B. hobbies.
C. games of chance.
D. competitive games.

57. **A child has poor independent sitting skills as a result of inadequate postural reactions. The FIRST activity the COTA would use to promote the development of independent sitting is:**

A. swinging on a playground swing with a bucket seat.
B. wide-base sitting on the floor while reaching for a suspended balloon.
C. straddling a bolster swing while batting a ball.
D. riding a "hippity-hop" while using only one hand for support.

58. **When a COTA plans a work-hardening program for a homemaker with severe back pain, the expected outcome is that the client will:**

A. acquire a part-time job out of the home.
B. resume previous leisure activities.
C. experience decreased pain levels.
D. resume the homemaker role.

59. **A COTA is planning to use remedial strategies to prepare individuals treated in a psychosocial setting for job hunting. The activity MOST consistent with this approach is:**
    A. reviewing an interest checklist.
    B. holding a class about job-seeking strategies.
    C. modifying the work environment to reduce stress.
    D. using an expressive group magazine collage using pictures of different types of jobs.

60. **An infant born 15 weeks prematurely has a history of multiple medical issues, including retinopathy of prematurity, mechanical ventilation for 5 weeks, and poor feeding skills. The infant is now a 43-week-old medically stable and engaging infant, with a G-tube and oxygen supplement of 2 liters by nasal cannula. The MOST appropriate intervention to provide at this time would be:**
    A. positioning and handling.
    B. PROM of all extremities.
    C. multisensory input.
    D. music therapy.

61. **An individual with weak grip strength and poor endurance wishes to bake something for a family member's birthday. The COTA wants to plan an activity during which the client can work on grasp/release for 5 minutes without becoming exhausted. The MOST appropriate activity for both purposes would be:**
    A. mixing blueberry muffins from scratch using a hand-powered mixer and scooping them into muffin tins with a cup.
    B. mixing an angel food cake from a box mix using an electric mixer and pouring the mix into a pan.
    C. mixing cold chocolate chip cookie dough using a spatula with a built-up handle and dropping dollops onto a tray using an ice cream scoop.
    D. slicing a prepared roll of sugar cookies at room temperature and placing them on a tray using a spatula.

62. **A COTA is planning to begin work on self-care activities with an individual who recently had a traumatic brain injury, and who has cognitive and visual perceptual impairments. The MOST effective way for the COTA to present directions during the activity would be to:**
    A. tell the patient about the activity he will be working on and ask him to begin.
    B. rely on facial expressions and body gestures, rather than words, to get the patient started.
    C. state simple, concrete directions allowing time for delayed responses.
    D. provide a written list of steps with pictures for the patient to follow.

63. **The COTA is working on dressing skills with a 7-year-old girl with limited balance. Which of the following would the COTA MOST likely recommend regarding socks?**
    A. Use socks with a wide opening.
    B. Attempt to use a sock aid.
    C. Purchase nylon tights because they slip on more easily than socks.
    D. Use socks with a narrow opening.

Treatment Implementation

64. **An auto mechanic is currently in a work-hardening program after being in a car accident that left him with numerous upper and lower extremity impairments. The ultimate goal for this individual is to return to full employment as an auto mechanic. Which of the following BEST represents a work-hardening activity for this individual?**
    A. Lifting weights
    B. Working on a mock car engine
    C. Visiting the work site garage
    D. Preparing a light lunch for mealtime

65. **A COTA is implementing cognitive rehabilitation interventions with a client. The client is given the task of finding telephone numbers of specific people in the telephone book. The client also has a card with a series of questions written on it such as, "Do I understand what I am supposed to do?" and "Do I have all the information I need?" Which intervention is the COTA MOST likely using with this client?**
    A. A self-management task with an environmental cue
    B. A task to improve visual scanning
    C. A memory task with external aid
    D. A problem-solving task with a "self-talk" cueing strategy

66. **A COTA is providing intervention for a 4-year-old child in a special needs pre-school. The MOST appropriate activity for the COTA to be working on with this child is:**
   A. practicing letter formation to develop dynamic tripod grasp.
   B. activities to promote mature cutting skills.
   C. working on simple puzzles to enhance attention span.
   D. practicing shoe tying.

67. **An individual who is several days s/p myocardial infarction experiences nausea during a bathing evaluation. Which of the following is the FIRST action the COTA should take?**
   A. Stop the activity.
   B. Document the symptoms.
   C. Instruct the individual to sit and then continue the activity.
   D. Ask the individual if he feels like he can continue the activity.

68. **The home health COTA is seeing a client in the middle stages of Alzheimer's disease. The family is very concerned that the client's memory loss is now interfering with performance of daily activities, even familiar self-care activities. The MOST relevant OT intervention at this point would be:**
   A. memory retraining activities for the client.
   B. ADL retraining program for the client.
   C. instructing caregivers in task breakdown.
   D. leisure activity planning.

69. **A COTA is working with a 4-year-old child who has significant hearing loss. The child also demonstrates decreased fine motor coordination for her age. Which of the following activities would the COTA MOST likely implement to address these needs?**
   A. Parachute activities to increase gross motor and sensory input.
   B. Visually color code the child's right and left shoes to compensate for decreased reception of verbal cues.
   C. Introduce the child to other children via socialization groups to increase social interaction and game playing.
   D. Digging in "Play Doh" to search for various coins and then placing them in a piggy bank.

70. **During a co-treatment, a COTA and speech therapist are working on feeding skills for an individual with amyotrophic lateral sclerosis who is in the late stages of the disease process. Which of the following is the MOST appropriate intervention for this individual?**
   A. Provide a rocker knife, plate guard, and nonskid mat.
   B. Implement a pureed diet and allow adequate time for eating.
   C. Emphasize upper extremity strengthening.
   D. Minimize the use of adaptive equipment.

71. **A nursing home resident with Alzheimer's disease has limitations in shoulder range-of-motion. The OT goal for this patient is to improve shoulder motion so that the person can resume self-care activities. Which strategy would be MOST effective in actively engaging the client?**
   A. Telling the resident to perform repetitions of active UE range-of-motion exercises independently
   B. Training the resident to use long-handled adaptive devices to compensate for decreased shoulder motion
   C. Incorporating simple, familiar activities such as hanging up clothing or catching a ball
   D. Performing PROM exercises on the resident

72. **The BEST position that the COTA can place a 15-month-old child to provide opportunity to further develop trunk rotation is in the:**
   A. supine position.
   B. prone position.
   C. sidelying position.
   D. sitting position.

73. **A client is experiencing acute right upper extremity and hand lymphodema after a recent mastectomy. The client's primary complaint is joint stiffness. The initial techniques the COTA can implement to alleviate joint stiffness would MOST likely be:**
   A. contrast baths, active and passive range of motion, and massage.
   B. ultrasound, electrical stimulation, and dynamic splinting.
   C. resistive exercises, weight bearing, and lifting.
   D. joint mobilization, serial casting, and dynamic splinting.

74. In an outpatient mental health facility, a depressed client gives a COTA a piece of valued jewelry so that the COTA will have something to remember her by, and asks the COTA if she personally believes in an afterlife. The MOST important action for the COTA to take is to:
    A. document the interaction with the client in detail.
    B. refuse the gift politely explaining that gifts to staff are inappropriate.
    C. use this as an opportunity to introduce and discuss spirituality issues with the client.
    D. inform medical team members immediately.

75. A COTA places an infant in the supine position and arranges attractive toys overhead to provide an opportunity to work against gravity. This position is MOST effective for developing which ability?
    A. Shoulder flexion and protraction
    B. Shoulder extension and retraction
    C. Development of head control
    D. Development of trunk control

76. A client with hemiplegia and her spouse are working on toilet transfer training activities with the COTA. The BEST way for the COTA to teach the couple to perform transfers will be:
    A. only to the unaffected side of the client's body.
    B. only to the affected side of the client's body.
    C. to both sides of the client's body.
    D. only to the side of the body from which the client will be approaching the toilet.

77. An intelligent inpatient with paranoid schizophrenia is starting in the OT program. Which activity would BEST engage this patient?
    A. Assembling a complex airplane model requiring use of detailed directions
    B. Finishing and painting a preassembled wooden box
    C. Playing a competitive game of chess
    D. Engaging in a reminiscence discussion

78. A child with a behavior disorder has an innately difficult temperament. Which of the following treatment approaches is MOST appropriate for the COTA to initiate?
    A. Emphasize limit setting with the child during activities.
    B. Help the child develop cognitive strategies for anxiety-producing activities.
    C. Help care providers develop an unpredictable routine for activities that disorganize the child.
    D. Provide a play environment in which the parent and child can demonstrate conflicts.

79. Which of the following is the FIRST step a COTA should take when initiating a safe wheelchair transfer?
    A. Have the patient scoot forward to the front of the seat.
    B. Position foot plates in the up position.
    C. Swing away the leg rests.
    D. Lock the brakes.

80. After one session with a new patient in a psychosocial treatment setting, it has become apparent that the patient is highly distractible and cannot complete a magazine collage when in a group. The BEST approach for the COTA to take is to:
    A. speak slowly and softly to the patient.
    B. coax and praise the patient until she completes the task.
    C. ask the rest of the group members to stop talking.
    D. position the patient so she is facing a blank wall.

81. Which adapted technique would the COTA MOST likely select in order to teach a 8-year-old girl with hemiparesis who wishes to dress independently?
    A. Encourage the child to do most of her dressing while lying in her bed.
    B. Teach the child to dress her hemiparetic extremities first.
    C. Educate the child's mother regarding how to assist with dressing skills.
    D. Teach the child to dress her non-hemiparetic extremities first.

82. A COTA is working with a client who experiences low back pain. During treatment the COTA observes the client engaging in poor body mechanics when lifting a box from the floor. The COTA instructs the client to do which of the following when lifting objects from the floor?
    A. Keep both knees straight, flex the back, and keep the object an arm's length away from the body when lifting.
    B. Bend both knees, keep the back straight,

and bring the object close to the body when lifting.

C. Keep both knees and back straight, and bring object close to the body when lifting.

D. Bend one knee while keeping the other leg straight, and keep the object an arm's length away from the body when lifting.

83. **A COTA is working on sequencing skills with a young patient who is s/p TBI. The MOST effective activity to promote development of these skills is:**

A. leather stamping using tools in a random design.

B. stringing beads for a necklace, following a pattern.

C. putting together a 20-piece puzzle.

D. playing "Concentration."

84. **A 13-year-old child with paraplegia wants to take a bath. Which of the following would the COTA recommend the boy use in the tub?**

A. A tub seat with a hand-held shower attached to the faucet

B. A hydraulic lift with a sling seat

C. An inflatable tub

D. A wheeled shower chair

85. **A COTA is reviewing dressing techniques with a young man with paraplegia. Which of the following would be MOST beneficial for this individual?**

A. A buttonhook zipper pull device

B. A clip-on tie

C. Adapted shoes

D. Loose-fitting clothing

86. **In a community mental health facility, a COTA is working on improving stress management skills with a group of patients with schizophrenia who have histories of psychotic behavior. Which of the following stress management strategies would be MOST appropriate for this group?**

A. The use of visual imagery as a relaxation method

B. Discussing one's problems with an empathetic listener

C. Engaging in a new, challenging activity

D. Progressive relaxation of muscles

87. **The COTA is educating the parents of a small child with sensory defensiveness regarding hair care. The parents report that each time they shampoo their child's hair she becomes anxious, restless and agitated. The COTA should recommend that the parents:**

A. wash the child's hair with water only, and to avoid shampoo.

B. have the child's hair washed thoroughly each time she gets a haircut.

C. use a calm and soothing voice, informing the child about each step of the hair wash prior to doing it.

D. use cool water when shampooing the child's hair.

88. **A COTA is working on feeding with an individual with a C3 spinal cord injury. The strategy that will enable the HIGHEST level of independence is for the individual to:**

A. clearly direct a caregiver in preferred head position, food portion size, and choice of food to eat.

B. use a mobile arm support.

C. use a wrist support with a utensil inserted into the cuff.

D. use a universal cuff with a utensil inserted into the cuff.

89. **An individual tells the COTA, "I don't know about going home tomorrow. I wanted to be discharged yesterday and the doctor suggested I stay in the hospital another day." Which of the following responses MOST accurately reflects the active listening approach in which the COTA should reply?**

A. "It sounds as if you're not sure whether you are ready to be discharged."

B. "You know, your doctor is a very intelligent person."

C. "How about calling your doctor when you get home if you feel a panic attack coming on."

D. "You've been doing extremely well, what are you afraid of?"

90. **The COTA is working on handwriting skills with a school-age child with decreased proprioception in the hand and wrist. Which of the following would the COTA recommend the child use to increase proprioception while writing?**

A. A wide pen

B. Attach rubber bands to the eraser and the child's wrist

C. A soft triangle grip

D. A pediatric weighted utensil holder

91. **A COTA is working with an individual who is about to be discharged from outpatient OT after rehabilitation for a hand injury. The client has not been able to work for 3 months and is unable to perform all of the job requirements as a sales manager in a clothing store. After discussing the case with his supervising OTR, the COTA and OTR agree that the client should receive which of the following at discharge?**

A. A home exercise program
B. Home health OT
C. Work hardening
D. No further OT services

92. **The COTA is using a five-stage group process for adults diagnosed with moderate levels of mental retardation. As a closure activity, which one of the following is the MOST appropriate?**

A. Reviewing the rules for appropriate behavior in the group
B. Discussing emotional reactions to the craft activity done earlier in the group
C. Walking through an obstacle course to music
D. Sitting in a circle and reciting a short poem

93. **A child with learning disabilities resulting in low frustration tolerance and poor self-esteem, is learning how to tie shoelaces. Which of the following methods would be MOST appropriate for the COTA to introduce to this child?**

A. Physical guidance
B. Verbal cues
C. Backward chaining
D. Forward chaining

94. **A patient who is being discharged from a rehabilitation center to home has Parkinson's disease and is at risk for aspiration (entry of food material into the airway). When instructing the primary caregiver in proper positioning during feeding, the COTA should recommend:**

A. feeding the patient in bed in a supine position.
B. seating the patient upright on a firm surface with the chin slightly tucked.
C. positioning the patient in a semi-reclined position in a reclining chair.
D. feeding the patient in bed in a sidelying position.

95. **A 78-year-old client who is ambulating with a walker in the home informs the COTA that a fear of falling while bathing concerns him. Although the client took showers in the past, his present fear of falling limits him to sponge bathing. The COTA tells the individual that it is wise to avoid situations in which the client feels the risk of falling is high. Which of the following should the COTA do next?**

A. Suggest bath tub bathing instead of showering.
B. Encourage the client to purchase a shower chair.
C. Demonstrate how using a shower chair improves safety.
D. Explain that therapy will boost his confidence level when showering.

96. **A COTA is reviewing bathing skills with a 13-year-old child when the client suddenly asks questions regarding his sexuality. What should the COTA do FIRST?**

A. Refer the teenager to someone who has increased knowledge regarding the subject of sexuality, such as a psychologist.
B. Tell the client that you don't mind appropriately discussing sexuality-related questions, as long as his parents are comfortable with the idea.
C. Attempt to change the subject because the child is too young to be educated on this topic.
D. Try to openly and honestly address the client's questions to the best of your knowledge.

97. **The COTA is treating a client for epicondylitis. Which of the following adjunct activities should the COTA use to treat the ACUTE symptoms of tennis elbow?**

A. PROM, weight bearing, and mobilization
B. Resistive exercises, heat application, and work simulation
C. Heat application, PROM, and strengthening
D. Ice application, immobilization, and splinting

98. **An elderly client likes to roam around the grounds of her assisted-living community each night after dinner, and frequently gets lost. Which of the following options is OPTIMAL?**

A. Install a gate that will prevent her from exiting the building and getting lost.

B. Provide clear, safe pathways for
   wandering.
C. Redirect the client to participate in group
   activities.
D. Implement a system that provides negative
   reinforcement for wandering.

99. **The COTA is working with a 6-year-old
    child who occasionally drops his utensils
    when eating because of a slight grasp
    limitation. Which piece of equipment
    would the COTA MOST likely recommend
    the child use?**
    A. Swivel utensils
    B. Pediatric universal holders
    C. Foam tubing around the utensils
    D. Weighted utensils

100. **A COTA who needs to transfer an obese
     man is not confident she can manage the
     transfer alone. The BEST action for the
     COTA to take is to:**
     A. use proper body mechanics.
     B. ask someone from PT to do the transfer.
     C. ask another OT/PT practitioner for
        assistance.
     D. refrain from transferring the patient.

101. **A young client who is diagnosed with
     depression tells a COTA about feelings
     associated with being alone and afraid.
     A chart review reveals that the individ-
     ual leads a very isolating lifestyle. The
     BEST way for the COTA to respond is to:**
     A. reassure the client that they can be
        friends.
     B. tell the client, "I know how you feel."
     C. encourage the client to socialize more
        often.
     D. use active-listening techniques.

102. **When preparing a home program with
     the goal of independent toileting for a
     young child with postural instability, the
     MOST important adaptation the COTA
     can recommend is:**
     A. replacing zippers and buttons on clothes
        with Velcro closures.
     B. mounting a safety rail next to the toilet.
     C. introducing toilet paper tongs.
     D. placing a colorful "target" in the toilet bowl.

103. **An individual with low endurance com-
     plains of becoming too fatigued during
     sexual activity to enjoy it. The BEST
     strategy for the COTA to recommend is
     for the individual to:**
     A. time sex for the end of the day.
     B. take the top, prone position.
     C. take the bottom, supine position.
     D. experiment with a variety of positions.

104. **When teaching deep breathing tech-
     niques to manage stress, the COTA
     should instruct the individual to:**
     A. make a fist, and then gradually relax it.
     B. focus on a rhythmic, repetitive word.
     C. walk rapidly until an increased heart rate is
        achieved.
     D. deeply inhale and slowly exhale.

105. **A child with a head injury is impulsive
     during self-feeding and frequently
     attempts to place too much food in her
     mouth at one time. Which of the follow-
     ing methods should the COTA recom-
     mend to MOST effectively control her
     rate of intake during self-feeding?**
     A. Cut her food into smaller pieces.
     B. Have her count to 10 between bites of
        food.
     C. Have her put the utensil down until she
        swallows.
     D. Serve the various food items in separate
        containers on the meal tray.

106. **An individual with MS reports extreme
     frustration because her house is so dir-
     ty. When she does attempt to clean it,
     she is too exhausted to do anything else
     afterward. She does not think she can
     afford to pay someone else to clean.
     Which of the following strategies is
     MOST appropriate for the COTA to rec-
     ommend to this individual?**
     A. Convince the individual to hire a house
        cleaner.
     B. Prescribe activities that will increase
        strength.
     C. Use the largest joint available for the task.
     D. Alternate tasks that require standing with
        those that can be performed sitting.

107. **During treatment the COTA responds to
     a client who recently lost her spouse in a
     car accident by paraphrasing. The COTA
     is MOST likely implementing this tech-
     nique in order to:**
     A. refocus or redirect the individual's
        comments.
     B. show acceptance and understanding re-
        garding the client's situation.
     C. persuade the individual to make a choice.

D. encourage the individual to provide additional information.

108. A child has mastered brushing her teeth with the COTA giving verbal and physical cues. What would be the NEXT step in the process of reducing the intrusiveness of cues?

A. Verbal cues

B. Verbal and gestural cues

C. Physical cues

D. Verbal and physical cues

109. A client with CP has severe motor impairment resulting in insufficient arm and hand motion, and insufficient grasp or prehension to access a computer keyboard. The COTA should recommend which of the following as the BEST low technology solution for improving the client's ability to access the keyboard?

A. A head pointer and slanted keyboard

B. A typing splint

C. An adapted mouse

D. A built-up pencil to press the keys

110. A client in a group home makes frequent sexual advances to a COTA. When group time arrives, he refuses to come down from his room. The MOST important action for the COTA to take is to:

A. avoid any physical contact with the individual.

B. go to his room and invite him to group.

C. agree to go with him on a community outing to the library.

D. agree to a date when he "gets better."

111. A school-age child has Duchenne's muscular dystrophy. Although he is able to use a manual chair for distances between classes, he is tired on arrival. What would be the BEST recommendation the COTA could make for wheelchair use at school?

A. Retain the manual chair to build up strength.

B. Change to an ultralight sports model because it requires less strength.

C. Change to a power wheelchair to reduce effort.

D. Encourage walking with a walker to alternate mobility methods.

112. A patient with Parkinson's disease has particular difficulty with both starting and stopping movements. The BEST strategy for the COTA to teach the person and the person's caregivers is to:

A. encourage the person to perform deep breathing exercise when movement is "frozen."

B. have the person practice the starting phase of the movement repeatedly.

C. have the person mentally identify the series of steps needed to initiate the movement.

D. provide a sensory cue, such as saying "stop!".

113. A COTA is planning treatment for individuals with a variety of personality disorders who have inaccurate perceptions of others and unrealistic perceptions of themselves. The treatment method that might BEST address these problem areas is a:

A. small group that provides a wide range of craft activities from which the members are encouraged to select.

B. session focused on understanding and changing the individual's way of relating with the COTA.

C. social skills training program completed in small groups.

D. cooperative group activity that both provides and elicits consistent and accurate feedback about interactions within the group.

114. A resident in a long-term care facility is being treated by the COTA to regain self-feeding skills. The MOST effective strategy for beginning self-feeding with a resident who is tactilely defensive around the facial area is to:

A. have the COTA clear food pocketed in the resident's cheeks.

B. use a guiding technique by placing food in the resident's hand and bringing it to the mouth.

C. wipe food particles from the resident's mouth and chin as he or she eats.

D. allow the resident to select whatever food or beverage he or she prefers.

115. The goal for a patient who has had a CVA is to be able to put on a shirt independently. The MOST effective way for the COTA to structure dressing training for maximum learning retention and generalization of this skill is:

A. teaching and practicing each segment of the dressing procedure during consecutive treatment sessions.

B. practicing the whole task of putting on a shirt in a setting similar to the real environment.

C. providing dressing simulation activities (button boards, etc.).

D. allowing the client to view a videotape on how to put on a shirt and providing written directions for completing steps for dressing.

116. **A man with a successful landscaping business is completing detoxification after many years of alcohol abuse. This is his first treatment experience. During a discharge planning group, he asks the COTA for community resources to "help me stay sober." Which is the BEST resource the COTA could provide for him?**

A. The YMCA
B. Vocational Rehabilitation
C. Alcoholics Anonymous
D. Volunteering to speak to high school students

117. **A child with CP tends to flex forward while riding her adapted tricycle, even though her lower extremities are correctly positioned. Which of the following adaptions should the COTA recommend to BEST enable the child to maintain an upright position while riding?**

A. Raising the seat height
B. Raising the handlebars
C. Lowering the seat height
D. Lowering the handlebars

118. **A child diagnosed with mental retardation has been participating in a craft group structured as a parallel group. The child is now developing skills such as sharing materials and interacting with other group members. The NEXT level of structured activity which the COTA would recommend for the child is in a(n):**

A. egocentric cooperative group.
B. project group.
C. cooperative group.
D. mature group.

119. **An adult with schizophrenia walks with a shuffling gait and hunched posture. Using a movement-centered frame of reference, which of the following activities would MOST effectively contribute to normalization of this individual's posture?**

A. Dancing with rapid alternating movements

B. Playing the game "Twister"
C. Digging a garden with a shovel
D. Rocking in a rocking chair

120. **A child with a diagnosis of athetoid CP would like to be able to dress herself independently. Which of the following clothing features could the COTA recommend that would be MOST useful in facilitating self-dressing?**

A. Mini tee shirts made of elasticized fabric
B. Dresses with side zippers and zipper pulls
C. Oversized tee shirts and elastic top pants
D. Shirts with front closures, such as snaps or large buttons

121. **A client with neurological deficits resulting from a head injury was performing the task of reaching for her brush on the shelf of her bathroom cabinet. During this task the COTA observed that the client located the brush, but became very distracted by the other items on the shelf. As a result of this observation, the COTA is MOST likely to provide activities that will improve:**

A. learning.
B. selective attention.
C. figure-ground perception.
D. problem solving.

122. **An individual with depression finishes making a poorly constructed Christmas tree ornament, and tells the COTA he wants to throw it away because it is "such a sorry looking thing." What is the BEST way for the COTA to respond?**

A. Suggest that he give it to a family member.
B. Tell him it is beautiful and ask to keep it.
C. Ask if it is OK to hang it on the tree on the unit.
D. Accept his decision.

123. **A child with a diagnosis of ADHD also exhibits perceptual deficits. The activity the COTA would MOST likely recommend for this child to train visual attention is:**

A. playing a game of "Memory" where images are matched by memory.
B. assembling a 200-piece puzzle.
C. finding "Waldo" against a complex visual background.
D. blowing cotton balls into a target.

124. **A COTA is working with a patient who has had a UE amputation to determine whether a hook terminal device or a**

functional prosthetic hand would be most appropriate for the patient. The patient's primary concern is his ability to return to work and function as a carpenter. The MOST important factor in the COTA's recommendation would be that:

A. a functional prosthetic hand has a better cosmetic appearance.
B. a hook provides better prehensile function and allows greater visibility of objects.
C. a hook weighs less than a hand.
D. a functional hand is covered by a rubber glove that stains easily.

125. While participating in the first session of a relapse prevention group, a client reports that he often misses a dose of his medication because he forgets when to take it. Which of the following actions should the COTA take FIRST?

A. Ask group members to discuss how they feel about taking their medications.
B. Suggest using a diary to record each dose of medication.
C. Instruct him in the use of a timer to assist in medication management.
D. Make sure he knows what his medication schedule is.

126. A COTA is working with a medically stable child who sustained bilateral upper extremity partial thickness burns 3 days ago while playing with a lighter. Which ADL intervention should the COTA introduce first?

A. Instruct the child to use all adapted equipment.
B. Encourage independent compression garment application.
C. Perform bilateral upper extremity PROM exercises twice a day.
D. Encourage independent self-feeding and dressing skills with minimal use of adapted utensils and tools.

127. A person with peripheral neuropathy exhibits loss of pinprick, light touch, pressure, and temperature sensation resulting in an absence of protective sensation. The COTA explains to the client that the most appropriate form of intervention to address this type of sensory loss would be a program of:

A. sensory re-education.
B. sensory desensitization.
C. sensory bombardment.
D. sensory compensation.

128. A COTA realizes that an adult worker with a developmental disability is having difficulty learning an assembly sequence during packaging a game box. The COTA decides to use backward chaining. The COTA can BEST implement this technique by:

A. encouraging the individual to reverse the packaging sequence.
B. having the worker put only the last piece into the game package.
C. putting only the pencil or the pad into the game box.
D. having the therapist demonstrate and repeat the correct sequence before each of the worker's attempts.

129. A child with a physical disability and poor postural stability is developmentally ready for toileting. Which of the following elements of the treatment plan should be considered FIRST?

A. Training in management of fasteners
B. Provision of foot support
C. Provision of a seatbelt
D. Training in climbing onto the toilet

130. A COTA making a bedside visit finds her patient poorly positioned with an edematous upper extremity caught between the mattress and the bed rail. The MOST appropriate intervention to address the edema in the upper extremity is to:

A. elevate the arm on pillows so it rests higher than the heart.
B. massage the arm gently, stroking toward the fingers.
C. instruct the patient to avoid active range of motion.
D. instruct the patient to avoid PROM.

131. An individual with mental illness has accepted a secretarial position, but is concerned about high levels of distractibility that may interfere with concentration and job performance. Which of the following interventions is MOST appropriate for this individual?

A. Arrange for the individual to have a job coach.
B. Ask the employer to provide more frequent breaks.
C. Explain the problem of distractibility to the employer.
D. Ask the employer to provide an isolated cubicle as the work space.

132. A COTA is working with a 17-year-old girl with impaired mobility, dexterity, and communication skills. The teenager is within function limits cognitively. Which of the following would the COTA MOST likely recommend to the family regarding emergency alert systems in the event of a fire?

A. Position a wireless cell phone within the child's reach.

B. Establish an exit routine in order to get out of the house quickly in the event of a fire.

C. Review "fire prevention within the home" literature.

D. Recommend that the child wear an emergency alert system pendant around her neck.

133. A COTA applies weights to the wrists of a woman who is making a macramé planter to improve strength in her shoulders. The COTA is MOST likely implementing which of the following treatment approaches?

A. Neurophysiological

B. Neurodevelopmental

C. Biomechanical

D. Rehabilitative

134. The PRIMARY functions of a COTA leading a therapeutic group in the beginning stages of group development will be to:

A. set the climate, provide structure, and offer support.

B. leave members to set the climate, provide structure, and offer support to each other.

C. aid group members in separation and reinforce gains made in the group.

D. work individually with group members until each is ready to join group activity.

135. While working with a child who has a neuromuscular disorder, the COTA places the child in a sitting position on a therapeutic ball, starts moving the ball, and asks the child to reach for a toy. The COTA's primary purpose for introducing this activity is MOST likely to:

A. increase upper extremity strength.

B. facilitate postural reactions.

C. decrease tactile defensiveness.

D. improve visual perception.

136. After wearing a new splint for 20 minutes, an individual develops a reddened area along the ulnar styloid process. The FIRST modification the COTA should make to correct the splint is to:

A. line the splint with moleskin.

B. line the splint with adhesive backed foam.

C. flange the area around the ulnar styloid.

D. reheat and refabricate the entire splint.

137. A COTA is working with an individual in a psychosocial partial hospitalization program who is having difficulty making decisions. The COTA has suggested a baking activity, but the client is unsure if she wants to do this activity. The OT practitioner's response that would BEST facilitate decision making is:

A. "I think baking would be a helpful activity to try. Baking something you like offers you several choices and decisions. You wanted to bake cookies today, didn't you?"

B. "I think baking would be a helpful activity to try. Baking something you like offers you several choices and decisions. What do you want to bake?"

C. "I think baking would be a helpful activity to try. Baking something you like offers you several choices and decisions. These choices and decisions can help you feel more positive about making other decisions. You can choose a cake mix or a cookie mix. Which would you like?"

D. "I think baking would be a helpful activity to try. Baking something you like offers you several choices and decisions. These choices and decisions can help you feel more positive about making other decisions. Do you want to bake cookies?"

138. When teaching children with moderate mental retardation to feed, groom, and dress themselves, the COTA is MOST likely to use which technique?

A. Chaining

B. Practice and repetition

C. Demonstration

D. Role modeling

139. A client who is s/p traumatic brain injury exhibits good strength with ataxia in both upper extremities. The writing adaptation that would be MOST appropriate in compensating for the patient's deficit areas would be:

A. using a keyboard.

B. a universal cuff with pencil holder attachment.

C. using a balanced forearm orthosis with built-up felt-tip pen.

D. a weighted pen and weighted wrists.

140. A client requests assistance with his ongoing memory problems. The MOST effective external compensation method of intervention the COTA can introduce is to:

A. teach the client to retrace steps mentally to stimulate memory.
B. teach the client to use a diary or log.
C. train the client to repeat important pieces of information aloud until memorized.
D. work with a memory training computer program.

141. To avoid overstimulation when handling a stable, 12-week premature infant in the NICU setting, the COTA must FIRST:

A. provide gentle human touch to enable the infant to slowly respond to intervention.
B. establish a calm state by utilizing an infant musical mobile.
C. swaddle the infant in a blanket and cuddle to provide containment and warmth to assist with self-regulation.
D. establish a bond through visual orientation to the therapist's face.

142. A mother of four teenage children who was diagnosed with a right CVA is receiving home care OT services. The treatment plan includes "activities to improve left upper extremity function" and "activities to improve balance in sitting and standing." The MOST appropriate activity for the COTA to recommend would be:

A. stacking cones.
B. door pulley.
C. folding laundry.
D. throwing a ball.

143. A client with cognitive deficits exhibits little transfer of skills from one activity to the next. Which intervention would be BEST to assist this client in performing the steps of doing his laundry?

A. Performing memory drills of the steps involved in doing in a laundry activity
B. Placing serial pictures of a laundry activity in sequence
C. Making a checklist of steps in the process, then consulting the list while doing laundry in the actual setting
D. Reading a story about a person doing laundry with the client, then discussing the story

144. During an oral motor treatment session, a COTA instructs the mother of a newborn infant regarding the facilitation of the rooting reflex. The COTA instructs the mother to facilitate this reflex prior to nursing her baby by:

A. touching the crowns of the infant's teeth.
B. touching the infant on the right or left corner of his mouth.
C. gently flexing the infant's neck approximately 5 degrees.
D. placing the baby supine on her lap while gently rocking the baby.

145. Which of the following is the MOST important adaptation to recommend to an individual returning home following a total hip replacement?

A. Move items from high cabinets to lower locations.
B. Obtain a raised toilet seat.
C. Place high contrast tape at the edge of each step.
D. Install a handheld shower head.

146. A COTA is working with a group of 2-½- to 3-year-old children in a preschool setting. The OTR has asked the COTA to initiate a group that facilitates symbolic play. Which of the following activities should the COTA introduce to the group?

A. Scissors and cutting activities with construction paper
B. Jump rope games
C. Make believe group with stuffed animals and imaginary friends
D. Building towers with blocks that resemble pictures in books

147. A COTA working with a person experiencing a manic episode would be MOST likely to select which type of activity?

A. Detailed needlepoint project requiring fine stitches
B. Using clay to mold an object of one's choice
C. A watercolor painting project
D. Finishing a prefabricated wood birdhouse from a kit

148. A patient is beginning to demonstrate return in the right upper extremity following a CVA, but has mildly impaired proprioception in the right hand, which results in uneven letter formation during writing activities. Which would be the BEST method to help improve letter formation?

A. The COTA verbally describes how to make a letter as the individual writes.
B. The individual watches her grip on a felt tip pen while writing.
C. The individual works with "theraputty" to strengthen her hand.
D. The individual traces letters through a pan of rice with her fingers.

149. The COTA is working with a child who has upper extremity weakness and incoordination. The child wishes to put on and take off her pants independently. Which of the following should the COTA recommend?

A. Pants with Velcro inserts placed in the zipper area
B. Pants with an elastic waistband
C. Cotton pants with large buttons inserted where the zipper area is located
D. Pants with an enlarged zipper pull attachment

150. A COTA in a long-term care facility is working with several residents who seem very isolated and disengaged from the other residents. The COTA has identified a need to provide these residents with a group activity that would enhance self-esteem, provide opportunities for social skills and assist residents in integrating past experiences with present life. The COTA should FIRST introduce a:

A. reminiscence group.
B. meditation group.
C. grooming activities group.
D. movement activities and games group.

151. An individual with Guillain-Barré syndrome was recently admitted to a rehabilitation unit and is expected to remain for 3 to 4 weeks. At what point in the rehabilitative process should the COTA recommend adaptive equipment for this individual?

A. After the patient and family have accepted the individual's disability
B. As soon as the insurance provider approves it
C. Within the first week of therapy
D. Just before discharge

152. A COTA in a psychosocial setting is documenting a client's responses to an activity. Which of the following should the COTA write in the chart in order to relay the objective portion of the note?

A. The client did not want to finish her stenciling activity.
B. The client was hostile to another client in the activity group.
C. The client independently selected one of six craft designs presented.
D. The client demonstrated an appropriate level of frustration tolerance during most of the activity.

153. COTAs working in the area of early intervention have frequent contact with a child's parents. Which of the following statements BEST describes how parents should be involved in the OT program?

A. Parents should not be present during OT sessions.
B. Parents should be trained as substitute therapists.
C. Parents should be considered as part of a collaborative partnership with OT practitioners.
D. Only one parent needs to be present when the OT program is discussed.

Effectiveness of Treatment and Discharge Planning

154. The family of an individual with paraplegia is moving into a new apartment and they need to select a floor surface for the living area. Finances are limited, but they are looking for the surface that will be easiest for maneuvering a wheelchair. Which of the following is the MOST appropriate surface for this situation?

A. Linoleum floor
B. Short pile carpeting
C. Deep pile carpeting
D. Several area rugs

155. A COTA is working with a client with mental retardation who engages in self-abusive behavior when anxious. After participating in a craft group for 2 months, the client has achieved the goal of engaging in a simple craft activity for up to 10 minutes, before demonstrating self-abusive behavior. Which of the following would be the MOST appropriate revised short-term goal for this individual?

A. The client will engage in a simple craft activity for 15 minutes without demonstrating self-abusive behavior.

B. The client will engage in a craft activity of moderate complexity for 10 minutes without demonstrating self-abusive behavior.

C. The client will engage in a craft activity of moderate complexity for 15 minutes without demonstrating self-abusive behavior.

D. The client will engage in a complex craft activity for 10 minutes without demonstrating self-abusive behavior.

156. **A young child has been wearing a left upper extremity prosthesis for 3 weeks. The MOST important activity recommendation that the COTA gives to the child's preschool teacher is to:**
    A. offer toys that the child can manipulate with one hand.
    B. stress bilateral play and school activities incorporating the prosthesis.
    C. teach the child one-handed manipulation techniques.
    D. involve the child in activities that do not require manipulation.

157. **A nonspeaking person who uses a wheelchair is suddenly making many errors on the augmentative communication device, but experienced no difficulty the previous day. Which of the following is the FIRST step the COTA should take in responding to this problem?**
    A. Refer the person to a physician for evaluation.
    B. Reposition the person in the wheelchair to allow optimal range of motion.
    C. Reassess the person's communication abilities.
    D. Replace the communication device.

158. **During discharge planning, a patient asks the COTA, "what should I do when people at work ask me where I have been all this time?" The BEST strategy to address this concern would be to:**
    A. arrange for the patient to discuss this with the social worker.
    B. suggest that the patient tell the truth.
    C. suggest that the patient report having been on an extended vacation.
    D. arrange for the patient to attend a discharge group to discuss these concerns.

159. **In a preschool setting, the COTA is providing information to the OTR concerning readiness for discharge of a 5-year-old**
    preschooler with mild developmental delay. The MOST important information for the COTA to focus on is:
    A. achievement of dressing independence.
    B. improved socialization and impulse control.
    C. attainment of kindergarten readiness skills.
    D. independence in toileting.

160. **A COTA has observed that his client has made gains in fine motor coordination in the past week. The MOST appropriate way to document this progress in the assessment section of the note is:**
    A. "Patient performed the Nine Hole Peg Test in 20 seconds."
    B. "Patient reports being able to button the buttons on most items of clothing."
    C. "Patient is demonstrating gradual improvement in fine motor coordination."
    D. "Family reports patient is performing more fine motor activities independently."

161. **An OT practitioner is considering possible topics for a discharge planning group for individuals on an inpatient psychiatric unit. Which of the following topics would be MOST important to cover because it is significantly related to the possibility of rehospitalization?**
    A. Managing family conflicts after returning home
    B. Living skills needed for keeping aftercare appointments
    C. Coping strategies for continuing medication compliance
    D. Education about alcohol and substance abuse

162. **A COTA is advising the parents of a 5-year-old child with athetoid cerebral palsy about the type of construction toy they should buy the child to facilitate play. The BEST type of construction toy to recommend for this child is a set with:**
    A. large, easily interlocking pieces.
    B. blocks that are small and have a firm surface.
    C. lightweight and soft-textured building blocks.
    D. colorful blocks in a variety of shapes.

163. **"The patient arrived without her walker 3 out of 3 days this week." The MOST appropriate section of a SOAP note for a COTA to place this statement is the:**
    A. subjective section.
    B. objective section.

C. assessment section.

D. plan section.

164. An individual with mental illness has been homeless for the past 4 years and recently began coming to a shelter. It has taken 3 weeks for the COTA to establish rapport, and the COTA believes attending a group is the next step. Which type of group is MOST likely to engage this individual?

A. Highly structured craft group

B. Volunteer activity group, such as stuffing envelopes

C. Simple meal preparation group

D. Social skills group

165. A school-age child with fine motor skill difficulties is ready for discharge from outpatient OT services. The MOST important information to include in the discharge summary concerns the:

A. child's interests and hobbies.

B. child's writing, dressing, and self-feeding skills.

C. child's academic achievement.

D. availability of the child's parents for follow-up services.

166. An individual with left hemiparesis and impaired balance wishes to vacuum floors upon return home. The BEST type of vacuum cleaner for the COTA to recommend is a(n):

A. canister vacuum cleaner.

B. upright vacuum cleaner.

C. self-propelled vacuum cleaner.

D. handheld cordless vacuum cleaner.

167. An OT practitioner is treating a client who has demonstrated a decrease in paranoid behavior. The statement which BEST documents this change is:

A. The patient is no longer as afraid of men.

B. The patient has not accused any men of attacking her this week.

C. The patient is participating more actively in beauty group.

D. The patient will tolerate sitting next to a man in group one time this week.

168. A COTA is discharging a 4-year-old child with athetoid cerebral palsy from a rehabilitation setting to home. The MOST appropriate instructions for the COTA to provide to the family for maintaining

correct jaw control while feeding the child from the side are:

A. "jaw opening and closing are controlled with your index and middle fingers; place your thumb on the child's cheek."

B. "jaw opening and closing are controlled with your index and middle fingers; place your thumb on the child's larynx for stability."

C. "jaw opening and closing are controlled with your whole hand on the child's jaw."

D. "jaw opening and closing are controlled with your index and middle fingers; place your thumb on the child's ear for stability."

169. An individual is about to be discharged to home following a hip arthroplasty. He is able to ambulate with a quad cane, but his balance remains slightly impaired. During the home evaluation, which is the MOST important safety recommendation for the COTA to make?

A. Remove all throw or scatter rugs.

B. Place lever handles on faucets.

C. Install a ramp if steps exist.

D. Install a handheld shower.

170. A COTA working in an acute psychiatric facility spends a portion of each day on documentation procedures. One of the MOST important purposes of documentation is to:

A. occupy the therapist's time between treatments.

B. satisfy accrediting agencies.

C. be used as a research tool.

D. facilitate effective treatment.

171. A COTA is educating the parents of a high-school-age patient who is being discharged from a burn center to his home environment after an 8-month inpatient stay for severe burns. In discussing common psychological reactions, the COTA would MOST likely address:

A. the possibility of decreased range of motion and sensation.

B. the potential for depression and low self-esteem.

C. the likelihood of violent behavior and sexual acting out.

D. the potential for delirium and fatigue.

172. A long-term goal for an individual with progressive weakness is for the family to carry out his feeding program. They have achieved the short-term goal of understanding how the individual's dis-

ability affects his ability to feed himself. Which statement is the BEST
revised short-term goal?

A. Patient will participate in feeding program.
B. Patient will feed himself with moderate
   assistance.
C. Family will feed patient safely and independently 100% of the time.
D. Family will demonstrate independence in
   current positioning and feeding techniques.

173. **A COTA is working with an elderly
     patient with early stage dementia who
     was admitted to the hospital after acci-
     dentally setting fire to his kitchen. The
     MOST appropriate follow-up services to
     identify relative to this patient's meal
     planning needs after discharge would
     be:**

A. OT services to teach the patient to cook
   safely.
B. volunteer companion services to supervise
   cooking at home.
C. transportation services to bring the person
   to a community meal site.
D. home-delivered meal services.

174. **The COTA has written the following
     statement: "continue social skills train-
     ing program and encourage client to at-
     tend one new after-school club acti-
     vity within the next week." The MOST
     appropriate section to place this state-
     ment is the:**

A. subjective section.
B. objective section.
C. assessment section.
D. plan section.

175. **An 18-year-old adolescent diagnosed
     with schizophrenia takes a neuroleptic
     drug that has caused him to experience
     extreme thirst, but he must continue
     taking the drug. At the time of dis-
     charge, it is MOST important to remind
     him to:**

A. limit sun exposure as much as possible.
B. drink coffee and caffeinated sodas whenever possible.
C. get up slowly from a standing, sitting, or lying position.
D. drink juices and caffeine-free colas when
   thirsty.

176. **Upon discharge, an individual will be per-
     forming sliding board transfers with
     assistance from family members. When**

ordering a wheelchair, which features
will be MOST important to include?

A. One-arm drive and low backrest
B. Reclining backrest and elevating footrests
C. Swing-away footrests and removable
   armrests
D. Elevating footrests and removable
   armrests

Occupational Therapy for Populations

177. **In a long-term care facility, a number of
     residents have Parkinson's disease and
     would benefit from regular group activi-
     ty which would help decrease muscular
     rigidity. The BEST activity the COTA
     could recommend for this purpose would
     be:**

A. weight training.
B. walking.
C. tai chi.
D. gardening.

178. **A COTA who has joined the staff of a
     drop-in shelter for homeless women is
     responsible for developing a leisure
     activity group. One of the goals of this
     group is to foster a sense of competence
     and mastery over the environment.
     Which of the following BEST addresses
     this goal?**

A. A small group collage activity
B. Leather lacing a change purse from a kit
C. Going to see a movie
D. Putting on a resident talent show

179. **As part of a university's community out-
     reach program, the OT program is devel-
     oping a club for youth at risk for vio-
     lence. The primary goal is to engage the
     children in meaningful occupations de-
     signed to protect and build the communi-
     ty. Which one of the following activities
     is MOST consistent with this goal?**

A. Develop "Community Olympics" competi-
   tions at group and individual levels.
B. Provide a psychoeducational intervention
   on anger management.
C. Plant flower seeds in small pots to be taken
   home once they sprout.
D. Convert an empty lot filled with trash into a
   garden.

180. **The goals of an occupational therapy
     health promotion program for a well eld-**

erly population include enhancing life satisfaction and preventing loss of physical and social function. What is the **MOST** important type of activity to include in this program?

A. Activities that promote home and community safety

B. Socialization activities

C. Balance and ambulation activities

D. Activities to promote the skills of caregivers

181. **A COTA has been hired to develop social skills training programs for persons with long-term mental illness in a community mental health facility. The COTA needs to select a behavior to assess as an outcome measure. Which would BEST indicate that the program was successful in achieving goals for this population?**

A. Improved ability to balance rest, work, play, and leisure

B. Improved verbal and nonverbal communication skills

C. Improved ability to identify areas for vocational exploration

D. Improved ability to perform daily self-care and home management activities

182. **After her own third-grade child was injured in a scooter accident, a COTA became interested in volunteering to develop a "Scooter Safety" program at her local elementary school. What is the FIRST step the COTA should take?**

A. Collect as much information as possible about injuries caused by scooter accidents.

B. Identify an OTR willing to supervise her while she develops and implements this program.

C. Emphasize the importance of protective clothing, such as helmets and knee and elbow pads, to children and parents.

D. Obtain permission from the school principal to implement the program.

183. **An OT practitioner is providing accessibility consultation services to a local library. In the back of the library there is a reference room with a doorway that has a threshold height of 1 inch. Concerning the threshold and accessibility according to the ADA guidelines, which of the following recommendations would be best?**

A. Keep the threshold as is, and place a sign near the door alerting people to the threshold.

B. Provide a throw rug that covers the threshold.

C. Remove the threshold altogether.

D. Ramp the threshold.

184. **An OT practitioner in a long-term care facility would like to provide an activity to engage a number of residents with dementia who wander and pace the halls throughout the day. The BEST type of activity to plan for these residents would be:**

A. reminiscing about previous jobs.

B. walking as part of a walking club.

C. singing oldies in a group.

D. a craft activity requiring concentration.

185. **OT practitioners employed by a school district provide consultation to a vocational instructor in a high school program for students with moderate mental disabilities. Which of the following activities would be MOST appropriately provided by the OT practitioners?**

A. Developing an in-house prevocational work program

B. Bringing in outside speakers from different job settings

C. Teaching the vocational instructor different assessment tools and scoring procedures

D. Meeting the vocational instructor weekly to discuss adaptations to work tasks

186. **A COTA/OTR team provides services to a large residential facility for adults with moderate to severe developmental disabilities. The team has been asked to develop an on site, paid employment program for individuals who are able to perform simple assembling and packaging tasks. Which of the following would be the MOST appropriate service delivery model?**

A. Sheltered workshop

B. Supported employment

C. Competitive employment

D. Supervised employment with job coaching

Service Management

187. **An entry-level COTA has joined the staff of a rehabilitation facility and requires "close supervision" for the first few months. As specified by AOTA, the COTA should have contact with the supervising OTR:**

A. once a day.

B. once a week.

C. once a month.

D. as needed.

188. **One week after a COTA begins a new job in a nursing home, the supervising OTR resigns, leaving no OTR onsite. The nursing home administrator advises the COTA to continue treating patients, and promises to hire an OTR within a week. The MOST acceptable action for the COTA to take is to:**

A. refuse to provide OT services to patients until an OTR has been hired to provide supervision.

B. agree to provide OT services to patients for 1 week, but not beyond that.

C. provide OT services only to patients who will suffer if they don't receive OT services.

D. report the nursing home to the AOTA.

189. **A COTA and OTR each carry out part of the initial evaluation of a newly admitted patient. Upon completion of the evaluation, each will write part of the initial note. The most appropriate part of the note for the COTA to write is the:**

A. treatment plan.

B. source of the referral, the reason for the referral, and the date the referral was received.

C. summary and analysis of the patient's assets and deficits.

D. projected outcome of treatment.

190. **An OT practitioner is about to begin hand rehabilitation activities with a client who has open dorsal hand wounds. The MOST appropriate way for the practitioner to protect himself from bloodborne pathogens is to:**

A. wear a mask.

B. wear gloves.

C. refuse to work with the patient.

D. wash hands before and after treating the patient.

191. **An OT practitioner is writing a job description for an aide position in the OT department. According to AOTA guidelines, which of the following is BEYOND the scope of practice of an aide?**

A. Cue an individual with schizophrenia to maintain attention to task during a weekly cooking group led by an OT.

B. Practice use of a sock aid and shoe horn in the OT department with a patient who has had a hip replacement and is able to perform the task safely but takes an excessive amount of time.

C. Help place food on the spoon for a patient practicing the use of a universal cuff in the patient's room at lunchtime, while the OT supervisor runs a lunch group in the dining room.

D. Help a child maintain correct positioning during paper and pencil activities, while the OT works with the child at the next desk.

192. **An OTR is working with an individual who tests positive for HIV. The individual is working on a copper tooling project when he cuts his finger on the edge of the copper. Which of the following are the MOST appropriate precautions to follow?**

A. Suicide precautions

B. Universal precautions

C. Escape from unit precautions

D. Medical precautions

193. **An OT practitioner completing a home assessment has recommended a hospital bed, lightweight wheelchair, bedside commode, reachers, long-handled sponge, shower chair, and hand-held shower. The family states they can only afford the items that can be billed as durable medical equipment. The OT practitioner should:**

A. explain to the family that they will need to pay for all items.

B. order only the reachers and long-handled sponge.

C. order only the shower chair and hand-held shower.

D. order only the lightweight wheelchair and hospital bed.

194. **A fieldwork supervisor is completing the final evaluation of a student who is in the last week of a level II fieldwork placement. In order for the student to complete the fieldwork experience successfully, the supervisor must:**

A. believe the student has the ability to work effectively with individuals with a wide variety of diagnoses.

B. determine that the student is functioning at or above the minimal entry level of competence.

C. have observed the student working with individuals of different ages and cultural backgrounds.

D. insure the student has a working knowledge of various health care systems.

195. OT services in a long-term care facility are provided by two OTRs and one COTA through a contract agency. When the absence of one of the OTRs creates a staffing shortage, the administration instructs the present OTR to perform evaluations only, and instructs the COTA, a new graduate, to perform all treatment planning and implementation until they are fully staffed again. No time is designated for supervision. What is the MOST appropriate way for the OT staff to respond?

A. Follow the administrator's instructions.

B. Express concern to the administrator about inadequate supervision and then follow administrator's instructions.

C. Express concern in writing to the contract agency and then carry out the administrator's instructions.

D. Explain to the administrator this is not an appropriate solution and then develop an alternate solution.

196. The OT department has been asked to provide information to the hospital administration regarding the cost effectiveness of services provided. Which of the following methods would MOST effectively obtain this information?

A. Outcomes measurement

B. Utilization review

C. Program evaluation

D. Productivity evaluations

Professional Practice

197. An OTR/COTA team begins to provide occupational therapy services through a Medicare-certified home health agency. What is the MOST critical component for establishing a successful collaborative relationship in this treatment setting?

A. Determining reimbursement when completing joint visits

B. Establishing a system for the OTR to countersign the COTA's documentation

C. Creating a written and specific supervisory

plan based on competency levels for both practitioners

D. Developing a handout to educate future clients regarding how the OTR/COTA team will provide services

198. On the way to lunch, an OT practitioner is stopped by a patient's spouse and questioned for 15 minutes about the patient's progress. What is the MOST appropriate action for the OT practitioner to take when determining how the patient will be treated and charged for the scheduled one hour treatment session?

A. Charge the patient for an additional 15 minutes of treatment for the time spent with family member.

B. Reduce the patient's therapy to 45 minutes and charge for 1 hour of treatment to cover the time spent with the family member.

C. Reduce the patient's therapy to 45 minutes and charge for 45 minutes of treatment.

D. Treat the patient as scheduled and charge only for the 1 hour of direct time spent with the patient.

199. An OT practitioner evaluating a child notices a bruise on the child's shoulder that looks like an adult's hand and fingerprint. Which of the following actions is MOST critical for the OT practitioner to take?

A. Discuss this with the family member who picks up the child.

B. Observe for additional injuries.

C. Make a report to appropriate authorities.

D. Avoid becoming involved in personal family matters.

200. An OT practitioner who has demonstrated service competency in the use of paraffin baths moves from one state to another to take a position in a hand rehabilitation center. The licensure act in the new state prohibits OT practitioners from using physical agent modalities. The MOST appropriate action for the therapist to take is to:

A. use PAMs only under the supervision of a licensed PT.

B. use PAMs only under the supervision of a medical doctor.

C. use only paraffin.

D. not use PAMs in the new state.

ANSWERS FOR SIMULATION EXAMINATION 3

1. (B) A pinch meter. A pinch meter is used to measure the strength of a three-jaw chuck grasp (also known as palmar pinch), in addition to key (lateral) pinch and tip pinch. These tests are performed with three trials that are averaged together and then compared with a standardized norm. Answer A, the aesthesiometer, measures two-point discrimination. Answer C, the dynamometer, measures grip strength. Answer D, the volumeter, measures edema in the hand. See reference: Pedretti and Early (eds): Kasch, M and Nickerson, E: Hand injuries.

2. (B) insecurity. Feelings of insecurity are often covered up by projecting difficulties as negative comments onto other objects (the collage) or other people. Hopelessness (answer C) involves negative statements about oneself or about changing. A comment or action which demonstrates the inability to choose between tasks typically reflects indecision, (answer D). Passivity (answer A) is often only "heard" through nonverbal communication. See reference: Posthuma: Observations and analysis.

3. (A) athetoid. Athetoid cerebral palsy is characterized by widely fluctuating tone. When tone rapidly shifts from hypertonic to hypotonic, movements appear writhing and uncontrolled. Hypertonic muscle tone, or spasticity (answers B and C), results in impaired ability to control movement or force of movement. Hypotonia, or low tone (answer D), results in flaccid muscles and floppy movements. See reference: Solomon (ed): Wandel, JA: Cerebral palsy.

4. (B) Demonstrate the procedure on the unaffected extremity, then occlude the client's vision while testing the affected extremity. Because visual cues can compensate for sensory deficits, it is necessary to occlude the individual's vision. The presentation of stimuli in sensory evaluation is extremely important. Stimuli should be presented in a random proximal-to-distal pattern. Picture cards are helpful in assessing individuals with expressive aphasia. Also, the unaffected extremity should be assessed before the affected extremity (the opposite of answer A) in order to ensure that the client understands the directions and to reduce anxiety. The OT practitioner should always establish rapport before beginning any of the evaluation procedures (also to reduce anxiety), which makes answer C incorrrect. An individual may not be aware of any deficit areas (answer D), so the OT practitioner should assess the entire extremity to ensure accuracy. See reference: Trombly (ed): Bentzel, K: Evaluation of sensation.

5. (B) Socialization, task performance, daily living skills, and time management. Evaluation of children who have psychosocial problems is centered on behavioral, affective or interpersonal areas, with visual motor and motor assessment following when screening suggests the need. However, specific emphases in evaluation vary according to the age of the client. Answer A reflects primary evaluation areas for toddlers and preschoolers. Answer C is more consistent with adult populations. Answer D reflects evaluation priorities for children with neurological, rather than psychosocial, dysfunction. See reference: Neistadt and Crepeau (eds): Florey, LL: Psychosocial dysfunction in childhood and adolescence.

6. (A) Visual-motor integration. Visual-motor integration skills "require coordination of eyes with hands....such that the eyes guide complex, precise movements" (p. 277). Visual acuity (answer B) refers to the ability to see clearly. A child with poor visual acuity would be observed bringing objects and papers close to his eyes in order to see them better. Visual tracking (answer C) is the ability to follow targets with smooth eye movements. "Children who have poor visual tracking skills often lose focus while trying to follow or find an object" (p. 276). Visual perception (answer D) refers to "the capacity to interpret sensory input, recognize similarities and differences and assign meaning to what is seen" (p. 276). Limitations in this area may result in difficulty matching and sorting (object perception); finding figures hidden in pictures, such as "Where's Waldo?" (figure-ground perception); and moving through small spaces (position in space perception). See reference: Solomon (ed): Jones, LMW: Occupational performance areas: Daily living and work and productive activities.

7. (B) figure-ground perception. Figure-ground perception is the ability to visually separate an object from the surrounding background. An example of this would be the ability to find a button on a plaid shirt. A problem with spatial relations (answer A) is seen in dressing when a person overestimates or underestimates reach because of an inability to judge the relationship between the object and the body. Body image (answer C) is a mental picture of the person's body that includes how the person feels about their body. Visual closure (answer D) is the ability to recognize an object even though only part of it is seen, e.g., recognizing a partially covered button. See reference: Zoltan: Visual discrimination skills.

8. (B) The child demonstrated tongue thrust. "Tongue thrust" is an objective, well-defined term. The other answers are less objective. Answer A infers the child's emotional reaction. Answer C implies voluntary control and judges behavior. Answer D interprets data based on insufficient evidence. See reference: Early: Medical records and documentation.

9. (A) Self-control demands, time management demands, self-expression opportunities, and interest in the activity. Components that are primarily within the psychosocial areas and skills of occupational performance are most important to consider with psychosocial populations. Answers B and C address performance components most commonly used with children. Answer D does not address performance components. See reference: Neistadt and Crepeau (eds): Crepeau, EB: Activity analysis: A way of thinking about occupational performance.

10. (D) Support. Answer D is correct because the term "support reaction" refers to the ability to coactivate muscle groups of the appropriate extremity or about the midline in order to support the body weight or posture in a certain position. Answer A is incorrect because protective reactions follow the development of support reactions in the arms (which protect the child when falling) and require that the body is free from support. Answer B is not correct because equilibrium reactions are compensatory movements used to regain stability, not to maintain stability. Answer C is not correct because rotational righting reactions involve turning of the head or trunk in order to maintain body alignment. See reference: Neistadt and Crepeau (eds): Kohlmeyer, K: Evaluation of sensory and neuromuscular performance components.

11. (C) anterograde amnesia. Anterograde amnesia is the inability to recall events after a trauma. Retrograde amnesia (answer D) is the inability to recall events prior to trauma. Long-term memory (answer B) is the storage of information for recall at a later time. Orientation (answer A) is the awareness of person, place, and time. See reference: Trombly (ed): Quintana, LA: Evaluation of perception and cognition.

12. (A) denial. "Defense mechanisms are unconscious intrapsychic processes by which anxiety producing information or wishes are kept out of conscious awareness" (p. 333). This individual may be having difficulty accepting her stroke and is using denial to avoid dealing with it (answer A). Projection (answer B) "is a process by which a person attributes to another person the feelings he is really having himself" (p. 333). Rationalization (answer C) is when an individual makes excuses for unacceptable behavior. Regression (answer D) is when an individual reverts to infantile or childlike behavior as a way of dealing with a difficult situation. See reference: Bruce and Borg: Appendix E: Defense mechanism.

13. (C) The infant is exhibiting ulnar palmar grasp. Ulnar palmar grasp precedes the other types of grasp. The infant first grasps on the ulnar side of the hand against the palm, then with all four fingers against the palm (palmar grasp), and finally the grasp moves to the radial side of the hand (radial grasp). The highest level of grasp is pincer grasp, in which the pad of the index finger meets the opposed thumb. See reference: Case-Smith (ed): Exner, CE: Development of hand skills.

14. (B) good (4). The individual's "available" range is the range through which the joint may be moved passively. Therefore, if an individual is able to move the joint actively through the entire movement, that is, completed passively and then take maximum resistance, the grade is normal (5). Good (4) is the grade given when an individual such as this client is able to move a part through the available range against gravity and is able to sustain moderate resistance. Fair (3) is the grade given when an individual is able to move a part through the full range against gravity, but lacks the strength for any resistance. Fair minus (3-) is the grade given when an individual moves a part against gravity through less than the full range of motion. Fair minus is the last graded range for movement against gravity. Grades poor (2) and trace (1) are for gravity eliminated movements. See reference: Trombly (ed): Evaluation of biomechanical and physiological aspects of motor performance.

15. (A) use of time. By comparing interests and actual participation, the OT practitioner may identify discrepancies between interests and actual play and leisure behavior. This information can help address the client's use of time, and facilitate temporal organization. The issues in answers B, C, and D are not directly addressed using this method. See reference: Case-Smith (ed): Cronin, AF: Psychosocial and emotional domains.

16. (B) Dressing habits. Certain dressing habits may indicate tactile defensiveness, e.g., the child may show poor tolerance of certain textures or avoid wearing turtlenecks, socks, or shoes. Conversely, some children may never take off their shoes in order to avoid tactile overstimulation. Reading skills (answer A), friendships (answer C), and the choice of hobbies (answer D), could be affected secondarily, as a result of intolerance of certain textures or human touch or the inability to concentrate. However, because of the close connection between dressing and tactile tolerance, knowledge of the child's dressing habits (answer B) will give the OT practitioner the most reliable information. See reference: Case-Smith (ed): Parham, LD and Mailloux, Z: Sensory integration.

17. (A) The doorway width needs to be expanded to have a minimum clear opening of 32 inches. According the ADA accessibility guidelines, a doorway needs to have a minimum clear opening of 32 inches with the door open 90 degrees, measured between the face of the door and the opposite stop. In an environmental evaluation process, according to ADA guidelines, the doorway rather than the individual's wheelchair (answer B) needs to be adapted. See reference: Americans with Disabilities Act: Accessibility Guidelines (ADAAG).

18. (D) The effect of personal traits and the environment on role performance. Evaluation according to the Model of Human Occupation would focus on the effect of personal traits and the environment on role performance. Evaluation according to the Behavioral frame of reference identifies problem behaviors that need to be extinguished (answer A). The Object Relations frame of reference attempts to clarify thoughts, feelings, and experiences that influence behavior (answer B). An OT using the Cognitive Disability frame of reference should evaluate cognitive function, including assets and limitations (answer C). See reference: Bruce and Borg: Model of human occupation.

19. (C) indicating initiative and beginning task-directed behavior. Because this child is very withdrawn, any spontaneous action should be seen as a very positive sign. It is important to encourage the child in independent exploratory behavior in order to develop task competence and to become less withdrawn. Her use of a toothbrush instead of a hairbrush may indicate cognitive limitations (answer B), possibly caused by a lack of exposure; it could also be caused by a visual deficit (answer D), but the primary importance of the observation lies in answer C. Attention-getting behavior (answer A) is unlikely in such a withdrawn child. See reference: Case-Smith (ed): Cronin, AS: Psychosocial and emotional domains.

20. (C) topographical disorientation. Topographical disorientation is difficulty in finding one's way in familiar surroundings, or in learning new routes, and would be exhibited by the patient's inability to find the therapy clinic. Spatial relations disorders (answer A) would be exhibited as difficulties in relating objects to each other. Figure-ground discrimination deficits (answer B) would be exhibited as difficulty in differentiating objects in the foreground from the background. Form discrimination deficits (answer D) would be exhibited as the inability to distinguish between different types of forms. See reference: Unsworth (ed): Arnadottir, G: Evaluation and intervention with complex perceptual impairment.

21. (C) attention span and social interaction skills. Conduct disorders often involve aggression toward people or animals and destruction of property. When working with this population, OT typically addresses the areas of attention span, impulse control, age appropriate social role performance, and social skills. Children with developmental delays typically require intervention for perceptual-motor skills (answer A). Multiple role performance (answer D) is more developmentally relevant to adulthood than to adolescence. Although leisure and vocational interests (answer B) may be relevant to the adolescent population, the issues of attention span and social interaction would be more significant for an individual with conduct disorder. See reference: Early: Understanding psychiatric diagnosis: The DSM-IV.

22. (C) gravitational insecurity. Gravitational insecurity is described as "excessive fear during ordinary movement activities" (p. 352). The child easily experiences a fear of falling and prefers to keep her feet firmly on the ground. Tactile defensiveness (answer A) is a term used to describe discomfort with various textures and with unexpected touch. Developmental dyspraxia (answer B) is a term used to describe a problem with motor planning. Intolerance for motion (answer D) refers to a very similar and often related problem of inhibition of vestibular impulses, but it is usually associated with sensory information received from the semicircular canals. Gravitational insecurity, on the other hand, is associated with the utricle and saccule. See reference: Case-Smith (ed): Parham, LD and Mailloux, Z: Sensory integration.

23. (B) radial-digital grasp. Children usually develop a radial-digital grasp at age 9 months; they use the grasp for precision control. A pincer grasp (answer A), or tip pinch, is characterized by opposition of the thumb and index fingertips to allow the child to make a circle with the fingers. The palmar grasp (answer C) is a power grasp, in which the individual flexes the fingers around an object while stabilizing it against the palm. In a lateral pinch (answer D), the individual places the pad of the thumb against the radial side of the index finger near the DIP joint. This pattern is used as a power grip on small objects. See reference: Case-Smith (ed): Exner, CE: Development of hand skills.

24. (B) Confusion. Medication side effects are typically observed and reported by OTs and OT assistants. Antianxiety medications often cause confusion. Akathisia, extrapyramidal syndrome, and tardive dyskinesia (answers A, C, and D, respectively) are adverse effects commonly linked to antipsychotic medications. See reference: Early: Psychotropic medications and other biological treatments.

25. (C) significantly delayed by several months. Answer C is correct because at 6 months of age, a child should initiate head flexion when pulled into a sitting position. The child assists with pulling of the arms and some trunk flexion or use of the abdominals at this age. Usually by 2 months of age, an infant is beginning to assist with being pulled to sit with some head flexion. Answers A, B, and D are not correct because they do not address the significance of the child's delay in head control. See reference: Neistadt and Crepeau (eds): Kohlmeyer, K: Evaluation of sensory and neuromuscular performance components.

26. (A) a cotton ball. When retesting, it is important to use the same method used initially in order to make an accurate comparison of status before and after treatment. In addition, evaluation results are more consistent when the individual who performed the initial evaluation performs subsequent reevaluations. An aesthesiometer (answer B) is used to measure two-point discrimination, not light touch. Semmes-Weinstein monofilaments (answer C) are a good tool for assessing light touch thresholds but the results may not be as useful for comparison purposes. A pin or straightened paper clip (answer D) is used for testing superficial pain. See reference: Pedretti and Early (eds): Pedretti, LW and Iyer, MB: Evaluation of sensation and treatment of sensory dysfunction.

27. (C) have the individual perform a simple cooking task, then use a different food at the next session. Giving the individual a functional task, then changing it and observing how he responds, will tell the therapist how well the individual can transfer learning to new situations. If the individual can't perform the activity when it is changed slightly, it suggests there may be difficulty transferring learning. If the patient can perform the activity with many changes and in a different setting, it suggests that he has more a for transfer of learning to new situations. Answers A, B, and D could be ways of assessing different aspects of cognition (judgment, perceptual problem solving and ability to calculate figures), but as described, would not provide evidence of transfer of learning. See reference: Neistadt and Crepeau (eds): Neistadt, ME: Theories derived from learning perspectives.

28. (A) further observation and evaluation of right-sided dysfunction is indicated. Answer A is correct because infants usually use a bilateral approach at this age. Although unilaterality occurs several months later, most children alternate hands in many activities until age 6 years. This means that this infant should be observed for possible right-sided dysfunction. Answer B is incorrect because unilaterality at age 4 months is not typical development. Answer C is incorrect because hand dominance begins to develop at age 3 to 6 months, and answer D is incorrect because bilaterality precedes unilaterality in the course of infant development. See reference: Neistadt and Crepeau (eds): Kohlmeyer, K: Evaluation of sensory and neuromuscular performance components.

29. (D) Strength. Exerting enough pressure to twist off a jar lid requires strength. The client demonstrates adequate range of motion (answer A) when he grasps the knife. He demonstrates adequate coordination (answer B) by spreading peanut butter on the bread and accurately positioning the lid onto the jar opening. He demonstrates adequate endurance (answer C) by standing during the entire activity of making a peanut butter sandwich. See reference: AOTA: Uniform Terminology for Occupational Therapy, ed 3.

30. (C) Briefly interview the individual using closed-ended questions, targeting the individual's premorbid and current self-care performance levels. Severely depressed individuals often exhibit low self-esteem, lack of interest in personal appearance and hygiene, difficulty concentrating, and low energy, in addition to many other possible symptoms. A brief assessment would be indicated for an individual with a short attention span, and closed ended questions are usually easier to answer and require less energy to answer than open-ended questions (answer B). Having to demonstrate self-care tasks (answer A) would likely be frustrating for this individual, and a poor performance level could reinforce feelings of low self-esteem. Basing an initial assessment on observation (answer D) could prove a valid method, however, many factors other than limited ability could account for this individual's appearance. For example, this appearance may be typical of this individual's premorbid appearance, or the individual may not have had time to prepare herself prior to the scheduled evaluation. See reference: Early: Responding to symptoms and behaviors.

31. (D) motor planning. Motor planning or praxis problems are often seen in young children when they are dealing with novel equipment. Motor planning requires an adequate body concept and the ability to cognitively plan movements. Fine motor skills (answer A) are required for dexterity and manipulation and are not required for mounting a rocking horse. In order to climb into the highchair and jump on a trampoline, the child must have integrated reflexes (answer C) and adequate gross motor skills (answer B). See reference: AOTA: Uniform Terminology for Occupational Therapy, ed 3.

32. (B) boutonnière deformity. A boutonnière deformity is typically characterized by PIP joint flexion and DIP joint hyperextension. Answer A, a mallet deformity, is characterized by DIP joint flexion and a loss of active extension. Answer C is not a typical description used to describe a deformity. Answer D, a swan neck deformity, is characterized by PIP joint hyperextension and DIP joint flexion. See reference: Pedretti and Early (eds): Belkin, J and Yasuda, L: Orthotics.

33. (C) Interview a reliable informant instead of the individual. Individuals who are unable to think clearly, or who are experiencing memory loss, are often disturbed or frightened by this change, and may confabulate stories or answers to cover themselves. When an individual is unable or unwilling to provide accurate information, it may be necessary to use a reliable informant (answer C). This is often someone who lives with the individual and is able and willing to provide the necessary information. Using closed-ended questions (answer A) with this individual would not necessarily yield more accurate information, but can be useful when specific information is being sought, or to more effectively structure or control an interview situation. This individual is unlikely to do any better with a written questionnaire than an oral interview. However, written questionnaires (answer D) may be used effectively with individuals with the requisite cognitive skills. There is no reason to think the individual would be any more reliable the next day (answer B). See reference: Early: Data collection and evaluation.

34. (A) Loosening nuts and bolts. Loosening nuts and bolts is the activity that most closely resembles a tip or lateral prehension activity. Prehension is a hand position that permits finger and thumb contact while facilitating the manipulation of objects. Answers B, C, and D are more closely related to grasping activities, which encourage contact of an object against the palm and the flexed digits. See reference: Pedretti and Early (eds): Breines, EB: Therapeutic occupations and modalities.

35. (A) sequencing of picture symbols. A person needs to use picture symbols to indicate a two or more part thought or sequence of activities. For example, pointing to pictures of a shoe and a closet would indicate the place to find a shoe in response to a question. Understanding letters or words (answers B and C), and then sequencing them (answer D), are significantly higher level skills than recognizing and sequencing pictures. See reference: Angelo and Lane (eds): Angelo, J: Written and spoken augmentative communication.

36. (A) Improve posture, then improve shoulder stability, then improve grasp. Because the proximal-to-distal approach begins at the center of the body, then proceeds to the extremities, answer A is correct. Postural stability would be developed first, then shoulder stability, and then grasping patterns. Answers B, C, and D are incorrect because they do not follow this order. See reference: Case-Smith (ed): Exner, CE: Development of hand skills.

37. (B) detachable arms. Armrests will need to be removed to allow the individual to move sideways out of the wheelchair. Footrests (answer A) may be swung away, but do not need to be detached to perform a transfer. Anti-tip bars (answer C) prevent a wheelchair from tipping over backwards when performing a wheelie or when going up or down a step, but not when transferring. Brake-handle extensions (answer D) allow the brakes to be locked more easily, but would be in the way of a board transfer. See reference: Pedretti and Early (eds): Adler, C and Titon-Burton, M: Wheelchair assessment and transfers.

38. (B) We will be working together to achieve your goals. The relationship that an OT practitioner develops with a client is "...a partnership which makes the client an active participant in the treatment process" (p. 282), exemplified by the statement in answer B, which reflects a collaborative therapeutic alliance. Answer A suggests that the central focus of OT treatment is the development of the therapeutic relationship. This relationship is instrumental in the therapy process, but not the central focus of the therapy. Although it shares a few characteristics of friendship, the therapeutic relationship is significantly different, because it requires the OT practitioner to understand the client's needs and values, as well as to understand and manage the OT practitioner's own reactions. Therefore, answer C is incorrect. Empathy, rather than sympathy, is recommended in therapeutic relationships, so the statement in answer D is also incorrect. See reference: Neistadt and Crepeau (eds): Peloquin, SM: The therapeutic relationship. Seymour, SG: Evaluation of psychosocial skills and psychological components.

39. (B) High contrast and defined borders. Visual material that is adapted as in answer B, high contrast and defined borders, provides the only combination of features that assist children with visual discrimination problems. High contrast of the stimuli (shape, letter, number, and so on) in relation to the background, and defining important areas of the stimuli with a border, attract the eye, and provide clear input. Answer A is incorrect because low contrast of the stimuli, such as blue ditto lettering, is difficult for the eyes to discriminate. Answer C, undefined borders around the important stimuli, make for less clear input. In answer D, both low contrast and unclear borders, would make visual discrimination difficult. See reference: Kramer and Hinojosa (eds): Todd, VR: Visual information analysis: Frame of reference for visual perception.

40. (A) Getting dressed without becoming fatigued. Prevention of fatigue is the primary purpose of energy conservation. Energy conservation techniques may often result in slower, not faster (answer D), performance. Using proper body mechanics may enable an individual with back pain to lift heavy cookware without pain (answer B). Using joint protection techniques may prevent further joint damage to arthritic hands when the patient is doing handicrafts (answer C). See reference: Pedretti and Early (eds): Buckner, WS: Arthritis.

41. (B) writing a soap opera. Although answers A, C, and D would benefit the self-confidence and stress management needs of women struggling with the issues associated with emotional and physical abuse, they are not expressive group activities. Writing a soap opera would most likely be a creative approach implemented to assist individuals in expressing their inner thoughts, feelings, anxieties, and beliefs. See reference: Early: Group concepts and techniques.

42. (D) weight bearing over a small bolster in prone. Weight bearing on the arms can help with overall inhibition of tone before participating in hand skill activities. Inhibition of flexor spasticity occurs through slow joint compression from weight bearing, as well as facilitation of ulnar to radial function in the hand. Answers A and B are incorrect because they require voluntary control of the release of objects without inhibition. Answer C is incorrect because traction on the finger flexors would increase spasticity in the flexor muscles, and make opening of the hand more difficult. See reference: Case-Smith (ed): Exner, CE: Development of hand skills.

43. (B) conditional reasoning. Conditional reasoning is a form of clinical reasoning that takes into account various systems and dynamics involved with the patient and his or her illness or injury. This approach is more "holistic," in that it takes into account the "whole patient" as he or she functions and interacts within his or her environment. Reasoning based on corresponding an individual's deficits and physical symptoms with a procedure that may benefit the area of need is referred to as procedural reasoning (answer A). Interactive reasoning (answer C) is a process by which the practitioner and patient collaborate so that the practitioner may better understand the patient's environment or situation. Narrative reasoning (answer D) is a form of "story telling" in which practitioners share similar experiences, allowing for problem solving to occur. See reference: Mattingly and Fleming: Fleming, MH: The therapist with the three-track mind.

44. (A) specific measurable statements with time frames. Goals can be either short term (i.e., in the immediate future) or long term (i.e., over an extended period). The purpose of a goal is to provide a specific statement that is measurable and indicates what is to be accomplished. Patients and significant others play vital roles in working with the therapist to establish goals that are meaningful and realistic. Time frames (answer B) may be only a part of a measurable goal or objective. Specific measurements of the patient's skill and performance (answer C) are parts of the assessment information that assists the therapist in establishing appropriate goals and objectives for treatment. Activities to be completed that correspond with the goals (answer D) are part of the objective and treatment plan. See reference: AOTA: The Occupational Therapy Manager: Acquaviva, JD: Documentation of occupational therapy services.

45. (A) Sit straddling a bolster with both feet on the floor. Once the child has learned to sit independently on the floor, an external stabilizing support is no longer necessary (answer D). After having developed independent postural reactions on a stable surface, that is, the floor, the child can further refine sitting skills by learning to maintain posture when placed on an unstable surface. At first, the child should be left in control of the movement on this surface, and she should have both feet on the floor for maximal stability. Later, these skills can be refined by placing the child on more challenging surfaces, such as on a "hippity-hop" (answer C) or on a scooter pulled by another person (answer B). See reference:

Case-Smith (ed): Nichols, DS: The development of postural control.

46. (C) Wrist splints to promote development of tenodesis. Hand splinting to promote tenodesis is implemented in the acute phase of rehabilitation. A tenodesis grasp is developed by allowing the finger flexors to shorten. The patient is then able to achieve a functional grasp by extending the wrist. This improves the ability of an individual with a C6 or C7 spinal cord injury to grasp and hold objects. A volar pan splint (answer A) would not allow finger flexors to shorten, and would interfere with the development of tenodesis. Interventions related to promoting independent performance (answer B) should begin as soon as possible, but issues related to positioning must be addressed first. An individual would not be instructed in bed mobility (answer D) until after the acute phase. See reference: Pedretti and Early (eds): Adler, C: Spinal cord injury.

47. (C) Implement compensatory strategies to manage the environment. Interventions directed toward improvement are typically unrealistic when working with individuals diagnosed with progressive cognitive disorders. "Since improvement is not generally expected, therapy seeks to maintain maximum functioning as long as possible through the teaching of compensatory strategies and by careful environmental management" (p. 131). These disorders are characterized by deteriorating courses. A social skills emphasis (answer A) is more appropriate for individuals with schizophrenia. Habit restructuring (answer B) is more appropriate for those with substance abuse disorders. Role resumption (answer D) is more appropriate for those with mood disorders. See reference: Early: Understanding psychiatric diagnosis: The DSM-IV.

48. (C) Design an individualized program directed at the underlying neurologic deficit. Sensory integration is a complex treatment modality that is a highly individualized form of treatment carried out by a therapist with advanced training and understanding in the area of neuroscience. Answer A is incorrect because the child's program is not being "individualized," but is included in a group program. Answer B is not correct because sensory integration treatment is active and requires an adaptive response from the child. Answer D is not correct because sensory integration is directed at improving underlying neurologic functioning rather than skill development. See reference: Neistadt and Crepeau (eds): Baloueff, O: Sensory integration.

49. (C) Passive ROM, positioning, and splinting. The initial phase of treatment for the individual with Guillain-Barré syndrome includes PROM, splinting, and positioning to protect weak muscles and prevent contractures. This should be followed by gentle, nonresistive activities and light ADLs (answer A) as tolerated. Resistive exercises, and balance and stabilization activities (answers B and D) should be implemented later after strength begins to improve. See reference: Pedretti and Early (eds): Lehman, RM and McCormack, GL: Neurogenic and myopathic dysfunction.

50. (A) a can of soup. Grading activities according to complexity is an important part of the therapist's selection of appropriate activities for each individual. Complexity increases as the number of steps, number of different ingredients or tools used, and time to complete the task increases. Answers B, C, and D all require more steps, materials, and time than preparing a can of soup. See reference: Neistadt and Crepeau (eds): Neistadt, ME: Overview of treatment.

51. (A) Drawing a picture entitled "This is me." Children who have trouble expressing their emotions verbally are sometimes able to express their feelings in open-ended drawing activities. Among the answers given, answer A is the only projective activity. Answers B, C, and D are highly structured activities with minimal potential for open-ended expression. See reference: Case-Smith (ed): Cronin, AS: Psychosocial and emotional domains.

52. (C) have the individual visualize the task first and then provide general statements such as "Let's get ready." Answer C is correct because visualizing a task and its movement sequences helps the individual with motor apraxia by giving a visual model to refer to during the activity. Using general comments such as "let's get ready", rather than specific step-by-step directions, is more effective because individuals with motor apraxia have difficulty imitating or initiating motor tasks on command, though they understand the concept of the task. Answer A, step-by-step commands, would add to the confusion for an individual with motor apraxia, but would be helpful for the individual with ideational apraxia who may not understand the concept of the task, but may be able to perform individual steps of the task on command. Removing visual distractions and enhancing the visual environment, as in answer C, is useful for individuals with visual perceptual deficits, rather than motor apraxia. Answer D, having the individual move slowly and touch objects during the task, is a method aimed at improving spatial relations' perception. See reference: Gillen and Burkardt (eds): Rubio, KB: Treatment of neurobehavioral deficits.

53. (C) Copper tooling using a template. When choosing activities to address self-competence and self-confidence, it is important first to choose activities that are relatively simple, structured, of short duration, and guaranteed to provide a successful experience to the patient. Answers A and B are fairly complex projects that require decision making, several sessions to complete, and have the potential for problems in any of the many stages of construction. Although they may be appropriate later in the treatment program, they are contraindicated at the beginning of treatment. Learning to play bridge (answer D) may be a good choice when addressing development of leisure activities, but it also involves learning a series of steps and interacting with others, requirements that are premature at this stage in treatment. See reference: Early: Responding to symptoms and behaviors.

54. (A) the therapist has the child play "sandwich" between heavy mats. The sandwich activity provides heavy touch pressure over the child's body, which can be inhibitory to a child experiencing sensory defensiveness. Answer B is incorrect because light use of a feather brush stimulates the light touch system, which is already impaired, and would be extremely uncomfortable for a child with tactile defensiveness. Answer C is not correct because the use of a blindfold, when a child is already reacting to unexpected touch, would most likely create a fearful response in a child with tactile defensiveness. Answer D, although not using a blindfold, has an unexpected touch from the back and this would also aggravate the child's existing problem. Answer A, the use of proprioceptive input to break through the protective response to light touch, will initially treat the child's defensiveness problem instead of stimulating further reaction. See reference: Kramer and Hinojosa (eds): Kimball, JG: Sensory integration frame of reference: Theoretical base, function/dysfunction continua and guide to evaluation.

55. (D) A volar pan splint for hand and wrist. A volar pan splint is indicated for the wrist, fingers, and thumb joints during acute synevitis. Answer B is indicated for wrist pain and to protect the extensor tendons from rupture. Answer C is a splint used to prevent ulnar drift, while maintaining joint alignment for grasp and pinch activities. Answer A assists in keeping the MP joints in normal alignment, while preventing volar subluxation. See reference: Pedretti and Early (eds): Buckner, WS: Arthritis.

56. (C) games of chance. Because winning a game of chance is based essentially on luck, individuals functioning at various functional levels have "equal" opportunities to win. Hobbies (answer B) are not considered to be a game category. Competitive and strategy games (answers A and D) both require specific skills to succeed. See reference: Early: Leisure skills.

57. (B) wide-base sitting on the floor while reaching for a suspended balloon. The child first practices skills in unsupported sitting on a stable surface, using a wide base of support. As skills improve, the wide base is reduced to a more narrow one. Reaching activities are used to promote postural reactions, because they involve displacement of the center of gravity and weight shifting. Answers A, C, and D are activities involving unstable support surfaces, typical of more advanced skills. See reference: Case-Smith (ed): Nichols, DS: The development of postural control.

58. (D) resume the homemaker role. The Commission on Accreditation of Rehabilitation Facilities defines work hardening as "a highly structured, goal oriented, individualized treatment program designed to maximize a person's ability to return to work" (p. 553). A homemaker's job is working in the home. A work-hardening program would not focus on obtaining employment outside the home (answer A), nor resuming leisure activities (answer B) for this individual. Although a work-hardening program may help to reduce pain levels (answer C), the emphasis is on a return to work in this case, resuming the homemaker role (answer D). See reference: Pedretti and Early (eds): Burt, CM: Work evaluation and work hardening.

59. (B) holding a class about job-seeking strategies. The purpose of applying remedial strategies is to enhance underlying abilities. Teaching and training methods are commonly used techniques. Answer A, an interest checklist, is a tool used to identify the degree of an individual's interest in a variety of leisure areas. Answer C is an example of a compensatory strategy. Answer D provides opportunities for exploration and expression. See reference: Early: Data collection and evaluation.

60. (C) multisensory input. Each of the possible four answers describes appropriate treatment interventions for infants in the NICU. However, an infant approaching full term or post term is now equipped with a maturing sensory system tolerant, and in demand of, a multisensory diet including oral stimulation, vestibular input, and auditory and visual orientation, to assist with age appropriate motor and behavioral skill acquisition. Often these very premature infants are limited in the amount of social interaction and appropriate sensory stimuli, because of necessary medical equipment and procedures (e.g., ventilators, IV catheters, isolettes, warmers, bililights, and nasogastric tubing). Therefore, stable, growing post-term premature infants would most benefit from a multisensory diet (answer C) to best meet the demands of their maturing sensory system and to capitalize on their socialization skills. Answers A, B, and D are all possible treatments for the 32 to 35-week-old infant who responds best to unimodal sensory input and minimal direct intervention, e.g., ROM and positioning, because of immature sensory systems and compromised respiratory systems. See reference: Case-Smith (ed): Hunter, JG: Neonatal Intensive Care Unit.

61. (D) slicing a prepared roll of sugar cookies at room temperature and placing them on a tray using a spatula. Answer D describes the lowest level of physical exertion and may be completed within the time frame designated by the therapist. The sugar cookie dough (answer D) would be soft enough to provide minimal resistance without causing immediate fatigue. In addition, the activity provides for isotonic contractions during the repetitive grasp and release of the knife and the spatula. Although muffin and cake batter (answers A and B) provide the least amount of resistance, the hand is using sustained isometric grasp on the electric or hand powered mixer, which combined with the minimal resistance of the batter and mixer weight, is fatiguing. The chocolate chip cookie dough (answer C) is resistive, whether it is warm or cold, and to maintain an isometric grasp while mixing with a spatula or scooping with an ice cream scooper, would cause the individual to fatigue before the activity is finished. If the individual becomes fatigued while performing any of the activities, only the sugar cookies or the chocolate chip cookies would allow the individual time to rest without affecting the final product. See reference: Trombly (ed): Stewart, C: Retraining housekeeping and child care skills.

62. (C) state simple, concrete directions allowing time for delayed responses. Answer C is correct because, "many patients with TBI exhibit concrete thinking, in which they are able to interpret information only at the most literal level" (p. 681). Since processing of information is also an area of difficulty, allowing time for delayed responses is frequently necessary. Answer A, telling the person what is expected and asking them to begin would require abstract thinking and initiation of activities—both areas that are likely to be impaired. Answers B and C, relying on gestures, and providing written directions with pictures, may not be effective if visual perception is impaired. See reference: Pedretti and Early (eds): Gutman, SA: Traumatic brain injury.

63. (A) Use socks with a wide opening. "A wide sock opening can prevent frustration during the most difficult part of putting on socks, which is inserting the toes" (p. 235). Answer B, a sock aid, may be a viable option, but at times, "these aids can be difficult to use...however, they may benefit children with limited reaching, coordination, and lower extremity functioning" (p. 235). Answer C, nylon tights, are typically more difficult to put on independently because of the elastic quality of the material and the high level of balance required. Answer D, utilizing a sock with a narrow opening, will also make it more difficult to put on because the child will not have as much room to insert her toes. See reference: Solomon (ed): Jones, LMW and Machover, PZ: Occupational performance areas: Daily living and work and productive activities.

64. (B) Working on a mock car engine. Working on a mock car engine provides a work simulation that would be required by the client's job. This activity would also assist with increasing his endurance, strength, and productivity. Answer A, lifting weights, is not a work hardening goal when performed in isolation of a simulated work task. Answer C, visiting the work site, would not be a work hardening activity, but rather part of the onsite analysis that is typically completed by the practitioner and vocational retraining counselor. Answer D, meal preparation, is not considered to be a demand required by this particular vocation. See reference: Pedretti and Early (eds): Kasch, MC and Nickerson, E: Hand and upper extremity injuries.

65. (D) A problem-solving task with a "self-talk" cueing strategy. Finding telephone numbers is a task that requires some problem solving, and the card is a strategy for providing cues for questioning oneself about the process of problem solving. Answer A is incorrect because self-management is a component of psychosocial, rather than cognitive performance. The task requires visual scanning (answer B) of the telephone book to accomplish, but that is not the primary focus of the task. Answer C, a memory task, is incorrect because the performance of this task is not primarily dependent on the use of memory skills and the questions posed relate to the problem solving process. See reference: Neistadt and Crepeau (eds): Toglia, JP: Cognitive-perceptual retraining and rehabilitation.

66. (C) working on simple puzzles to enhance attention span. "The role of the occupational therapist is to support the child's ability to successfully perform the occupations related that to environment", and to "...increase independence in daily activities such as play, self-care, classroom maintenance and preacademic skills" (p. 734). Enhancing a child's attention span is an important preacademic skill. Activities listed in answers A and B are not activities that are more appropriate for school age children. Answer D, practicing shoe tying, is a self-help skill, but one not which is typically achieved until a child is older. See reference: Case-Smith (ed): Gartland, S and Dubois, SA: Occupational therapy in preschool and childcare settings.

67. (A) Stop the activity. Activity should be stopped immediately when symptoms occur during treatment of an acute cardiac patient. Symptoms, including confusion, shortness of breath, profuse sweating, cold skin, clammy skin, chest pain, nausea, and lightheadedness, should be reported to the physician. After the session is over, symptoms should be documented (answer B). Continuing the activity, whether seated or with the patient's permission (answers C and D), is dangerous and may result in further cardiac damage. See reference: Dutton: Introduction to biomechanical frame of reference.

68. (C) instructing caregivers in task breakdown. Instructing the client's caregivers in task breakdown, or breaking down tasks into simple steps and then providing step-by-step instructions, will allow the client to perform activities as capabilities decline. At this stage of the disease, memory retraining (answer A) and ADL retraining (answer B)

will probably not be effective. Leisure activities (answer D) structured to meet the needs of the client with Alzheimer's disease could be helpful, but will not address the primary problem of performance of self-care activities. See reference: Pedretti and Early (eds): Schultz-Krohn, W, Foti, D, and Glogoski, C: Degenerative diseases of the central nervous system.

69. (D) Digging in "Play Doh" to search for various coins and then placing them in a piggy bank. The most appropriate selection the COTA can make is to encourage the child to work on fine motor skills since this child will most likely rely on signing as a way to communicate. "The movements of the hands of a fluent signer require opposition, finger and thumb flexion and extension, and finger and thumb abduction and adduction. The hand's coordination seems to be related to its sensory abilities, particularly tactile discrimination" (thus introducing the "Play Doh") (p. 784). "The therapist can enhance kinesthetic, tactile, and visual processing through multi-sensory activities" (p. 783). Answer A, parachute activities, are indicated for gross motor and/or kinesthetic needs, but are not necessarily related to the child's fine motor limitations. Answer B, visually coding the child's shoes, is an appropriate choice when attempting to encourage self-care skills. "Adapting techniques or assistive devices may be needed. At times self-care skills involve concrete concepts that require concrete cues for the child to learn" (p. 784). While answer C, introducing the child to socialization groups, would be appropriate to address because many children with hearing impairments feel isolated from the hearing community, the goal of the COTA in this scenario is to address the child's fine motor limitations. See reference: Case-Smith (ed): Snow-Russel, E: Services for children with visual or auditory impairments.

70. (B) Implement a pureed diet and allow adequate time for eating. As ALS progresses, speaking and swallowing become more difficult and a pureed diet becomes necessary. The individual runs the risk of aspiration or choking if meals are rushed. Adaptive equipment (answers A and D), are provided much earlier in the disease process. The independence achieved with adaptive equipment has a positive psychological effect on the individual who most likely sees his or her independence slipping away. Answer C, upper extremity strengthening, would be contraindicated in the late stages of the disease. See reference: Pedretti and Early (eds): Schultz-Krohn, W, Foti, D, and Glogoski, C: Degenerative diseases of the central nervous system.

71. (C) Incorporating simple, familiar activities such as hanging up clothing or catching a ball. Incorporating simple activities would be most effective for gaining active cooperation participation from a person with Alzheimer's. Telling the person to perform repetitions of active exercises (answer A) might not be effective because the patient may not be able to remember to perform repetitions of exercises or may not understand the purpose and become confused. Training in the use of adaptive devices (answer B) would not increase active shoulder motion and could be confusing if cognitive deficits were present. PROM exercises (answer D) would not lead to improvement of active range of motion. See reference: Hellen: Communication: Understanding and being understood.

72. (D) sitting position. Answer D is correct because an upright sitting position provides the child with the opportunity not only to further control head movement (stability has developed in horizontal positions), weight bearing, and weight shifting, but also to rotate the trunk as he or she reaches towards the opposite side of the body. Answers A and B are not correct because head and neck stability have most likely developed primarily in the prone and sidelying positions, before the child's attaining a seated position. See reference: Kramer and Hinojosa (eds): Schoen, SA and Anderson, J: Neurodevelopmental treatment frame of reference.

73. (A) contrast baths, active and passive range of motion, and massage. Contrast baths, active and passive range of motion, and massage are all initial techniques considered for the prevention or relief of joint stiffness. Answers B and D, ultrasound, electrical stimulation, dynamic splinting, and joint mobilization are all considered treatment techniques for more established joint stiffness. Answer C, resistive exercises, weight bearing, and lifting could all potentially contribute to increasing joint stiffness and pain. See reference: Pedretti and Early (eds): Kasch, MC and Nickerson, E: Hand and upper extremity injuries.

74. (D) inform medical team members immediately. Giving away personal items and discussing issues related to death can be signs of suicidal intent. Any indication that a person is considering suicide is extremely serious and must be reported to other medical team members immediately so that the potential for suicide can be psychiatrically evaluated and addressed. Answers A, B, and C are actions that may be appropriate under other circumstances, but none is critical to the immediate safety of the client, which is the most important priority in this case. See reference: Early: Safety techniques.

75. (A) Shoulder flexion and protraction. Answer A is correct because the infant changes from extensor influences on posture to development of flexion in the supine position. This requires the ability to flex and protract the shoulders against gravity in order to reach forward and upward to grasp toys. Answer B is not correct because shoulder extension and retraction would not be encouraged during supine activities when the toys are placed overhead. Answers C and D are not correct because most activities of

looking and reaching can be accomplished without using head or trunk control against gravity in the supine position. See reference: Kramer and Hinojosa (eds): Colangelo, CA: Biomechanical frame of reference.

76. (C) to both sides of the client's body. Answer C is correct because the client must be able to transfer to both sides of the body. It is usually difficult, or impossible, to arrange the home environment so that the all transfers can be done from one side only. For instance, if the toilet at home is close to the wall, getting on and off the toilet will require transfer first to one side of the body and then to the opposite side. The family also needs to know the different kinds, and amounts of support, they must use on each side of the client's body. Thus, answers A, B, and D are incorrect because they all involve transfer to only one side. See reference: Trombly (ed): Retraining basic and instrumental activities of daily living.

77. (A) Assembling a complex airplane model requiring use of detailed directions. Assembling a complex airplane model would be the best choice, because it has many of the activity characteristics that appeal to a person with paranoid schizophrenia (e.g., it is complicated enough to engage the person intellectually and sustain his interest), and it uses controllable materials and requires organization to complete. Answer B, finishing and painting a reassembled wooden box, would be insufficiently challenging. Answer C, playing a game of chess, is intellectually challenging, but presents an element of competition that can be threatening to a person with this diagnosis. Answer D, engaging in a reminiscence discussion, requires a degree of self-disclosure through the sharing of previous experiences and feelings that might prove disturbing for this patient. See reference: Early: Responding to symptoms and behaviors.

78. (B) Help the child develop cognitive strategies for anxiety-producing activities. Children with innate temperament problems need cognitive strategies to help them overcome anxiety in order to approach and participate in activities. Parents need to understand the innate temperament problem and the discomfort the child feels during activities, and limit setting (answer A) will not promote understanding. Children find a predictable routine helpful when activities are disorganized, so answer C is not correct. Answer D is not correct because the parent and child need to learn mutual play in an environment that promotes positive engagement. See reference: Kramer and Hinojosa (eds): Olson, LJ: Psychosocial frame of reference.

79. (D) Lock the brakes. Brakes should be locked first to stabilize the wheelchair. Answers A, B, and C involve movements that could cause loss of balance or wheelchair movement unless the brakes are locked. See reference: Pedretti and Early (eds): Adler, C and Tipton-Burton, M: Wheelchair assessment and transfers.

80. (D) position the patient so she is facing a blank wall. One way to modify the environment for this individual who is easily distracted is to position her facing a blank wall (answer D), thereby lessening possible distracters. It may also be necessary to speak loudly to get the patient's attention, which is why answer A is not recommended. If the patient is still unable to participate in the activity successfully, the COTA should direct her to a simpler activity. Coaxing and praising (answer B) will not increase her skill level. Asking the rest of the group members to stop talking (answer C) would probably interfere with the goals of the rest of the group. See reference: Early: Responding to symptoms and behaviors.

81. (B) Teach the child to dress her hemiparetic extremities first. Occupational therapy practitioners, "help children compensate for delays or deficits in performance by adapting activities or applying assistive technology...A child with hemiparesis is taught to dress his or her affected extremities first" (p. 10). Answer A (dressing in bed) is also considered to be an adapted technique, but would be most appropriate for an individual with poor balance. While answer C, educating the child's mother regarding dressing, is something the COTA would do at some point in the occupational therapy process dependent upon the child's age, it is not something the COTA would do to encourage independent dressing skills for an 8-year-old child. Finally, answer D, teaching the child to dress her non-hemiparetic extremities first, is not considered an adaptive skill, since this technique will typically interfere with independent dressing skill development. See reference: Case-Smith (ed): Case-Smith, J: An overview of occupational therapy for children.

82. (B) Bend both knees, keep the back straight, and bring the object close to the body when lifting. Bending with both knees while keeping the back straight and the object close to the body (answer B), will prevent low back bending and strain. Answers A, C, and D are all incorrect methods for lifting and carrying objects. Answers A and C will actually increase an individual's chance of increasing low back strain. See reference: Pedretti and Early (eds): Smithline, J and Dunlop, LE: Low back pain.

83. (B) stringing beads for a necklace, following a pattern. This is the only activity of those listed that requires the individual to follow a sequence to achieve the desired outcome. Leather stamping in a random design (answer A) does not require sequencing skills, but does require coordination, visual-motor integration, and strength. Putting together a puzzle (answer C) requires perception of spatial relations. Playing "Concentration" (answer D) requires memory and attention span. See reference: AOTA:

Uniform Terminology for Occupational Therapy, ed 3.

84. (A) A tub seat with a hand-held shower attached to the faucet. Answer A would be the most appropriate choice, because an individual with paraplegia would most likely be able to transfer himself out of the wheelchair and onto a tub seat. Because the child will not have use of his legs, a hand-held shower would permit the child to wash without having to adjust the faucet overhead. Answer B, a hydraulic lift, would be indicated for an obese individual or for someone who has very limited function of both the upper and lower extremities. Answer C would also be used for an individual with limited function, in that the child can be rolled onto the tub prior to its inflation. Answer D, a wheeled shower chair, would be a choice made for washing in a shower, not a tub. The chair can simply be rolled into a stall. See reference: Solomon (ed): Jones, LMW and Machover, PZ: Occupational performance areas: Daily living and work and productive activities

85. (D) Loose-fitting clothing. Individuals with paraplegia can dress independently. The process is somewhat easier when loose fitting clothing and dressing loops are used. Buttonhook zipper pull devices and clip-on ties (answers A and B) are useful for individuals without the hand function required to button, pull a zipper, or tie a tie. Individuals with C6 through C8 quadriplegia usually require assistance to put on shoes, but may be able to put on specially adapted shoes independently. See reference: Christiansen (ed): Garber, SL, Gregorio, TL, Pumphrey, N, and Lathem, P: Self-care strategies for persons with spinal cord injuries.

86. (B) Discussing one's problems with an empathetic listener. One goal of stress management intervention is to identify "...behaviors that in the past have been effective in making us feel more relaxed, less anxious, and generally more secure about ourselves" (p. 437). Verbalization of stressful feelings and problems (answer B) is an effective stress coping strategy that also serves to reinforce connection with reality. Answers A and D, visual imagery and progressive relaxation of muscles, are effective relaxation techniques, but are typically performed with the eyes closed, which may increase psychosis and the effect of hallucinations. Engaging in a familiar activity may help relieve stressful feelings, but engaging in a new or too challenging activity (answer C) could add stress. See reference: Stein and Cutler: Stress management, biofeedback and relaxation techniques.

87. (C) use a calm and soothing voice, informing the child about each step of the hair wash prior to doing it. "Even if the child does not yet understand language, each time hair is shampooed and dried, use a soothing voice to repeat what will happen next. The rhythmic repetition of words can be calming. If the child understands the words, knowing what is going to happen next can lessen anxiety" (p. 245). Answers A and B would not be appropriate strategies, because washing the hair with only water or waiting until the child goes to the barber, would not be efficient techniques to maintain proper hygiene in a young child. Answer D, the use of cool water, can actually be contraindicated. Water temperature should be warm, not hot, to increase relaxation. See reference: Solomon (ed): Jones, LMW and Machover, PZ: Occupational performance areas: Daily living and work and productive activities.

88. (A) clearly direct a caregiver in preferred head position, food portion size, and choice of food to eat. An individual with C3 quadriplegia lacks the strength necessary to use an MAS or any cuff device (answers B, C, and D). It remains important for this individual to be able to instruct a caregiver how to assist with feeding in a manner that is pleasant and enjoyable. See reference: Christiansen (ed): Garber, SL, Gregorio, TL, Pumphrey, N, and Lathem, P: Self-care strategies for persons with spinal cord injuries.

89. (A) "It sounds as if you're not sure whether you are ready to be discharged." Paraphrasing is repeating what someone has said in your own words. Chitchat (answer B) is a conversational response unrelated to what the individual said. Confrontation (answer D) is a response that requires the individual to acknowledge difficult or painful issues. Proposing a solution (answer C) does not help the individual improve his or her decision making skills or sense of competence. See reference: Denton: Effective communication.

90. (D) A pediatric weighted utensil holder. "Children who lack sensory discrimination skills in the hands use the weighted holder. The weight increases proprioceptive (deep-pressure) feedback to the joints and muscles in the hand and wrist, adding to children's awareness of the position and movement of the hand, fingers, and wrist in relation to the pencil and paper" (p. 264). Answers A and C, a wide pen and soft triangle grip, would assist a child with decreased grip, while answer B, rubber bands, would assist a child who has difficulty opposing their thumb into the web space. See reference: Solomon (ed): Jones, LMW and Machover, PZ:Occupational performance areas: Daily living and work and productive activities

91. (C) Work hardening. Work hardening programs are designed to include and/or simulate job related tasks that gradually progress the client to obtain the skills that meet the actual demands of a job. Continuing to perform a home exercise program, and discontinuing OT services, (answers A and D), would probably not enable the client to return to the work force after a 3 month absence. Home health OT (answer B) is only appropriate for individuals who

are unable to leave their homes to attend outpatient occupational therapy. See reference: Pedretti and Early (eds): Burt, CM: Work evaluation and work hardening.

92. (D) Sitting in a circle and reciting a short poem. The purpose of a closure activity in a five-stage group is to provide a familiar activity to end the group on a positive, affirming note. Answer A is an orientation activity (stage I). Answer B is typical of an activity that would be used to transition from visual perceptual (stage III) to cognitive activities (stage IV). Answer C is a movement activity (stage II). See reference: Ross and Bachner (eds): Ross, M: A five-stage model for adults with developmental disabilities.

93. (C) Backward chaining. In backward chaining, the COTA completes all of the steps of a task except the last one. As the child becomes competent, the COTA completes all but the last two steps, and so on, until the child is able to perform the entire activity. This method provides immediate gratification, and is particularly useful for children with low frustration tolerance and poor self-esteem. Physical guidance (answer A) requires the least amount of cognitive ability, and provides the child the opportunity to learn through a sensory motor experience. Verbal cues (answer B) may be perceived as intrusive and critical by children with low self-esteem. Forward chaining (answer D) begins with the child completing the first step and the practitioner completing the rest. When competent, the child progressively takes on more of the steps. This method is beneficial for individuals who have difficulty with sequencing and generalizing skills. See reference: Case-Smith (ed): Shepherd, J: Self-care and adaptations for independent living.

94. (B) seating the patient upright on a firm surface with the chin slightly tucked. The best position for feeding an individual with a swallowing disorder is upright and symmetrical, with their chin slightly tucked (answer B). Supine, semi-reclined, and sidelying positions (answers A, C, and D) all place the patient at greater risk for choking and aspiration. See reference: Pedretti and Early (eds): Nelson-Jenks, K: Dysphagia.

95. (D) Demonstrate how using a shower chair improves safety. Educating the client is the first response the COTA should make. By describing and demonstrating the shower chair and how it makes showering safer, the COTA is conveying the concept that occupational performance is based on the interaction of performance contexts (physical environment) and performance components (the confidence to execute tasks safely). The COTA would then inquire about the client's desire to purchase a shower chair (answer B). Getting into a bathtub is even more dangerous than getting into the shower (answer A), so this is not a viable option. Answer D, explaining the therapy, will increase the client's confidence level is a subjective belief of the COTA's that may not be embraced by the client due to his very valid fear of falling. See reference: Piersol and Ehrlich (eds): Seibert, C: The clinic called home.

96. (B) Tell the client that you don't mind appropriately discussing sexuality-related questions, as long as his parents are comfortable with the idea. "While working with adolescents on personal self-care tasks such as bathing or personal hygiene, sexuality questions may arise. Children and adolescents of all disabilities are sexual beings. Their parents may be receptive to discussing their child's sexuality, or they may feel unprepared to address these issues. When the child is less than 18 years of age, parental permission to discuss sexuality issues is necessary" (p. 518). Answer A, referring the client to a psychologist, would be an appropriate response if the parent's agreed to the idea, and if the treating clinician did not feel comfortable or knowledgeable regarding the topic of sexuality. Answer C, attempting to change the subject, may encourage the child to feel inadequate, frustrated or more confused regarding his sexuality. It is important to remember that "children of all disabilities are sexual beings" (p. 518). Answer D, answering the client's questions, would only be appropriate after seeking the permission of the child's parents to discuss the topic of sexuality. See reference: Case-Smith (ed): Shepherd, J: Self-care and adaptations for independent living.

97. (D) Ice application, immobilization, and splinting. Ice application, immobilization, and splinting (answer D) are all interventions that are considered to be appropriate adjunct activities to be used during the acute stages of tennis elbow. Answers A, B, and C, are all contraindicated because of their potential to increase edema, pain, and immobility, during an acute flare up of epicondylitis. See reference: Cailliet: Elbow pain.

98. (B) Provide clear, safe pathways for wandering. Environments designed to allow individuals to wander safely at will can be a source of satisfaction for the client, while at the same time eliminating the need for constant supervision by staff. Gates and redirection (answers A and C) will not satisfy the individual's desire to pace or roam. Negative reinforcement (answer D) in this situation would be counterproductive. See reference: Neistadt and Crepeau (eds): Holm, MB, Rogers, JC and James, AB: Treatment of activities of daily living.

99. (C) Foam tubing around the utensils. Foam tubing would be the best choice because it increases the diameter of the utensils, thus permitting an easier grip. Answer A, swivel utensils, are most appropriate for children who experience incoordination or tremors, while answer B, pediatric universal holders, are commonly introduced when a child has no grip at all. In this case, the cuff can be directly attached to the child's hand while the utensils, are inserted into the sleeve of the cuff. Answer D, weighted utensils would not assist the child with decreased grip, but may assist a child with motor incoordination. See reference: Solomon (ed): Jones, LMW and Machover, PZ: Occupational performance areas: Daily living and work and productive activities.

100. (C) ask another OT/PT practitioner for assistance. Trying to attempt this transfer alone could result in injury to the patient and/or the OT practitioner, even if she uses proper body mechanics (answer A). It is often necessary to get assistance when transferring obese individuals. Asking someone else to do a difficult task answer B) is not professional. If the patient needs to be transferred, not transferring him (answer D) is not an option. See reference: Pedretti and Early (eds): Adler, C and Tipton-Burton, M: Wheelchair assessment and transfers.

101. (D) use active-listening techniques. Active listening (answer D) is an effective listening response that enables the patient to know that his or her message has been communicated. Behaviors listed in answers A, B, and C can be counterproductive to developing a therapeutic relationship. Answers A and B may be perceived as enhancing a friendship, rather than a therapeutic relationship, and answer C may be considered inappropriate for someone who does not have adequate social skills. See reference: Sladyk, K and Ryan, SE (eds): Tufano, R: Applied group dynamics and therapeutic use of self.

102. (B) mounting a safety rail next to the toilet. In order to sit independently on the toilet and relax sufficiently to control muscles needed for elimination, the child has to feel posturally secure. Safety rails next to the toilet, low toilets that allow the child to put both feet on the ground, and reducer rings to decrease the size of a toilet seat, all help to provide maximal stability for the child with unstable posture. Answers A, C, and D describe adaptations used for other deficits. Replacing zippers and buttons with Velcro closures (answer A) is helpful for a child with reduced strength or fine motor coordination. Introducing toilet paper tongs (answer C) helps increase reach in a child with limited range of motion. Placing a colorful "target" (answer D) helps boys aim into the bowl, a difficulty associated with perceptual or cognitive limitations. See reference: Case-Smith (ed): Shepherd, J: Self care and adaptations for independent living.

103. (C) take the bottom, supine position. This position requires the least amount of energy expenditure and should be the primary recommendation. In addition, the COTA may encourage experimentation with a variety of positions (answer D). Having sex at times when there is most energy would also be beneficial, but the individual will most likely be more fatigued at the end of the day (answer A). See reference: Pedretti and Early (eds): Burton, GU: Sexuality and physical dysfunction.

104. (D) deeply inhale and slowly exhale. Deep breathing can be learned quickly and may be effective in reducing tension in the shoulders, trunk, and abdomen. Progressive relaxation exercises, another method of stress reduction, involve a series of isometric exercises of systematically contracting and relaxing selected muscle groups (answer A). Meditation, which may take many months to learn, involves focusing on a word or phrase to reduce stress (answer B). Aerobic activity (answer C), which can reduce pain and relieve stress, involves repetitive contraction of the large muscles of the arms and legs. See reference: Neistadt and Crepeau (eds): Giles, GM and Neistadt, ME: Treatments for psychosocial components: Stress management.

105. (C) Have her put the utensil down until she swallows. The child needs to learn to pace herself during feeding. A child with problems relating to the rate of intake tends to put too much food in her mouth despite the size of the pieces (answer A). An impulsive person who eats too fast will also have difficulty counting slowly enough (answer B) to clear her mouth by the time she reaches the count of 10. Putting the various items of food in separate containers (answer D) would slow the meal down if items were presented one at a time, but would not necessarily slow the rate of food intake. See reference: Neistadt and Crepeau (eds): Holm, MB, Rogers, JC and James, AB: Treatment of activities of daily living.

106. (D) Alternate tasks that require standing with those that can be performed sitting. The performance component at issue in this question is fatigue. When fatigue impedes occupational performance, energy conservation techniques should be considered. Alternating sitting and standing activities is one method that can be applied to conserve energy; others include avoiding bending and stooping, avoiding unnecessary trips, using an appropriate work height, and relaxing homemaking standards. Convincing the individual to do something she can't afford (answer A) may not be in her best interests, and it is not an example consistent with the OT concept of collaborative decision making. Although increasing strength (answer B) may ultimately be useful, endurance is typically a more pressing issue for individuals with MS. Using the largest joint available for the task (answer C) is a joint protection technique more appropriate for an individual with arthritis. See reference: Pedretti and Early (eds): Buckner, WS: Arthritis.

107. (B) show acceptance and understanding regarding the client's situation. Paraphrasing is used to clarify and relay acceptance of what an individual has communicated. The COTA paraphrases by repeating in her or his own words what the client has said. Redirection (answer A) is used to promote healthier thoughts and behaviors. Forcing the individual to make a choice (answer C) may be accomplished by providing a question that includes two pos-

sible choices. A client is encouraged to provide additional information (answer D) when the COTA asks open ended questions. See reference: Denton: Treatment planning and implementation.

108. (B) Verbal and gestural cues. The next least intrusive level of cues consists of the combination of verbal and gestural cues. Physical cues (answers C and D) are the most intrusive, and only verbal cues (answer A) are the least intrusive. See reference: Case-Smith (ed): Shepherd, J: Self-care and adaptations for independent living.

109. (A) A head pointer and slanted keyboard. The use of a head pointer on a slanted keyboard would be the best solution because it requires no hand use. Answer B, a typing splint, which can be used if there is adequate wrist control, but inadequate finger control, and answer D, using a built-up pencil, are incorrect because they both require some upper extremity or hand function. Answer C, an adapted mouse would not improve ability to access keys, and would also require some UE movement. See reference: Angelo and Lane (eds): Angelo, J: Low-technology interface devices.

110. (A) avoid any physical contact with the individual. When working with individuals who act out sexually, it is important for the practitioner to avoid physical contact with the individual, avoid being alone with the individual (answers B and C) and discourage discussion about a possible sexual relationship between them (answer D). See reference: Early: Responding to symptoms and behaviors.

111. (C) Change to a power wheelchair to reduce effort. Considering the progressive nature of the child's disease, as well as strength and endurance, the best recommendation would be to change to a power wheelchair. The child would be better able to participate in the cognitive tasks of school if less effort was required for mobility. Answer A, retaining the manual chair, would be counterproductive to functioning well at school, and strength will not improve with this child's condition. Answer B might make mobility slightly easier, but will not solve the long-term problem of decreasing strength and endurance. Answer D would still make demands on strength and energy that would appear inappropriate considering the nature of Duchenne's muscular dystrophy. The team's recommendation should also be integrated with the family's needs and resources. See reference: Case-Smith (ed): Case-Smith, J, Rogers, J and Johnson, JH: School-based occupational therapy.

112. (D) provide a sensory cue, such as saying "stop!". The use of auditory, visual, or tactile sensory cues can help the person with Parkinson's disease to change the motor program in which they are engaged. Deep breathing exercises (answer A), practicing of movements (answer B), and mentally reviewing steps in the sequence of movement (answer C) will not provide the sensory information needed at the moment to evoke movement or change a "frozen" movement pattern. See reference: Trombly (ed): Newman, EM, Echevarria, ME, and Digman, G: Degenerative diseases.

113. (D) cooperative group activity that both provides and elicits consistent and accurate feedback about interactions within the group. Because the underlying issues for most personality disorders are related to inaccurate perceptions of the self and others, this treatment approach should directly address these problems. A cooperative group format offers a wide variety of feedback about the specific interactions that occur. The group activity should be based on a central goal of reducing misperceptions. Social skills groups (answer C) are often used to address the interaction difficulties experienced with cluster C personality disorders. The question does not specify that cluster C personality disorders are included in this group. Answer B is best used for problems of individuals, not groups. Answer A addresses decision making in regard to the selection of craft modalities, and does not typically focus upon individual patient perceptions. See reference: Sladyk, K and Ryan, SE (eds): Tufano, R: Applied group dynamics and therapeutic use of self.

114. (B) use a guiding technique by placing food in the resident's hand and bringing it to the mouth. Use of a guiding technique (answer B) is particularly effective because the person receives sensory cues that something is approaching the face ahead of time. This can facilitate opening of the mouth. Answer C, wiping food particles from a person's face, is not recommended until after the person swallows, because this can start a reflexive opening of the mouth which would interfere with eating. Answer A, clearing food pocketed in the resident's cheeks, should be performed by the resident themselves, not the COTA. Allowing the resident to select what food or beverage they prefer (answer D), would not have any particular effect on a resident who is tactilely defensive. See reference: Larson, Stevens-Ratchford, Pedretti, and Crabtree (eds): Foti, D: Evaluation and interventions for the performance area of self-maintenance.

115. (B) practicing the whole task of putting on a shirt in a setting similar to the real environment. Retention of a skill will be enhanced if the task is practiced in its entirety during each performance trial, because whole task performance is easier to recall than separate steps. Generalization of skills is enhanced when an activity has been acquired in a setting that resembles the natural environment where the skill will be performed. Answer A, practice of each segment of the process, may be useful for improving performance of the activity segments practiced, but will not enhance retention and generalization of the skill. Providing simulation activities

(answer C) may improve some performance components involved in the dressing process, but will not enhance learning of the whole task of putting on a shirt. Answer D, showing a videotape and providing written directions, is a useful instructional technique for client education from a cognitive perspective, but does not provide the motor component necessary for learning a motor skill. See reference: Gillen and Burkardt (eds): Application of learning and environmental strategies to activity-based treatment.

116. (C) Alcoholics Anonymous. This is a self-help group whose purpose is to help members achieve and maintain sobriety. The meetings are free, available at varied times and locations, and there is no limit on the number of meetings one can attend. The YMCA (answer A) is a good resource for leisure activities, but does not offer a sober support model. Vocational rehabilitation (answer B) could be an effective resource for someone in recovery who is having difficulty with employment, but this man has no such difficulty. Because he is in the early stages of recovery, speaking to high school students (answer D) about his addiction and recovery is not yet recommended. See reference: Early: Understanding psychiatric diagnosis: The DSM-IV.

117. (B) Raising the handlebars. The correct answer is B because raising the handle bars demands that the arms are raised, thus bringing the child to an upright posture. Answers A and C are not correct because the hips and lower extremities are already positioned correctly. Answer D is not correct because the arms would be lowered, and trunk forward flexion would be increased. See reference: Kramer and Hinojosa (eds): Colangelo, CA: Biomechanical frame of reference.

118. (B) project group. The next level of structured activity is termed project group, because the group members are now able to share the completion of a group project, however, they still require strong group leadership to guide them. Following a project group, the next level of group interaction is the egocentric cooperative group (answer A), followed by the cooperative group (answer C), and the then mature group (answer D), which is the most advanced. See reference: Sladyk, K and Ryan, SE (eds): Tufano, R: Applied group dynamics and therapeutic use of self.

119. (C) Digging a garden with a shovel. Activities that include bilateral use of tonic muscles against resistance, such as digging a garden, playing volleyball, or playing tug of war, can help to normalize tone in this population. Dancing with rapid alternating movements (answer A) may heighten arousal. Playing "Twister" (answer B) may facilitate balance and promote interpersonal skills. Rocking in a rocking chair (answer D) may reduce the level of arousal. See reference: Bruce and Borg: Movement-centered frame of reference.

120. (C) Oversized tee shirts and elastic top pants. For a child with difficulty in self-dressing due to incoordination (as seen with athetoid CP), clothing should be loose fitting with simple or no fasteners. Oversized clothing is preferred to tight fitting garments (answers A and B). Garments with elasticized waist bands are better than those using zippers (answer B), or snaps and buttons (answer D). See reference: Neistadt and Crepeau (eds): Erhardt, RP and Merrill, SC: Neurological dysfunction in children.

121. (B) selective attention. The client demonstrated difficulty in attending to the activity because the presence of other environmental stimuli was distracting. This suggests a deficit in selective or focused attention. The client's performance of the activity provides no observable information about learning (answer A) or problem solving skills (answer D). Since the client visually located the brush initially, the problem would not be perceptual in nature, so answer C, figure-ground perceptions is not correct. See reference: Unsworth (ed): Unsworth, C: Evaluation and intervention with concentration impairment.

122. (D) Accept his decision. Individuals with depression are aware they are not performing at their usual level, and recognize when they have not done a good job. It is important to accept his decision and not pursue it further. He will recognize the implied praise (answers B and C) as false, and may be too ashamed or embarrassed to give a poorly executed project as a gift (answer A). See reference: Early: Responding to symptoms and behaviors.

123. (D) blowing cotton balls into a target. Children with ADHD have difficulty with sustained attention and effort. Answers A, B, and C require sustained visual vigilance and involve delayed gratification. In contrast, blowing cotton balls into a target is a short-term activity with immediate reward for successful completion; therefore, it responds to the child's dual needs. See reference: Neistadt and Crepeau (eds): Florey, L: Psychosocial dysfunction in childhood and adolescence.

124. (B) a hook provides better prehensile function and allows greater visibility of objects. The fact that a hook TD provides better prehensile function and allows greater visibility of objects would be the most important consideration for a person whose primary concern is functioning as a carpenter. Answers A, C, and D are incorrect because although they can be important considerations for some people with UE amputations, they are not as relevant to this person's goals. See reference: Pedretti and Early (eds): Keenan, DD and Rock, LM: Body-powered protheses.

125. (A) Ask group members to discuss how they feel about taking their medications. "Any effort to help a client manage medication independently should begin with a discussion of his or her feelings about it" (p. 421). Also, clients can often benefit from hearing about the experiences of others. Using diaries (answer B), timers (answer C), lists, and other environmental supports can also increase success in independent medication management. Knowledge of the medication schedule is critical, but the first action the COTA should take is leading the discussion on feelings about taking medications. See reference: Early: Activities of daily living.

126. (D) Encourage independent self-feeding and dressing skills with minimal use of adapted utensils and tools. Encouraging independent self-feeding and dressing skills with minimal use of adapted utensils and tools is the most appropriate ADL intervention. It is important to avoid an overreliance on adapted equipment so the child can experience full active range of motion when engaged in ADL. Answer A, instruct the child to use all adapted equipment, may interfere with the achievement of reaching full AROM when engaging in ADL. Answer B, encourage independent compression garment application, is typically contraindicated with open wounds and is not implemented until wound closure. Answer C, perform bilateral upper extremity PROM exercises twice a day, is not considered an ADL intervention. See reference: Neistadt and Crepeau (eds): Rivers, EA and Jordan, CL: Skin system dysfunction: Burns.

127. (D) sensory compensation. When protective sensation is severely decreased or absent, the primary focus of intervention becomes protection of the insensate part through educational methods, to increase awareness of potential injury dangers, teach safety procedures, and train in the use of vision, to compensate for sensory loss. Sensory reeducation (answer A) is a remedial retraining technique which focuses on helping the patient correctly interpret sensory impulses through a program of graded sensory stimuli. Sensory desensitization (answer B) involves a program of graded sensory stimuli to gradually decrease hypersensitivity to sensory stimuli. Sensory bombardment (answer C) is a sensory retraining method of stimulating many senses. See reference: Pedretti and Early (eds): Iyer, MB and Pedretti, LW: Evaluation of sensation and treatment of sensory dysfunction.

128. (B) having the worker put only the last piece into the game package. Working backwards from the last successful step of a sequence is known as "backward chaining." Answer A represents the opposite of backward chaining. Answer C is more descriptive of shaping behaviors, and answer D is more descriptive of modeling behaviors. See reference: Pedretti and Early (eds): Sabari, JS: Teaching activities in occupational therapy.

129. (B) Provision of foot support. Adequate foot support would be the first concern of the practitioner for the child to feel secure on the toilet and to be positioned for bowel control. Answer A is not correct because management of fasteners can be developed later, after positioning for stability has been achieved. Answer C is not correct because provision of a seatbelt may not be necessary if foot support (or back support) is provided. Answer D is not correct because climbing onto the toilet independently may be developed later (as occurs with normal developmental progression). See reference: Case-Smith (ed): Shepherd, J: Self care and adaptations for independent living.

130. (A) elevate the arm on pillows so it rests higher than the heart. Elevation, contrast baths, retrograde massage, pressure wraps, and active range of motion are effective methods for managing edema. When massaging an edematous extremity, stroking should be performed from the distal area to the proximal, not the reverse (answer B). Because active and PROM can both be beneficial to managing edema, instructing the patient to avoid range of motion activities (answers C and D) would be incorrect. See reference: Pedretti and Early (eds): Kasch, MC and Nickerson, E: Hand and upper extremity injuries.

131. (D) Ask the employer to provide an isolated cubicle as the work space. An isolated cubicle is a reasonable accommodation to request for an individual who is highly distractible. The Americans with Disabilities Act (ADA) requires employers to provide reasonable accommodations for individuals with documented disabilities that will enable them to work despite the disability. A job coach (answer A) is more appropriate for an individual who needs frequent cueing or assistance to perform their job. Frequent breaks (answer B) are a reasonable accommodation suitable for individuals with anxiety who need to manage stress. Although explaining the problem of distractibility to the employer (answer C) may open the lines of communication with the employer, it does not offer a solution. See reference: Early: Work, homemaking and childcare.

132. (D) Recommend that the child wear an emergency alert system pendant around her neck. An emergency alert system would be the most likely solution for the COTA to recommend to the family. "Emergency alert systems, worn as pendants or stabilized on wheelchairs, are available for purchase with a service that places emergency calls when the system is activated" (p. 518). This intervention would be most effective because it can be placed on the client's body and does not require a great deal of dexterity to manipulate. This would also be especially appropriate if the teenager's parents were not home when the fire occurred. Answer A, positioning a wireless cell phone near the child, may be an effective solution, but would not be of much assistance if the child's dexterity is limited, in that she may not be able to push the buttons effectively. Answer B, establishing a quick exit routine in the event

of a fire, is something that the COTA and the client's family should address, but in the event that no family members are home with the client when a fire occurs is potentially hazardous. While answer C, educating the client regarding fire prevention within the home, is something that should be reviewed by the COTA, it does not address the immediate needs of responding to an actual fire via an emergency call system. See reference: Case-Smith (ed): Shepherd, J: Self-care and adaptations for independent living.

133. (C) Biomechanical. The biomechanical approach uses voluntary muscle control during performance of activities for individuals with deficits in strength, endurance, or range of motion. The biomechanical approach focuses on decreasing deficits in order to improve performance of daily activities. The neurophysiological approach (answer A) is applied to individuals with brain damage. Emphasis is on the nervous system and methods for eliciting desired responses. The neurodevelopmental approach (answer B) also focuses on the nervous system, but emphasizes eliciting responses in a developmental sequence. The rehabilitative approach (answer D) teaches an individual how to compensate for a deficit on either a temporary or permanent basis. See reference: Trombly (ed): Zemke, R: Remediating biomechanical and physiological impairments of motor performance.

134. (A) set the climate, provide structure, and offer support. Answer A reflects typical leadership involvement in OT groups. Answer B is incorrect because it reflects minimal direction from the leader which is uncharacteristic of OT groups. Answer C is incorrect because the group leader performs these functions at the termination stage, rather than the initial stages of group development. Working individually with group members (answer D) is incongruous with current OT group treatment formats that use properties of the group to achieve therapeutic goals. See reference: Neistadt and Crepeau (eds): Schwartzberg, SL: Group process.

135. (B) facilitate postural reactions. By placing a child in the sitting position on a therapeutic ball, "the therapist can facilitate postural reactions using activities that displace the center of gravity and require corrective or protective responses" (p. 284). The addition of the reaching activity will cause the child to change his or her center of gravity during the reaching phase, which will require a further postural response to compensate for the change of position. See reference: Case-Smith (ed): Nichols, D: Development of postural control.

136. (C) flange the area around the ulnar styloid. Reddened areas indicate the splint is too tight in a particular spot. To reduce pressure, it is often helpful to flange splint edges. Lining the splint with any material, whether moleskin or foam (answers A and B), will only make a tight area tighter. Remaking the splint (answer D) is unnecessary and a waste of the COTA's time. See reference: Neistadt and Crepeau (eds): Fess, EE and Kiel, JH: Neuromuscular treatment: Upper extremity splinting.

137. (C) "I think baking would be a helpful activity to try. Baking something you like offers you several choices and decisions. These choices and decisions can help you feel more positive about making other decisions. You can choose a cake mix or a cookie mix. Which would you like?" Answer C limits options and provides the rationale for the choices. Answer A is a leading question that really offers only one choice. Answer B does not provide any options. Answer D is a closed question, offering no real choice for the individual. See reference: Denton: Effective communication.

138. (A) Chaining. Chaining with a child who demonstrates a cognitive disability shows all sequences in the entire process of a task. Initially, the child performs only the beginning or end of a task. Thus, the child initially concentrates on only a small part of the task and gradually increases participation in all sequences in their correct order. Answers B, C, and D are other methods that can be used, but forward and backward chaining are instructional methods that have been particularly successful with individuals who are mentally retarded. See reference: Early: Medical and psychological models of mental health and illness.

139. (D) a weighted pen and weighted wrists. Weighting body parts and utensils (e.g., writing tools) are effective for individuals with ataxia to improve control during performance of a task. Hitting the keys on a keyboard (answer A) would be difficult for such a client, although weighting the wrists could make performance of the activity possible. A keyboard is a good alternative for individuals with difficulty writing due to weakness, limited range of motion, or incoordination. A universal cuff with a pencil holder attachment (answer B) would be appropriate for an individual with hand weakness who uses a universal cuff for other tasks. A balanced forearm orthosis (answer C) is appropriate for individuals with severe muscle weakness. In addition, individuals with muscle weakness find felt tip pens easier to write with than ballpoint pens. See reference: Pedretti and Early (eds): Gutman, SA: Traumatic brain injury.

140. (B) teach the client to use a diary or log. Compensation techniques are used to work around a deficit area by using alternative methods to accomplish the same task. Teaching the use of a diary or log (answer B) is an example of an external memory aid which provides cues to compensate for memory deficits. Answers A and C are incorrect because they are examples of internal memory strategies (retracing and rehearsal) which rely on mental effort. Answer D, use of a memory training computer program, is a technique for remediation of memory

skills and, therefore, is not an example of a compensation method. See reference: Trombly (ed): Quintana, LE: Remediating cognitive impairments.

141. (A) provide gentle human touch to enable the infant to slowly respond to intervention. Although all answers are possible examples of applied calming techniques, the tactile system is the first to develop, and the most sophisticated, in the young NICU patient. Therefore, answer A is the most suitable for initial interaction contact. Answers B and C could be overstimulating because they involve the auditory and vestibular systems, which are fully operational during the youngest possible gestation viable for life, but are still immature. The visual system is the last to develop. Answer D is an optimal visual strategy for early infancy after 30 weeks' gestation, when the infant's visual sensory system for visual interaction is maturing. See reference: Case-Smith (ed): Hunter, JG: Neonatal Intensive Care Unit.

142. (C) folding laundry. Sorting and folding laundry (answer C) challenge balance and upper extremity function in ways that are more functional than stacking cones or throwing a ball. Rather than seeking contrived activities (answers A, B, and C) that challenge single component deficits, the focus of home care is to find ways for the patient to actually perform the daily activities that are presenting the challenges. Because this patient is the mother of four teenagers, it is presumed that her occupational role includes homemaking activities. See reference: Piersol and Ehrlich (eds): Seibert, C: The clinic called home.

143. (C) Making a checklist of steps in the process, then consulting the list while doing laundry in the actual setting. Making a checklist and having the person use the checklist during the activity, would provide an external memory aid during practice of the functional activity. This would provide compensation for cognitive deficits during task training in the specific context where it will be performed. Answers A, B, and D are methods that require a person to be able to transfer learning of skills from one context to another. See reference: Pedretti and Early (eds): Wheatley, CJ: Evaluation and treatment of cognitive dysfunction.

144. (B) touching the infant on the right or left corner of his mouth. The rooting reflex can best be facilitated by applying a stimulus (touching the baby on either corner of the mouth). The desired response is to have the baby move his or her lips in the direction of the stimulus. This reflex should become integrated by approximately 4 months. Answers C and D, placing the child in various positions, may assist with breast and bottle feeding, but do not contribute to the facilitation of the rooting reflex. Answer A, touching the crowns of the infant's teeth, is typically performed to facilitate the bite reflex between the age of four to seven months. See reference: Pedretti and Early (eds): Nelson-Jenks, K: Dysphagia.

145. (B) Obtain a raised toilet seat. The individual will most likely continue to require a raised toilet seat for several months in order to avoid flexing the hip past the designated range. A handheld shower (answer D) is not always necessary, however, a shower chair with adjustable legs and grab bars could be helpful. High contrast tape (answer C) may help to make ascending and descending stairs safer for individuals with limitations in vision. Moving items from low cabinets to higher locations may help this individual comply more readily with the necessary hip precautions, but moving objects from high to lower cabinets (answer A) would not. See reference: Pedretti and Early (eds): Coleman, S: Hip fractures and lower extremity joint replacement.

146. (C) Make believe group with stuffed animals and imaginary friends. Encouraging a drama/make believe group with 3-year-old children is the most suitable answer. Symbolic play is typically imaginative in nature, thus making any activity that involves pretending that dolls and stuffed animals are real is appropriate. "The child may also imitate the actions of parents, teachers, and peers. At age 3 to 4 years, pretend play becomes more abstract, and objects, such as a block, can be used to represent something else" (p. 85). Answer A, scissors and cutting tasks, would most likely be used to facilitate fine motor and in-hand manipulation skills, while answer B, jumping rope, would involve gross motor skills typically seen in older children. Answer D, building towers to resemble an actual picture, is an activity that would be more representative of constructive play and/or manipulation skills. See reference: Case-Smith (ed): Case-Smith, J: Development of childhood occupations.

147. (D) Finishing a prefabricated wood birdhouse from a kit. A person experiencing a manic episode is likely to exhibit high energy levels, short attention span, poor frustration tolerance, difficulty delaying gratification, and making decisions. Finishing a prefabricated wood birdhouse would be the most appropriate activity because it is a short-term, predictable activity with few steps. It also can be carried with the person if he or she needs to get up and move around during the activity. Answer A, a needlepoint project, would require too high a degree of attention to detail for guaranteed success. Answer B, making a clay object, uses an unpredictable material and requires creative decisions, both of which are qualities that should be avoided. Answer C, watercolor painting, would not be a good choice because it is an unfocused activity involving artistic skill performance that could lead to frustration. See reference: Early: Responding to symptoms and behaviors.

148. (D) The individual traces letters through a pan of rice with her fingers. This method involves greater input of sensory information to the brain by performing a gross movement in a more stimulating environment. A verbal description of how to make a letter (Answer A), watching her grip (answer B), or performing strengthening exercises (Answer C), would not give the individual proprioceptive feedback on her letter formation through tactile input. See reference: Trombly (ed): Bentzel, K: Remediating sensory impairment.

149. (B) Pants with an elastic waistband. According to Solomon "pants or skirts with elastic waistbands are the easiest to put on and remove. Waistbands may need to be fairly loose for children with severe weakness, abnormal movement patterns, or incoordination" (p. 232). Answers A, B, and C typically make dressing and undressing easier, but due to this particular child's incoordination and weakness, elastic waistbands would be the most effective method to introduce in order to promote independence with this particular dressing skill. See reference: Solomon (ed): Jones, LMW and Machover, PZ: Occupational performance areas: Daily living and work and productive activities

150. (A) reminiscence group. In a reminiscence group, the focus is on providing social opportunities for sharing life stories and feelings, expressing pride in past life experiences, and gaining support for past life difficulties, all of which would enhance self-esteem and help the residents achieve acceptance of past and present life. Answers B, C, and D would address some of the goals stated, but not as comprehensively as a reminiscence group. See reference: Hellen: Appendix 9-10: Activity therapy care conference report form information: Therapeutic value.

151. (D) Just before discharge. Because the prognosis for patients with Guillain-Barré syndrome is usually good, equipment should be ordered just before discharge to accurately determine the individual's needs. Equipment ordered during the first week of therapy, or as soon as approved (answers B and C), may not be necessary at the time the individual is discharged. Although collaborating with the patient and family on decisions about ordering equipment is essential, acceptance of the disability (answer A) may not necessarily correspond with the appropriate time for ordering equipment. See reference: Pedretti and Early (eds): Lehman, RM and McCormack, GL: Neurogenic and myopathic dysfunction.

152. (C) The client independently selected one of six craft designs presented. The notation of the client's response to treatment that contains the most objective information is answer C. The notations that address the client's wants and hostility (answers A and B) are interpretations of behavior versus directly observable responses. The use of the word "appropriate" (answer D) reflects the OT practitioner's judgement. See reference: Early: Medical records and documentation.

153. (C) Parents should be considered as part of a collaborative partnership with OT practitioners. "The first interactions of the therapist with a family open the door to establishing a partnership" in which "the family and therapist collaborate using agreed upon roles to obtain agreed upon goals for the child" (p. 117). Parents should be encouraged to observe their child in therapy so that they may better understand the program, and their child's problems, therefore, answer A is incorrect. Answer B is incorrect because, although some parents may carry out therapy programs at home, "the goal is not for parents to become quasiprofessionals" (p. 117). It is also recommended that both parents be present when an OT program is discussed (unlike answer D), so that one does not become dependent on the other for information and communication. See reference: Case-Smith (ed): Humphry, R and Case-Smith, J: Working with families.

154. (A) Linoleum floor. Linoleum floors are the easiest and least expensive surface over which to maneuver a wheelchair. Although it is possible to find inexpensive short pile carpeting (answer B), a smooth, uncarpeted surface is still the easiest to maneuver over. The friction provided by deep pile carpets (answer C) makes them difficult to push a wheelchair across, and wheeling over the edge of an area rug (answer D) also increases the level of difficulty for wheelchair users. See reference: Christiansen (ed): Bates, PS: The self-care environment: Issues of space and furnishing.

155. (A) The client will engage in a simple craft activity for 15 minutes without demonstrating self-abusive behavior. It would be a higher priority for the client to reduce the amount of self-abusive behavior, than to learn increasingly complex craft activities. After a significant reduction in self-abusive behavior has been achieved, attempting to maintain that level while gradually raising the level of stress, through increasingly complex tasks, may be attempted. This would progress the client toward tolerating greater levels of stress without becoming self-abusive. Answers B, C, and D all emphasize increasing the complexity of the task, rather than extending the length of time without self-abusive behavior. See reference: Early: Analyzing, adapting, and grading activities.

156. (B) stress bilateral play and school activities incorporating the prosthesis. Two-handed activities for play, school and self-care should be used to incorporate the prosthesis into the child's body image and to help develop bilateral skills. Activities that avoid the use of the prosthesis, as in answers A, C, and D, would not help the child to integrate the prosthesis into normal patterns of use. See reference: Case-Smith (ed): Rogers, SL, Gordon, CY, Schanzenbacher, KE, Case-Smith, J: Common diagnoses is pediatric occupational therapy practice.

157. (B) Reposition the person in the wheelchair to allow optimal range of motion. When a person in a wheelchair who uses an augmentative communication device suddenly begins making errors, it is necessary to first check the position of the individual. Improper positioning could result in the wheelchair interfering with access or with range of motion needed to use the communication device. A person may eventually need to be referred to a physician for a physical examination (answer A). However, it is best for the therapist to first problem solve and seek a solution if the person's medical status has not changed. The person's communication abilities would not be reassessed (answer C) until the person has been optimally positioned in the wheelchair. A communication device would only need to be replaced (answer D) if there were a mechanical problem within the system could not be fixed. See reference: Angelo and Lane (eds): Taylor, SJ and Kreutz, D: Powered and manual wheelchair mobility.

158. (D) arrange for the patient to attend a discharge group to discuss these concerns. A discharge planning group can be structured to encourage patients to share similar concerns regarding adjustment after hospitalization. The group can provide support and encouragement for fellow patients, as well as opportunities for brainstorming and problem solving issues related to the return to community living. Answers A and B do not provide opportunities for the patient to gain the insight and perspective of other patients who may share similar concerns. Suggesting that the patient lie (answer C) is unethical. See reference: Early: Psychosocial skills and psychological components.

159. (C) attainment of kindergarten readiness skills. The primary focus of intervention for a 5-year-old preschooler is to prepare the child for transition to kindergarten. The child's ability to perform the occupations related to that environment comprise readiness for kindergarten and include academic skills, as well as ADL (answers A and D) and social skills (answer B). A child who has achieved age-level skills in all these areas may benefit fully from the educational program and OT services can then be discontinued. See reference: Case-Smith (ed): Gartland, S and DuBoise, SA: Occupational therapy in preschool and childcare setting.

160. (C) "Patient is demonstrating gradual improvement in fine motor coordination." The assessment portion of the note "contains the analysis of plans and goals for the patient...and involves the professional judgment of the therapist" (p. 110). It is also where the OT practitioner draws conclusions and justified decisions, as described in answer C. The objective portion of the SOAP note should contain information that is measurable or based on specific observations, such as answer A. The subjective portion contains information gained from communication with the patient, his or her family (answers B and D), or other staff members. This information is not measurable, and is therefore considered subjective. See reference: Kettenbach: Writing assessment (A).

161. (C) Coping strategies for continuing medication compliance. Medication noncompliance (answer C) is a primary factor related to frequent readmissions for individuals with psychiatric conditions. The other strategies (answers A, B, and D) listed are also important, but are not the primary issue. See reference: Early: Activities of daily living.

162. (A) large, easily interlocking pieces. For the child with fluctuating muscle tone, efforts should be made to provide a means of stabilizing toys and equipment. The interlocking quality of such toys as "bristle blocks" and magnets will provide some stability and assist with controlled release. The large size of the blocks will facilitate a more effective grasp. Small or lightweight blocks (answers B and C) are more difficult to manipulate and are therefore, not recommended for constructive play for a child with coordination difficulties. Colorful blocks (answer D) may stimulate some interest, but have no direct bearing on the child's ability to engage in construction efforts. See reference: Case-Smith (ed): Morrison, CD and Metzger, P: Play.

163. (B) objective section. Measured results based on an individual's performance are included in the objective section. The subjective portion (answer A) of the SOAP note contains information provided by the patient or family. Analysis of the measurements is recorded in the assessment area (answer C) of the SOAP note. Plans for future sessions are included in the plan section (answer D). See reference: Sabonis-Chafee and Hussey: Treatment planning and implementation.

164. (C) Simple meal preparation group. Obtaining food is a basic survival need and is often the focus of a homeless individual's day. Therefore, while all the above groups may meet a need, activities related to food are likely to be more highly valued by this individual. Craft groups (answer A) may be useful in developing healthy leisure interests. Volunteer activities (answer B) can help develop necessary work habits. Social skills groups (answer D) address interpersonal skills necessary for living in society. See reference: Early: Who is the consumer?

165. (B) child's writing, dressing, and self-feeding skills. Because the child was being treated for difficulties with fine motor skills, discharge information should focus on fine motor function. Answers A, C, and D describe information that is relevant in overall discharge planning, but is not specifically relevant to the performance problems the child was treated for in OT. See reference: Case-Smith (ed): Case-Smith, J, Rogers, J, and Johnson, JH: School-based occupational therapy.

166. (A) canister vacuum cleaner. A canister vacuum cleaner may be managed by someone with weakness and balance problems while the person is sitting. The hose is light enough to be easily pushed, and the canister is on wheels and may be moved by a seated person pushing it with the foot, or having someone move it for him or her. An upright vacuum cleaner (answer B) is too heavy for repetitive pushing and pulling, and its use can cause exhaustion or pull the person off balance. A self-propelled vacuum cleaner (answer C) could also pull a person off balance by moving too fast for the person to respond with appropriate postural adjustments. A handheld vacuum cleaner (answer D) requires too much stooping to do anything but a very small area of the floor, because repetitive bending can cause fatigue quickly and challenges decreased balance. See reference: Trombly (ed): Stewart, C: Retraining housekeeping and child care skills.

167. (B) The patient has not accused any men of attacking her this week. The number of times the patient demonstrates one aspect of paranoid behavior (fear of men) is objectively stated in the correct answer. Answer A indicates improvement, but does not provide substantiation for the statement. Answer C may be indicative of improved interpersonal skills and self-esteem, but does not reflect decreased paranoid behavior. Answer D is a statement of a goal, not of improvement. See reference: Early: Medical records and documentation.

168. (A) "jaw opening and closing are controlled with your index and middle fingers; place your thumb on the child's cheek." The correct position of the adult's hand for jaw control when the child is fed from the side is described in answer A. Answers B and D are incorrect because the thumb should be placed on the child's cheek to provide joint stability. Answer C is incorrect because controlling the child's jaw movement with the adult's whole hand provides less control of the child's jaw than the recommended method. Placing the adult's thumb on the child's ear (answer D) is also incorrect because of discomfort for the child, and because thumb placement should be near the fulcrum of jaw movement (at the temporomandibular joint). If the child is fed from the front, the adult's thumb is placed on the chin, with middle finger under the chin to control opening and closing of the jaw. The index finger then rests on the side of the child's face to provide stability. See reference: Case-Smith (ed): Case-Smith, J and Humphry, R: Feeding intervention.

169. (A) Remove all throw or scatter rugs. Regardless of whether an individual with instability walks with the help of a walker, cane, or no equipment, the floor should be cleared of any obstacles that could cause them to slip or trip. A person's foot or on the tip of an assistive device may catch on scatter or throw rugs. Also, rugs may not be firmly taped down or secured with nonskid backing, causing a further safety hazard. Installing lever handles, a ramp, or a handheld shower (answers B, C, and D) would make certain tasks easier for a patient, but they would not be necessary for safety. See reference: Pedretti and Early (eds): Foti, D: Activities of daily living.

170. (D) facilitate effective treatment. The primary purpose of documentation is to facilitate the treatment process. By defining the problem, goals and objectives, and a treatment plan, the practitioner's thoughts are organized in order to carry out goal-directed services. Additional purposes of documentation are to serve as legal documentation, to report services provided for reimbursement, and to provide communication among the team, patient, or family. Answers A, B, and C are incorrect in that they are not part of the primary reasons for documentation. However, some forms of documentation may be necessary to meet accrediting agency guidelines or to be used in research. See reference: AOTA: Effective documentation for occupational therapy.

171. (B) the potential for depression and low self-esteem. The potential for depression and low self-esteem is commonly associated with the long-term psychological mode of recovery. Answer A, the possibility of decreased range of motion and sensation, is a physical response to a burn. Answers C and D are psychological reactions typically associated with the early and intermediate stages of recovery. See reference: Richard and Staley (eds): Moss, BF, Everett, JJ, and Patterson, DR: Psychologic support and pain management of the burn patient.

172. (D) Family will demonstrate independence in current positioning and feeding techniques. Goals should be functional, measurable, and objective. In addition, short-term goals must relate to the long-term goal being addressed. Answer D meets those criteria. Answer A does not provide measurable criteria, nor does it directly relate to the long-term goal of family training. Answer B, while measurable, does not relate to the long-term goal. Answer C describes the long-term goal of family independence in the feeding program. See reference: AOTA: Effective documentation for occupational therapy. Moorhead, P and Kannenberg, K: Writing functional goals.

173. (D) home-delivered meal services. Answer A, continued OT services to teach the patient to use the kitchen appliances safely, is incorrect because individuals diagnosed with dementia tend to decline over time, and interventions aimed at improvement are unrealistic. Volunteer companions (answer B), provide companionship to elders at home, but not skilled supervision of activities. Transporting to a community site for meals (answer C) on a daily basis could be inconvenient, overly challenging and taxing for an elder with beginning dementia. Answer D, in-

home meal delivery services such as Meals-on-Wheels, would be the best and safest option for providing consistent access to food in the home. See reference: Larson, Stevens-Ratchford, Pedretti, and Crabtree (eds): Aitken, MJ and Lohman, H: Health care systems: Changing perspectives.

174. (D) plan section. The plan section of a SOAP note includes statements related to continuing treatment; the frequency and duration of the treatment; suggestions for additional activities or treatment techniques; the need for further evaluations; and, when needed, recommendations for new goals. The subjective portion of a SOAP note (answer A) refers to what the patient comments about the treatment. The objective portion of the SOAP note (answer B) focuses on measurable and/or observable data obtained by the OT practitioner through specific evaluations, observations, or use of therapeutic activities. The assessment part of a SOAP note refers to the effectiveness of the treatment and any changes needed, the status of the goals, and any justification for continuing OT treatment. See reference: Borcherding: Writing the "P"-Plan

175. (D) drink juices and caffeine-free colas when thirsty. Continual dry mouth and thirst are a common side effect of many drugs. Juices and caffeine-free drinks are preferable for preventing dehydration. Caffeinated drinks (answer B) can intensify the dehydrating effects of this medication. Photosensitivity, an increased sensitivity to the sun, is another side effect often associated with neuroleptic medications, and can be addressed by limiting sun exposure (answer A). Answer C is a strategy that can be used to avoid postural hypotension, a sudden drop in blood pressure resulting in feeling faint, or loss of consciousness when moving from lying or sitting to standing. All of the answers are strategies for managing possible side effects of neuroleptic medications, but answer D is most important because it addresses the only side effect the individual has experienced. See reference: Early: Psychotropic medications and somatic treatments.

176. (C) Swing-away footrests and removable armrests. After swinging away footrests and removing armrests, the individual can perform a sliding board transfer without being blocked by a wheelchair. Answers A and B include nothing that would facilitate a sliding board transfer. One-arm drive (answer A) is useful for individuals with the use of only one upper extremity. A low backrest (answer A) is useful for those who require minimal trunk support, because it allows greater freedom of movement for the arms and shoulders. A reclining backrest (answer B) benefits individuals who are unable to sit upright for prolonged periods of time, or who need to recline for weight shifts. Elevating footrests (answer D) are desirable for individuals with lower extremity edema. Answer D is incorrect because although removable armrests may make transfers easier, elevating footrests would not. A footrest would need to be a detachable or swing-away type for it to be moved out of the way. See reference: Pedretti and Early (eds): Creel, TA, Adler, C, Tipton-Burton, M, and Lillie, SM: Mobility.

177. (C) tai chi. Tai chi would be the best activity because it incorporates slow stretching movements. This type of movement can help improve balance which is often affected when muscles become rigid, particularly muscles of the neck and trunk. Answer A, weight training, would not be recommended because resistive activity can increase rigidity. Answer B, walking, is a good general exercise, but would not provide stretching movement. Answer D, gardening, would not be particularly useful because it can be performed without requiring stretching movements. See reference: Pedretti and Early (eds): Schultz-Krohn, W: Parkinson's disease.

178. (B) Leather lacing a change purse from a kit. All of the choices are good leisure group activities. However, activities that can be completed in one session, are structured for success, and yield a tangible end product (such as a kit) are very likely to turn out well regardless of the individual's skill level. They are best for promoting a sense of competence and mastery over the environment. Collages (answer A) are useful for expressing thoughts or feelings about a particular theme, such as nutritional foods or leisure activities one enjoys participating in, however, the end product is not always predictable. Going to the movies (answer C) can incorporate goals related to community mobility and money management, however, there is no tangible end product. Putting on a resident talent show (answer D) can promote self-esteem and self-expression, however, it usually requires more than one session to prepare. See reference: Cottrell (ed): Kearney, PC: Occupational therapy intervention with homeless women.

179. (D) Convert an empty lot filled with trash into a garden. Activities based on the concepts of building and creating and that result in one shared outcome are more effective for team building than those involving competition (answer A) or individual reward (answer C). Anger management skills are important for children at risk for violent behavior, however, a psychoeducational format (answer B) will not contribute to protecting or building the community. See reference: Fazio: Programming examples within the community of clubs.

180. (A) Activities that promote home and community safety. The "Well Elderly Study," conducted at the University of Southern California, demonstrated that individuals who participated in an occupation-based program that included the relationship between activity and health, joint protection and energy conservation education, use of adaptive equipment, use of public transportation, and home and community safety, experienced significant health benefits compared to those who participated in a socialization intervention (answer B) or no intervention. A physical therapy program would be more likely to focus on balance and ambulation activities (answer C). While caregiver training (answer D) is important, it would not be the emphasis of a health promotion program. See reference: Scaffa, ME (ed): Scaffa, ME, Desmond, S, and Brownson, CA: Public health, community health, and occupational therapy.

181. (B) Improved verbal and nonverbal communication skills. Improved verbal and nonverbal communication skills would be the most relevant behavioral outcome indicating program effectiveness in the area of social skills development. Answers A, C, and D may all indirectly benefit as a result of improved social and communication skills, but these would not directly reflect positive outcomes for measuring effectiveness of social skill training programs. See reference: Cottrell (ed): Salo-Chydenius, S: Changing helplessness to coping: An exploratory study of social skills training with individuals with long-term mental illness.

182. (A) Collect as much information as possible about injuries caused by scooter accidents. The first step in new program development is to obtain as much information as possible about the topic (e.g., frequency and severity of injuries, causes, and prevention). An idea for a new program should not be presented to the people in charge (answer D) until the COTA is well versed in the topic. Use of protective clothing (answer C) is an intervention technique that will be part of the program once it is implemented. It is not necessary for the COTA to be supervised by an OTR (answer B), because she is not being hired by the school as a COTA. See reference: Sladyk, K and Ryan, SE (eds): Sladyk, K: Wellness and health promotion.

183. (C) Remove the threshold altogether. Removing the threshold altogether would be the simplest and safest solution. Door thresholds may have a maximum height of half an inch and these must be beveled; keeping it as it is (answer A) would provide a barrier to wheelchair accessibility and a safety hazard for people with visual deficits. Placing a throw rug to cover the threshold (answer B) would not improve accessibility and would present a slipping hazard. Because the threshold height is greater than 0.5", placing a ramp over the threshold (answer D) would be required if the threshold could not be removed. The best solution would still be to remove the threshold altogether to provide the most accessible surface. See reference: Americans with Disabilities Act: ADA Accessibility Guidelines.

184. (B) walking as part of a walking club. Walking as part of a walking club throughout a facility can provide an outlet for the movement needs of some people with dementia. Walking in a structured way can be calming, provide an activity of exploration, and help to refocus the resident. Answers A, C, and D are good activities but would not provide the element of movement to the same degree. See reference: Hellen: Meaningful activities: Daily life stuff.

185. (D) Meeting the vocational instructor weekly to discuss adaptations to work tasks. Effective consultation involves ongoing communication that helps team members problem solve more effectively. Answers A and B are activities typically done by the vocational teacher. A vocational instructor should already be able to perform assessments (answer C). See reference: Case-Smith (ed): Spencer, K: Transition services: From school to adult life.

186. (A) Sheltered workshop. Sheltered workshops are segregated settings designed to help individuals master basic work skills. Supported employment (answer B) typically occurs in regular work sites, and provides intensive, ongoing support to individuals with disabilities. Job coaching (answer D) is one form of supported employment. Competitive employment (answer C) does not provide for supervision, and individuals at this level of disability would not be successful in competitive employment. The sheltered workshop is the only on-site alternative listed. See reference: Ross and Bachner (eds): Wysocki, DJ and Neulicht, AT: Adults with developmental disabilities and work.

187. (A) once a day. The *Guide for Supervision of Occupational Therapy Personnel* provides definitions for levels of supervision. Close supervision is defined as "daily, direct contact at the site of work" (p. 592). Other levels of supervision are routine, general, and minimal. Routine supervision is provided when direct contact is made every 2 weeks with "interim supervision occurring by other methods such as telephone or written communication." Under general supervision, contact is made monthly (answer C). Minimal supervision is provided on an "as needed" basis as in answer D. It is possible that this may be less than once a month. Requirements for supervision are often specified in state licensure laws, and supercede AOTA guidelines. See reference: AOTA: Guide for supervision of occupational therapy personnel in the delivery of occupational therapy services.

188. (A) refuse to provide OT services to patients until an OTR has been hired to provide supervision. A COTA cannot provide OT services without supervision from an OTR. Doing so could result in disciplinary action. Providing services for a limited period of time and treating only a few select patients (answers B and C) are both violations of certification, state licensure, the *Code of Ethics* and the *Standards of Practice*. Answer D is incorrect because the AOTA has no authority over nursing homes. See reference: Sladyk, K and Ryan, SE (eds): Ryan, SE and Sladyk, K: OTA supervision.

189. (B) source of the referral, the reason for the referral, and the date the referral was received. The initial note is used to record basic information, results of initial evaluations and, often, the treatment plan. In addition to documenting the items in answer B, the COTA may also contribute data collected from assessments she or he has performed. The OTR is responsible for analyzing an individual's assets and deficits, developing a treatment plan, and for projecting the outcome of treatment (answers A, C, and D). See reference: Early: Medical records and documentation.

190. (B) wear gloves. Wearing gloves places a barrier between the practitioner and any possible infective agent on the patient's hand. A mask (answer A) is more effective as a barrier for airborne pathogens, or for protection from splashes of bodily fluids. Refusing to work with the patient (answer C) is not an option, as indicated in the *OT Code of Ethics*. Individuals fearful of infection should educate themselves about appropriate precautions and procedures, and should seek employment in environments in which they can provide intervention to all patients served by the facility. Although handwashing before and after treatment (answer A) should be the rule with all patients, and is effective in protecting the patient and practitioner from contamination, that precaution would not be effective in protecting the practitioner during patient treatment. See reference: Pedretti and Early (eds): Buckner, WS: Infection control and safety issues in the clinic.

191. (C) Help place food on the spoon for a patient practicing the use of a universal cuff in the patient's room at lunchtime, while the OT supervisor runs a lunch group in the dining room. An aide may be delegated client-related tasks when (1) the outcome of the task being delegated is predictable; (2) the situation is stable and will not require judgment or adaptation; (3) the client has previously demonstrated the ability to perform the task; (4) the aide has demonstrated competence in the specific task; (5) the aide has been instructed in how to carry out the task with the specific client; (6) the aide knows the relevant precautions; and (7) continuous supervision is provided. When these conditions are met, answers A, B, and C are all acceptable. Although answer C may meet the other criteria, continuous supervision is absent, because the supervising OT is in the dining room. See reference: AOTA: Guidelines for the Use of Aides in OT practice.

192. (B) Universal precautions. Health care personnel should follow universal precautions when blood or body fluids are present. Suicide, escape, and medical precautions (answers A, C, and D) are guidelines developed for individuals identified with risks that are not noted in this question. See reference: Early: Safety techniques.

193. (D) order only the lightweight wheelchair and hospital bed. Durable medical equipment is defined by Medicare as "that which can withstand repeated use, is primarily and customarily used to serve a medical purpose, and generally is not useful to a person in the absence of illness or injury." Answers B and C are incorrect because they include items that are not considered "durable medical equipment" (e.g., reachers, a shower chair, or a hand-held shower). Depending on the patient's medical condition, a bedside commode may be covered. See reference: AOTA: The Occupational Therapy Manager: Thomas, VJ: Evolving health care systems: Payment for occupational therapy services.

194. (B) determine that the student is functioning at or above the minimal entry level of competence. A student must demonstrate the ability to function at or above entry level competence in order to pass level II fieldwork. For the OTA student, this includes adequate skills in the areas of evaluation, treatment, communication and professional behavior. Fieldwork experiences are designed to provide students with exposure to individuals across a lifespan, with a variety of diagnoses and in a variety of practice settings. The student must demonstrate competence with the population at the fieldwork setting, not all ages, diagnoses and cultural backgrounds (answers A and C). Likewise, the student must have a working knowledge of the system where the fieldwork experience is occurring, not all systems (answer D). See reference: AOTA: Purpose and value of occupational therapy fieldwork education.

195. (D) Explain to the administrator this is not an appropriate solution and then develop an alternate solution. OT departments frequently are understaffed and need to operate as efficiently as possible. The collaborative teamwork between an OTR and a COTA is vital in treatment planning and implementation. When a collaborative relationship is operational, the COTA may participate in evaluation and treatment planning, provide treatment, and carry out documentation. Complying with the administrator's instructions (answers A, B, and C) would result in inadequate supervision and would violate both the *Standards of Practice* and *Code of Ethics*. It is not within the OTA's scope of practice to carry out treatment planning and implementation without supervision. See reference: Neistadt and Crepeau (eds): Sands, M: Practitioners' perspectives on the occupational therapist and occupational therapy assistant partnership.

196. (D) Productivity evaluations. "Productivity is the ratio between the output and the resources expended to obtain the desired output" (p. 780). High productivity is often associated with cost-effectiveness. Analysis of productivity data can contribute to program development, improving staff effectiveness and containing costs. Outcomes measurements (answer A) are taken at the completion of service intervention and are used to evaluate the effectiveness of the intervention. Utilization reviews (answer B) assess the care that is provided to ensure that services were appropriate and not overutilized or underutilized. Program evaluation (answer C) is a method used to determine how well the program's goals have been achieved. See reference: Neistadt and Crepeau (eds): Perinchief, JM: Management of occupational therapy services.

197. (C) Creating a written and specific supervisory plan based on competency levels for both practitioners. Medicare certified home health agencies have extensive requirements for OT supervision of the OTA. In addition to requiring adequate competency on the part of the supervising OT and the practicing OTA, Medicare may request to see specific supervisory plans that detail the type and frequency of supervision provided. Supervision options include documentation review, joint visits or telephone consultation. Countersignature alone for documentation (answer B) does not necessarily constitute adequate supervision. Individual states may have additional specific guidelines. A handout (answer D) may provide useful information to the client and caregivers about OT services, but is not a critical component is establishing a collaborative relationship. See reference: Glantz and Richman:

198. (D) Treat the patient as scheduled and charge only for the 1 hour of direct time spent with the patient. This answer is correct in that this meeting was not part of the planned intervention and occurred spontaneously and without measurable goals. Based on the *Standards of Practice*, only if collaboration with the individual or family was included as a part of the intervention plan, the patient could be billed for the time. See reference: Kornblau and Starling: Legal issues in ethical decision making.

199. (C) Make a report to appropriate authorities. In many states the OT practitioner, as a health professional, is in the position of being a "mandated reporter" who must make a report if there is any reason to believe a child has been abused. A report of the injury should be made to appropriate authorities. Answers A, B, and D delay or prevent proper assistance to a family involved in the occurrence of child abuse. All agencies serving children have policies and procedures for reporting injury in these situations. See reference: Neistadt and Crepeau (eds): Davidson, DA: Child abuse and neglect.

200. (D) not use PAMs in the new state. Although AOTA policy supports the use of PAMs by qualified practitioners as an adjunct to, or in preparation for, purposeful activity, state laws supersede AOTA policies. Answers A, B, and C all violate state law as well as the *OT Code of Ethics* and could result in loss of licensure, loss of NBCOT certification, a fine, or imprisonment. See reference: AOTA: Occupational therapy code of ethics.

SIMULATION EXAMINATION 4

Directions: Circle the correct answer to the following questions. When you have completed this examination, check your answers against the answer key that follows. As you will see, an explanation is given for each answer along with a reference for further study. The book author is listed as well as the chapter author. See the bibliography for complete references. Study the areas in which your comprehension was low, then test yourself again by taking Simulation Examination 5.

Pediatrics

1. A child is lacing a series of geometric beads from a stimulus card and is unable to identify a moon-shaped bead when it is turned sideways on the table. This **MOST** likely indicates difficulty with:
   A. figure-ground perception.
   B. form constancy perception.
   C. position in space perception.
   D. visual sequencing.

2. An individual with underreactive sensory processing has been referred to OT. Based on a sensory integration frame of reference, activities for this individual should have which of the following facilitory characteristics?
   A. Arrhythmic and unexpected
   B. Arrhythmic and slow
   C. Sustained and slow
   D. Unexpected and rhythmic

3. The COTA is working with the parents of a 4-year-old boy who demonstrates a strong tonic bite reflex when eating. What type of utensils will the COTA **MOST** likely recommend to the child's parents?
   A. Pediatric weighted universal grips
   B. Curved utensils
   C. Swivel utensils
   D. Rubber-coated spoons

4. A child with poor sitting balance is unable to put on and remove lower extremity clothing. Which of the following approaches would the COTA recommend to **BEST** address this functional issue?
   A. Teach the child to dress in a sidelying position.
   B. Add loops to the waistbands of pants and skirts.
   C. Use Velcro fasteners in place of zippers.
   D. Teach the child to dress in a standing position.

5. Setting up an obstacle course that provides several options for allowing a child to choose the direction he will take (unstructured) would be **MOST** appropriate if the COTA wished to encourage:
   A. exploratory play.
   B. symbolic play.
   C. creative play.
   D. recreational play.

6. A COTA and an OTR are working on discharge plans for a child with paraplegic spina bifida who has just started using a powered wheelchair. The community resource that would be recommended as **MOST** critical for this child is:
   A. the local social service agency.
   B. a local wheelchair equipment vendor.
   C. the family physician.
   D. an early intervention program.

7. A COTA is demonstrating bathing techniques for a child with hypertonic muscle tone. Which of the following suggestions would be **MOST** appropriate for the

COTA to recommend to the child's parents?

A. Avoid the use of adaptive equipment.

B. Avoid explanations of the procedure.

C. Handle the child slowly and gently.

D. Stand and lean over the tub to support and wash the child.

8. **During the evaluation of a 6-month-old baby the COTA gently pulls the infant from a supine position into a sitting position by the hands. The child demonstrates the ability to hold her head and trunk in alignment against gravity. This observable movement can MOST accurately be described by the COTA as a(n):**

A. protective reaction.

B. flexion righting reaction.

C. body righting on body reaction.

D. optical righting reaction.

9. **A child with athetoid CP demonstrates a jaw and tongue thrust when a food filled spoon is placed in his mouth. To decrease this problem, the COTA is MOST likely to recommend a positioning strategy that includes increased:**

A. neck flexion.

B. shoulder retraction.

C. hip extension.

D. neck extension.

10. **A COTA observes a 5-year-old child with Down syndrome who has low muscle tone sitting on the floor exclusively using a "W" sitting position. This observation MOST likely indicates that the child is:**

A. developing atypically.

B. using a noncompensatory position to achieve stability.

C. demonstrating typical development for a child with Down syndrome.

D. using a position normal for a younger child, not for a 5-year-old child.

11. **A child is on a pureed diet because of an inability to chew food. The MOST effective method for the COTA to facilitate the child's ability to chew would be to:**

A. encourage the child to remove food from the spoon with his teeth.

B. stimulate the management of texture by using vegetable or beef soup.

C. increase the management of texture by slowly increasing texture of food with a baby food grinder.

D. stimulate biting and chewing by placing a raisin between the child's teeth.

12. **An OT practitioner is administering a standardized test to a young client who suddenly becomes uncooperative and complains that the test is "too hard." The MOST appropriate response would be to:**

A. switch to easier items to improve the child's self-esteem.

B. terminate the session and schedule another session to administer the remainder of the test.

C. follow administration instructions and note changes in behavior.

D. adapt the remaining test items to ensure success.

13. **A child with poor anticipatory postural control demonstrates inadequate playground skills, losing her balance when trying to anticipate movement. Which of the following activities will BEST promote the development of these skills?**

A. Ballet

B. Soccer

C. Basketball

D. Ping-pong

14. **A 3-year-old child with a diagnosis of mental retardation is dependent in all areas of dressing. If the COTA uses a developmental approach with this child, which skill should FIRST be addressed?**

A. Putting on garments with the front and back of clothing correctly placed

B. Putting on a tee shirt

C. Removing pants

D. Buttoning and tying bows

15. **The COTA has fitted a 6-year-old child for an adapted seat for use in the home for mealtime and other tabletop activities. Which of the following instructions is MOST appropriate to convey to the parents?**

A. Change the seat as needed.

B. Bring the seat in for each weekly therapy session in order to adjust it according to the child's growth.

C. Bring the seat in for reevaluation within 6 months.

D. Keep the seat until the end of the IEP.

16. **The BEST activity to encourage the bilateral use of a child's hands is:**

A. finger painting.
B. playing clapping games.
C. turning pages in a story book.
D. making "Play Doh" "meatballs" using the index finger and thumb.

17. A COTA is working with a child who has mild spastic cerebral palsy. The evaluation has shown that the child has poor in-hand manipulation skills. Practicing what type of activity would be BEST to improve this inability?

A. Grasping blocks to build a building
B. Placing pegs from one pegboard to another
C. Carrying a bag of Lego blocks with a handle
D. Removing a nut from a bolt

18. A preschooler is having difficulty performing tasks requiring eye-hand coordination as a result of poor visual tracking skills. The FIRST activity the COTA uses to promote visual tracking skill is:

A. tossing and catching a water balloon.
B. catching and bursting soap bubbles.
C. throwing and catching a beach ball.
D. playing softball.

19. A 1-year-old child is working on increasing neck flexor strength. At this time, the child can maintain head alignment when tilted backward from an upright supported sitting position, to a 45-degree incline, but loses control when tilted further back. The COTA recommends that the NEXT important step in the intervention is to work on head and neck alignment:

A. in a sidelying position while batting a toy.
B. in a prone position while watching a peek-a-boo game.
C. by tilting backward up to 60 degrees while rocking.
D. in a supine position while watching an overhead mobile.

20. A COTA learns that a young child receiving OT is easily aroused because of a sensory-modulation disorder. Which of the following describes the MOST effective environmental adaptation for assisting the child to fall asleep?

A. A mini-trampoline in the bedroom to tire the child out before going to bed
B. A noise machine producing white noise at bedtime
C. A lightweight, fuzzy blanket providing light touch

D. Shutters on the windows to produce total darkness

21. To promote play skills and self-expression in a child who is withdrawn, a COTA should FIRST select activities that:

A. promote open-ended symbolic play, such as using action figures, puppets, and dolls.
B. provide a defined structure, such as simple craft activities with instructions.
C. promote social interaction, such as a game of tag with peers.
D. provide a means of tension release, such as leather tooling or wedging clay.

22. A child has poor sitting balance, which interferes with seated tabletop activities. Which of the following should the COTA suggest to the child's teacher for the promotion of ongoing postural adjustments in sitting?

A. Use a sturdy chair with lateral trunk supports while the child is doing homework.
B. Use a corner floor seat with built in desk surface while the child is self-feeding.
C. Provide a bolster for back support while the child is coloring.
D. Provide a therapy ball to sit on while the child is playing a game of checkers.

23. A toddler diagnosed with developmental delays does not finger feed when presented with food in the clinic. The BEST way to obtain further information about his feeding skills is to:

A. interview his parents to determine his favorite foods.
B. observe him in his home during feeding time.
C. review his chart for food allergies.
D. repeat the observation in a quiet area to minimize distractions.

24. During an initial visit with a 5-year-old child with a suspected learning disability, the COTA observes the child run across the room, hop around on one foot, pick up a pencil, and draw a stick figure using a tripod grasp. When asked to complete a 4-piece puzzle, the child gives up after several unsuccessful attempts. Which type of assessment would MOST effectively address this child's area of difficulty?

A. Fine motor
B. Gross motor
C. Developmental

D. Visual perceptual

25. **A child with athetoid cerebral palsy is learning to use augmentative communication and is frustrated because it takes so long to produce a sentence. Which of the following would the COTA recommend as the BEST solution for this problem?**
    A. A larger monitor
    B. A voice output tool
    C. Word prediction software
    D. Masking inappropriate keys

26. **Which of the following is the BEST position for promoting isolated head control in a child with very limited postural control and significant upper and lower extremity weakness?**
    A. Standing in a standing frame with knee and hip support
    B. Quadruped with chest supported in a sling
    C. Prone over a wedge
    D. Sitting on a therapy ball with hips supported by the therapist

27. **An 8-year-old boy is being treated in OT for social withdrawal and depression. At the time of discharge, the BEST recreational activity for the COTA to recommend is:**
    A. swimming lessons.
    B. Boy Scouts.
    C. computer games.
    D. piano lessons.

28. **A child with CP demonstrates poor head control, high lower extremity extensor tone, and high upper extremity flexor tone. The COTA should recommend which of the following to BEST position the child for feeding?**
    A. A prone stander with lateral trunk supports
    B. A corner chair with head support and padded abductor post
    C. A wedge that positions the hips in 115 degrees of flexion when the child is supine
    D. A bolster chair without back support

29. **When developing a self-care program for a 3-year-old child with significant visual impairment, the home care COTA would MOST likely implement which of the following?**
    A. Create a reliable route to the bathroom, encouraging the child to familiarize herself

with the smells and sounds of the bathroom.
    B. Have the child practice various obstacle courses at a local playground to improve body image/awareness.
    C. Practice hand writing and fine motor skills with a "Lite Brite" activity board.
    D. Introduce the child to other children who have visual impairments.

30. **A COTA is working on prewriting skills with an 11-month-old child. Which of the following activities would be MOST appropriate for the COTA to instruct the child to perform?**
    A. Scribble on a piece of paper.
    B. Copy a triangle.
    C. Copy a horizontal line on a chalkboard.
    D. Copy numerals on a sheet of paper.

31. **A COTA positions an infant in the prone position to provide an opportunity to work against gravity. This position is MOST effective for developing which ability?**
    A. Retraction of the shoulders in weight bearing
    B. Stability of the head and neck
    C. Development of trunk flexion
    D. Mobility in the upper extremities

32. **A COTA is working with a school-age child to improve her power grasp technique. Which of the following activities would the COTA MOST likely request the child perform in order to elicit the power grasp position?**
    A. Pegboard activities
    B. Brushing her own hair
    C. Carrying a light weight briefcase
    D. Throwing a ball

33. **A child with limited upper extremity range of motion is being prepared for discharge. The MOST important home adaptation for the COTA to recommend concerning use of the toilet is:**
    A. installation of safety bars next to the toilet seat.
    B. mounting of a wide base toilet seat.
    C. placement of a skidproof stepping stool next to the toilet.
    D. installation of a bidet with a spray wash and air drying mechanism.

34. **The COTA is planning treatment to promote developmental acquisition for an**

infant in the neonatal intensive care unit. Which of the following actions will have the most **PERMANENT** impact?

A. Modify the environment to protect the infant from additional stressful stimuli.

B. Recommend early intervention referral to assess the infant upon discharge home.

C. Complete the neurobehavioral assessment and identify interventions emphasizing developmental skill acquisition.

D. Create a comfortable foundation for fostering parent skills through parent-therapist collaboration.

35. **A third-grader's readiness for discharge from direct OT, as a related service, has been determined on the basis of:**

A. whether the areas of concern to the OT interfere with the child's education.

B. the degree of functional skills possessed by the child.

C. the level of independence in ADL.

D. the degree of accessibility of the learning environment.

36. **A COTA is working with a 3-year-old child who has spastic diplegia. The mobility device which would be MOST appropriate to use in assisting this child to explore space would be:**

A. a body length prone scooter.

B. an airplane mobility device.

C. a tricycle.

D. a power wheelchair.

37. **A preteen with a history of TBI is relearning to prepare simple foods, but has been having difficulties with sequencing, so the COTA has provided the patient with a chart of steps to follow. The child has just learned to prepare his favorite sandwich without "losing his place" in the process, but continues to need occasional verbal reminders to look at the chart and to ensure safety. At this point, the child's MOST recent level of independence would be documented as:**

A. independent.

B. independent with setup.

C. supervision.

D. minimal assist.

38. **A child has difficulty controlling food in her mouth when swallowing. In helping the parents plan snacks, the COTA would be MOST likely to recommend:**

A. chicken noodle soup.

B. peanut butter.

C. carrot sticks.

D. applesauce.

39. **A fifth grade child with hypertonicity adducts her legs and extends her hips and spine when seated to do schoolwork. The BEST way for the COTA to encourage better postural control in sitting would be to position the child:**

A. in a 20- to 30-degree forward tilt.

B. upright.

C. 45 degrees reclined.

D. in a 45-degree lateral tilt.

40. **A COTA and OTR are planning for the discharge of a child from an early intervention program. What advice to the parents will MOST likely result in effective carryover of a therapeutic home program?**

A. Set aside a certain time daily to focus on therapeutic activities.

B. Incorporate therapeutic activities into family routines.

C. Provide therapeutic activities on an as needed basis.

D. Do therapeutic activities daily, but vary the time of day.

41. **The BEST way for a COTA to utilize sensory stimulation for a child with tactile defensiveness is to:**

A. apply intense light touch stimulation, such as tickling on the abdomen, for desensitization.

B. avoid all forms of tactile stimulation to accommodate the child's preferences.

C. allow the child to self-apply tactile stimuli to maximize the child's tolerance.

D. avoid all deep pressure tactile stimuli to decrease defensiveness.

42. **A COTA is planning treatment activities to use for a child with an underreactive vestibular system. The activities selected would MOST likely address:**

A. poor postural responses.

B. discomfort with motion activities.

C. anxiety when his or her feet are off the ground.

D. gravitational insecurity.

43. **During assessment of a 10-month-old child with Down syndrome, the COTA notes hyperextensibility of all joints, which MOST likely reflects:**

A. increased muscle tone.
B. decreased muscle tone.
C. anterior horn cell disease.
D. muscle and joint disease.

44. **While standing and holding onto furniture, a 3-year-old boy with delayed motor development shifts his weight onto one leg and steps to the side with the other. This movement pattern is BEST described as:**
    A. creeping.
    B. crawling.
    C. cruising.
    D. clawing.

45. **A COTA is using a visual perceptual frame of reference to plan intervention for a child with visual perceptual problems. The FIRST activities planned should address which type of visual skills?**
    A. Visual memory skills
    B. Visual attention skills
    C. General visual discrimination skills
    D. Specific visual discrimination skills

46. **A young child with hypertonicity is unable to bring his hands to midline to reach for a toy while in the supine and sitting positions. The BEST position to use in order to reduce the effects of abnormal patterns and facilitate midline grasp is:**
    A. the standing position.
    B. the prone position.
    C. the sidelying position.
    D. the quadruped position.

47. **When providing occupational therapy for children who have been diagnosed with a terminal illness, the PRIMARY focus for OT intervention would be:**
    A. educational activities.
    B. play and self-care activities.
    C. socialization activities.
    D. motor activities.

48. **A young boy with hemiplegia has difficulty putting on his socks each morning before school. Which of the following should the COTA recommend?**
    A. Encourage the child to wear tight fitting socks.
    B. Teach the child to sit in a chair and lift and place the affected foot up on a small stool.
    C. Encourage the child to lay on his back in bed when putting on socks.
    D. Teach the child to sit in a chair and lift and place the unaffected foot up on a small stool.

49. **A student is unable to focus on a blackboard 20 feet away and then refocus on the book on her desk to copy a mathematics problem. This MOST likely indicates a problem with:**
    A. ocular motility.
    B. binocular vision.
    C. convergence.
    D. accommodation.

50. **A COTA observes a child with autism waving his right hand in front of his eyes repeatedly in an apparently purposeless manner. This behavior MOST likely indicates:**
    A. the child is able to focus his eyes at close range.
    B. that wrist mobility is WNL.
    C. right hand dominance.
    D. the presence of self-stimulatory behavior.

51. **The COTA is working on dressing skills with a 7-year-old child with limited pincer grasp. The child wishes to zip his own pants in school, and mentioned that he "feels embarrassed" that he sometimes needs to ask his teacher for assistance after using the bathroom. Which of the following should the COTA recommend the child try FIRST?**
    A. A large key ring
    B. Oversized fasteners
    C. Colored zippers
    D. Velcro fasteners

52. **The COTA is selecting activities for a young school age child with postural control deficits. Which activity would BEST promote postural control?**
    A. Sliding down a playground slide
    B. Playing "Simon Says"
    C. Swimming
    D. Playing on a trampoline

53. **A COTA is working on hand function with a school-age child diagnosed with juvenile rheumatoid arthritis. Which of the following devices should the COTA recommend to MOST effectively prevent hand fatigue?**
    A. Reacher

B. Jar opener
C. Pencil gripper
D. Plate guard

54. A COTA is discussing discharge plans with the parents of a 7-year-old child with sensory defensiveness problems. The MOST appropriate activity the COTA could recommend to provide proprioceptive input for this child would be to:
A. walk barefoot on textured surfaces.
B. rock over a large therapy ball.
C. play in a large box full of styrofoam pellets.
D. perform slow push-ups against the wall.

55. The COTA is setting up a feeding session with a normally developing 24-month-old boy. The COTA should encourage the child to eat a bowl of peas and carrots with which of the following?
A. A small spoon
B. His fingers
C. A swivel spoon
D. A small fork

56. Which of the following would the COTA recommend to a 12-year-old child with mild visual impairments who desires independent use of the telephone with-in his home?
A. A speaker phone
B. A hands-free phone
C. A phone with extra large buttons
D. A phone with a receiver holder

57. Which of the following activities should the COTA introduce FIRST when treating a child for tactile defensiveness?
A. Gentle brushing of the child's face and neck
B. Rubbing lotion on the child's arms
C. Having the child roll around in a carpeted barrel
D. Swinging the child in a hammock swing

58. A child with cerebral palsy has tongue thrust. Prior to feeding, the COTA should do which of the following FIRST?
A. Position the child's trunk, head, neck, and shoulders in proper alignment.
B. Hyperextend the child's head.
C. Place his digits directly under the child's chin, facilitating tongue retraction.
D. Provide upward pressure under the child's lower jaw prior to chewing.

59. The COTA is attempting to increase dressing independence with a 13-year-

old boy with hemiplegia. The child has been unsuccessful for the past 2 months with buttonhooks and zipper pulls and appears frustrated with his performance. He also complains about the time that it takes to fasten his pants after toileting while in school. Which of the following should the COTA suggest NEXT?
A. Encourage the child to work with a dressing stick.
B. Have the child practice with fastening boards.
C. Encourage the child's mother to assist with buttoning and zippering.
D. Place Velcro fasteners in the child's clothing in place of zippers and buttons.

Mental Health

60. An OT practitioner has been asked to design a series of stress management sessions for individuals with multiple sclerosis. The first session should include:
A. time management techniques.
B. self-assessment.
C. aerobic exercise.
D. progressive resistive exercise.

61. A patient with mild mental retardation and schizophrenia received OT services in a mental health facility to improve his daily living skills. In developing the discharge summary for this patient, which section of the summary would be the sole responsibility of the OTR to complete?
A. Discharge recommendations
B. Summary of the OT process, including number of sessions
C. Patient's discharge disposition
D. Patient's current level of functioning in grooming and hygiene

62. An OT practitioner is working as a consultant to a long-term care facility that is designing a dementia care unit. The OT practitioner would MOST likely recommend which type of environmental attributes as therapeutic?
A. Controlled stimulation with meaningful sensory cues
B. High sensory stimulation, to encourage active engagement
C. Subdued, low sensory stimulation environment, to prevent agitation

D. Stimuli that are very similar to those found in the residents' home environments

63. The goal for an adolescent with anorexia is to improve self-concept. Which component of a meal preparation activity BEST addresses this goal?

A. Participate in a nutrition group and plan a healthy meal.

B. Develop a budget and shop for ingredients with three other group members.

C. Delegate tasks and prepare the meal with three other group members.

D. State strengths and limitations regarding performance in the activity.

64. A COTA is running a group for individuals who have difficulty managing anger. Based on a cognitive-behavioral frame of reference, which of the following steps would the COTA BEGIN with?

A. Discuss the benefits of alternative beliefs about anger and alternative responses to anger.

B. Develop awareness about what produces anger and how the clients respond to anger.

C. Role play a situation that presents minimal difficulty to group participants.

D. Role play a situation that presents significant difficulty to group participants.

65. An individual with a history of substance abuse lives in a group home. The residential manager has asked the COTA to work with the individual to develop house-cleaning skills. Which of the following interventions is MOST appropriate when a cognitive approach is desired?

A. Reward the individual with a snack bar token when chores have been successfully completed.

B. Praise the individual when chores have been successfully completed.

C. Post a schedule of each individual's chore responsibilities in a highly visible location.

D. Conduct a group discussion about responsibilities people have when living in a group home.

66. A COTA working in a group home with individuals with serious mental illness is developing a program to promote healthier eating habits. Which of the following activities BEST represents a psychoeducational approach?

A. Each client makes a healthy food collage.

B. Plan and shop for a meal as a group.

C. Designate 1 day a week for the residents to be responsible for cooking dinner.

D. Show a video about nutrition and keep a meal diary for a week.

67. An individual with a cognitive disability has recently joined a sheltered workshop setting and has been referred to OT for assignment to an appropriate group. The individual demonstrates the ability to copy demonstrated directions when presented one step at a time. The individual can visualize an end product, but is unable to recognize errors, and may not be able to correct them when they are pointed out. According to Allen's Cognitive Disability Theory, the MOST appropriate group for this individual is one involved with:

A. sorting plastic utensils into separate containers.

B. assembling packets that include a knife, fork, spoon, and napkin based on a sample.

C. selecting matching shoelaces from a mixed pile and lacing them onto a display card.

D. gluing labels onto cans and placing them in an appropriate container according to color.

68. A COTA is evaluating self-care skills with an individual who has recently come out of a coma following a TBI. The individual is able to pick up a toothbrush and apply toothpaste independently. He takes 15 minutes to brush his teeth. This behavior most likely indicates difficulty in which of the following areas?

A. Sequencing

B. Following directions

C. Problem solving

D. Termination of activity

69. An individual with a history of anxiety is in an OT group that meets twice a week. However, he frequently interrupts the COTA during other OT groups of which he is not a member. What is the MOST effective approach for the COTA to use in this situation?

A. Listen to what the individual has to say and schedule a time to meet after the group.

B. Set a time to meet with the individual after group and let him know that you will hear what he has to say at that time.

C. Allow the individual remain in the group and encourage him to express his needs.

D. Tell the individual that his behavior is inappropriate and refuse to listen to him.

70. **While observing a group of individuals eating lunch, a COTA observes one individual who grabs the ketchup away from her neighbor, chews with her mouth open, and does not make eye contact with those around her. The other clients seem to be trying to avoid her. The behaviors exhibited by this individual MOST likely indicate a deficit in which of the following?**

A. Social conduct

B. Self-esteem

C. Self-control

D. Coping skills

71. **An individual diagnosed with substance abuse has recently begun attending a partial hospitalization program and the COTA has received a request to evaluate the individual's leisure performance. Which of the following methods would MOST effectively evaluate how this individual spends his leisure time?**

A. Administer an interest checklist.

B. Administer a time-use assessment.

C. Assess his ability to play a sport.

D. Observe him playing a game.

72. **A COTA is working in a psychosocial setting with clients who are classified as being at risk for suicide. In selecting craft media, the activity that would MOST likely be the safest is a:**

A. leather checkbook cover with single cordovan lacing.

B. macramé plant hanger.

C. ceramic ashtray.

D. stenciling project on poster board.

73. **An individual with borderline personality disorder has been referred to occupational therapy. Which of the following would be MOST important to evaluate?**

A. Activities of daily living

B. Instrumental ADL's

C. Relationships with others

D. Sensorimotor skills

74. **An individual in an adult day program demonstrates poor social skills and frequent sexual acting out. The activity that would MOST effectively provide re-** lease for this individual's sexual tension is:

A. jogging.

B. macramé.

C. reading a pornographic magazine.

D. ballroom dancing.

75. **While in the hospital, a 48-year-old roofing contractor experienced extrapyramidal syndrome after being placed on neuroleptic medications. The patient is to continue taking the medication after discharge from the hospital. It is MOST important to advise the patient to:**

A. limit sun exposure as much as possible.

B. avoid use of power tools and sharp instruments.

C. get up slowly from a standing, sitting, or lying position.

D. be aware of the dehydrating effects of caffeinated drinks and alcohol.

76. **A COTA is running a sensorimotor group for individuals diagnosed with severe depression who tend to withdraw from social activities. Which of the following would be the MOST appropriate opening activity?**

A. Group members take turns introducing themselves.

B. Group members toss a ball to each other.

C. Each group member describes his or her day.

D. Group members pass around and smell a basket of scented potpourri.

77. **An individual with depression is ready to return to the job held before taking a leave of absence. Which of the following is the FIRST action the OT practitioner should take?**

A. Perform a job analysis.

B. Request reasonable accommodation.

C. Emphasize activities that promote a sense of self-efficacy.

D. Encourage the individual to participate in a weekly support group.

78. **A COTA is evaluating the decision-making, problem-solving, and sequencing skills of a woman with a long-standing history of mental illness as she makes brownies from a mix. He observes the individual put the whole egg, shell and all, into the bowl. Which of the following actions should the COTA take FIRST?**

A. Evaluate the individual's cognitive function.

B. Determine that the individual is interested in meal preparation as a goal, then develop short- and long-term goals and a treatment plan.
C. Schedule the individual for meal preparation group sessions to improve skill level.
D. Determine the individual's home environment and her need for meal preparation skills.

79. In planning intervention for an adult with schizophrenia who has tactile defensiveness, a COTA has selected a ceramics activity. Which element of ceramics would be MOST difficult for the client?
A. Wedging the clay
B. Imprinting a design with a rolling pin
C. Glazing the clay
D. Firing the clay

80. A COTA has been asked to develop a program of self-awareness activities for a group of substance abusers. A graded program to develop an individual's self-awareness MUST include activities that:
A. encourage self-awareness.
B. are structured by the COTA to encourage self-reflection and feedback.
C. provide opportunities for the patient to be self-aware.
D. allow for increasing social interaction.

81. An elderly client was hospitalized for an episode of acute depression after the death of his spouse. The client is preparing for discharge and would like to return to his home, but is fearful of spending his days alone. The BEST environment for the client to continue socialization and participation in meaningful occupation would be:
A. partial hospitalization.
B. adult daycare.
C. home health care.
D. psychosocial rehabilitation center.

82. A COTA is running a parallel group. What level of assistance should the COTA offer to address the needs of this particular group?
A. Encourage experimentation among group members.
B. Observe from the sidelines and not act as an authority figure.
C. Participate as an active member.
D. Assist clients in the selection of simple, short-term tasks.

83. A COTA is selecting treatment activities to use with a young adult diagnosed with schizophrenia (undifferentiated type) that would help to increase the patient's ability to receive, process, and respond to sensory information. The MOST suitable activities for this patient would include:
A. social skills training.
B. vestibular stimulation and gross motor exercise.
C. role playing.
D. discussion groups.

84. The goal of an arts and crafts group for chronically mentally ill individuals is to improve their decision-making abilities. The MOST appropriate approach to initiating a mosaic tile activity would be to:
A. provide each patient with an individual project and have him or her choose a tile color.
B. have the patients choose from a variety of projects.
C. have the patients decide on a design, size, shape, and color for a group mosaics project.
D. have each patient decide on a pattern and two tile colors to use in his or her mosaic project.

85. An individual with strong dependency needs is able to lace a leather wallet only with consistent verbal cueing. Which is the BEST way to grade this activity to decrease dependency?
A. Provide written instructions on lacing techniques and ask the individual to continue on her own.
B. Ask the individual to try some lacing with distant supervision and praise her for what she has been able to do.
C. Ask the individual to take the lacing to her room and continue without the OT's assistance.
D. Tell the individual to complete a small amount of lacing while the OT assists another patient in the same room.

86. A young woman with bulimia is approaching readiness for discharge and is able to eat individually sized portions from the cafeteria without binging or purging. What is the BEST way to upgrade her next meal experience?
A. Dine as a group using a family style dining format.

B. Offer her double portions.

C. Ask her to provide a calorie count of the entire meal.

D. Emphasize the need to exercise aggressively if she chooses to eat a dessert.

87. An adolescent boy is admitted to an acute psychiatric facility after several uncontrollable violent outbursts toward his mother. He admits to experimenting with marijuana and beer since he was 16 years old in order to be accepted by his peer group. Which of the following activities would MOST effectively address the goal of emotional expression?

A. Tell his peers what makes him angry.

B. Learn karate techniques.

C. Participate in writing a group rock song using "I" statements.

D. Learn relaxation techniques he can use when feeling angry.

88. A patient diagnosed with an anxiety disorder tells a COTA that he can't go with his therapy group on a planned shopping trip because he feels fearful. The FIRST appropriate response for the COTA is to:

A. change the topic of conversation or redirect the person's attention to an activity.

B. be relaxed but firm, reinforcing that the person needs to, and should, go on the trip.

C. encourage the patient to describe what makes him fearful about going on this trip.

D. clearly state the reasons why there is nothing to fear in going on the trip.

89. During a group movement activity, a female client begins to pull at her clothes and move seductively around the room. She does not stop, despite repeated attempts by the group leader to end this behavior. Which response is MOST appropriate?

A. Dismiss her from the group.

B. End the movement activity.

C. Direct her toward the back of the room.

D. Encourage her to express herself using a different medium, such as painting.

90. An individual with a history of substance abuse is working on skills she will need to take public transportation to an office where she will be working as a volunteer. She has successfully demonstrated the ability ride the bus to her destination and return home again without assis-

tance. What is the next challenge the COTA should introduce?

A. Develop the ability to take the bus to the "Y" where her AA group meets.

B. Require that she ride the bus according to a designated schedule.

C. Have her identify strategies to use in case of bad weather.

D. Work on the ability to count out exact change for bus fare.

91. An individual who demonstrates compulsive behaviors is unable to complete a cookie baking activity because he spends so much time measuring and remeasuring ingredients. Upon observing this, how should the COTA respond?

A. Tell him that measuring so many times is unnecessary.

B. Encourage him to talk about his fears.

C. Acknowledge that he uses rituals to cope with anxiety.

D. Discontinue group work and treat him individually.

92. A COTA is working with an individual who has just broken up with his girlfriend. He spends most of his day in bed and reports feelings of helplessness and hopelessness. How should the COTA respond upon hearing about these feelings?

A. Listen to what the individual says and reflect back to him.

B. Redirect the individual to more positive thoughts.

C. Emphasize his positive qualities and tell him he's bound to find another girlfriend soon.

D. Tell him he needs to pull himself together.

93. A COTA has been working with a young adult client with mental retardation and is providing information to assist the OTR in making work placement recommendations for the client. The COTA reports that the client functions best when performing simple, highly structured tasks in a closely supervised environment. The MOST appropriate recommendation would be for work placement in a:

A. supported employment program.

B. volunteer work program.

C. transitional employment program.

D. sheltered work program.

94. A COTA asks a manic client what he would like to do in craft group. The client

answers, "I'm a really good carpenter, so I'm going to build my kids a club house." The BEST response is to:

A. support him in this choice.
B. tell him he doesn't have the necessary attention span at this time.
C. redirect him toward an activity that doesn't require sharp tools.
D. suggest a more realistic activity.

95. **An individual with mental illness attends group on a regular basis, but interrupts others, grabs tools and supplies, and bosses others around at almost every group session. What is the BEST way to respond to this disruptive behavior?**

A. Have the individual contribute to a discussion identifying the "rules" for the group.
B. Tell the individual he may not return to the group until he is able to treat others with respect.
C. Ignore the behavior during the group and speak to him about it afterwards.
D. Explain to him that this type of behavior is unacceptable.

96. **An elderly man with chronic schizophrenia is frequently observed with his hand in his pants, sexually stimulating himself. The BEST approach is to:**

A. tell him to stop the behavior.
B. involve him in activities with physical contact.
C. revoke his cigarette privileges.
D. provide him with regular forceful gross motor activities.

97. **The initial short-term goal for a client working on improving socialization skills is, "patient will verbally respond to others during performance of a common task three times per session with minimal verbal cues within 1 week." After several sessions, the COTA observes that the client is responding to others three times or more per session without cueing, but does not maintain eye contact or initiate conversation. Which of the following would be the MOST appropriate action for the COTA to take next?**

A. Continue following the treatment plan exactly as written.
B. Collaboration with the OTR to change the short-term goal.
C. Begin a formal re-evaluation of the client.
D. Revise the long-term goal and report the change to the OTR.

98. **A young woman with anorexia nervosa is participating in a lunch preparation and cooking group. What should the COTA do when the woman asks to go to the bathroom following the meal?**

A. Tell her she needs to remain in the group.
B. Allow her to go to the bathroom.
C. Pull her aside and ask her if she is upset.
D. Call her floor nurse for advice.

99. **An extremely withdrawn individual has developed the ability to tolerate interaction with one other group member while glazing slip molds in an ongoing ceramics group. Which of the following steps should be taken NEXT in order to develop this individual's ability to interact with others?**

A. Involve the individual in a three-member task group.
B. Progress the individual from glazing slip molds to building coil pots.
C. Instruct the individual in how to pour the molds in addition to glazing them.
D. Encourage the individual to choose his own project and glazes.

100. **A COTA is providing instruction to caregivers in a long-term care facility concerning assisting a resident whose severe attention span deficits impair the ability to participate in self-feeding. The COTA is MOST likely to recommend which method?**

A. Demonstration of feeding process for the resident
B. Providing verbal feedback to the resident about how he or she is progressing
C. Hand-over-hand assistance
D. Chaining

101. **A COTA is preparing to complete part of an initial evaluation on an individual diagnosed with obsessive-compulsive disorder. Which of the following environmental modification strategies is likely to be MOST effective?**

A. Limit the time available to answer each question.
B. Instruct the individual to take her time and not rush.
C. Utilize open-ended questions.
D. Minimize environmental distractions.

102. **A COTA is using a functional skill, or task-specific training approach, with an individual with severe memory impair-**

ment who is learning to brush his teeth. This approach will rely on:

A. forward chaining.
B. negative reinforcement.
C. generalization of learning.
D. gradual fading of cues.

103. An individual with moderate cognitive limitations lives in a group home and has difficulty telling the difference between his toothbrush and everyone else's. This individual will benefit MOST from:

A. using an electric toothbrush.
B. having the only red toothbrush.
C. putting a built-up handle on his toothbrush.
D. having a caregiver brush his teeth twice a day for him.

104. A young adult who sustained a severe TBI has begun participating in a community re-entry program. The OTR will evaluate self-care skills, and the COTA will evaluate the individual's ability to perform work and productive activities. Which of the following are MOST appropriate for the COTA to address?

A. Health maintenance, socialization, and community mobility
B. Feeding, eating, and sexual expression
C. Clothing care, cleaning, and volunteering
D. Reading, watching television, and doing small handicrafts

105. A COTA is leading a social skills group for clients in a community mental health center. The group members have learned about social skills and their components, and the COTA has spent time in modeling and demonstrating ways to perform social skills. Which of the following would be the NEXT step in the process of learning social skills?

A. Practicing how to self-evaluate one's social behavior
B. Independent practice in real life situations
C. Role playing of social situations
D. Providing feedback on the client's hygiene and physical appearance

106. Which one of the following interventions will most successfully enable an individual to develop and maintain good coping skills?

A. Describe how it feels to have limitations.
B. Eat well, exercise, and participate in meaningful occupations.
C. List personal accomplishments.

D. Identify values and interests.

107. An individual with chronic pain from a back injury is participating in a work hardening program. At what point should the COTA instruct the individual to take a break?

A. When pain becomes intolerable
B. Right before the individual feels pain is about to begin
C. When the individual has worked to tolerance
D. After 30 minutes

108. A patient with schizophrenia is leaving a half-way house (community mental health setting) and will return home to live with his family. Which area of education would be MOST beneficial to address with the family prior to discharge?

A. The need for environmental adaptations in the home to ensure safety
B. Encouraging the client to attend twelve-step self-help programs
C. Monitoring of nutrition, physical activity, and rest
D. Information about the disease, its management, and communication strategies

109. A COTA is working with a group of individuals with substance abuse disorders. The COTA wants to use an activity that will allow the clients to experience success after making a mess and one that will delay gratification. The activity process that BEST provides this experience is:

A. working in a group with three other individuals.
B. selecting the design pattern for a tile trivet.
C. applying grout to a tile trivet and waiting for it to dry.
D. encouraging the individual to clean off the table at the end of the group.

110. A patient who sustained head trauma is receiving an OT program of repetitive pegboard, paper and pencil tasks, and computer activities to remediate attention and memory deficits. The COTA is implementing these cognitive remediation tasks because the patient is MOST likely demonstrating which of the following?

A. Cognitive deficits that must be treated within a short treatment time frame

B. Awareness, minimal deficits, and learning potential

C. Difficulty transferring learned skills to new situations

D. A history of cognitive deficits resulting from a head trauma years ago

111. **The OTR has asked the COTA to administer the last portion of an assessment to an individual who was recently admitted to an inpatient psychiatric unit. When presented with the standardized evaluation, a checklist to determine the individual's interests in various leisure activities, the individual is unable to read the evaluation because he does not have his glasses with him. Which of the following options is MOST appropriate?**

A. Instruct the individual to bring his glasses to the next session and complete the evaluation then.

B. Ask the OT aide to read the evaluation to the individual and check off his answers.

C. Include the individual in the group session that is about to begin and remind the individual to bring his glasses to the next session.

D. Read the questions to the individual and check off his responses.

112. **A COTA is planning to run a coping skills group for individuals diagnosed with bulimia for the primary purpose of:**

A. decreasing the sense of alienation among group members.

B. bringing about change among the members.

C. enabling members to experience several points of view.

D. effectively managing the economic forces within the health care setting.

113. **Upon completion of the initial interview and chart review, the NEXT step to be taken in the OT process is to:**

A. analyze the data.

B. develop a treatment plan.

C. perform selected assessments.

D. select appropriate evaluation procedures.

114. **An older adult with schizophrenia lives in a group home for individuals with chronic mental illness. During a socialization activity in the community living room, the COTA notices beginning signs of agitation. Which of the following methods is MOST likely to decrease agitation?**

A. Have the individual lie down on a sofa.

B. Have the individual sit in a rocking chair.

C. Direct the individual to leave the room immediately.

D. Give the individual prescribed anti-anxiety medication.

115. **A COTA is training an adult worker with a developmental disability to put a pencil in a box before putting a score pad in the box for a game packaging task in a sheltered workshop assembly line. The employee has not done this task before. Which of the following reinforcement schedules would MOST likely achieve the goal of learning this task sequence?**

A. Intermittent reinforcement with correct responses

B. Reinforcement every 10 minutes

C. Reinforcement for every fourth correct response

D. Continuous reinforcement of correct responses

116. **During a craft group comprised of individuals diagnosed with substance abuse, a COTA observes one individual having difficulty gluing two pieces of a birdhouse together. The individual becomes increasingly agitated. As the COTA approaches him, he storms out of the room and heads to the smoking area for a cigarette. This behavior MOST likely indicates a problem in which of the following?**

A. Eye-hand coordination

B. Stress management

C. Visual perception

D. Fine motor skills

117. **While running a discussion group, the COTA encounters a group member who frequently monopolizes the discussion and interrupts other members. The COTA has unsuccessfully attempted various subtle and indirect methods to decrease the client's behavior. Which direct intervention should the COTA implement NEXT to modify the client's behavior?**

A. Sit beside the person who is monopolizing the discussion and touch his or her hand or arm as a reminder not to interrupt others who are talking.

B. Confront the individual's behavior and ask, "Are you aware that your frequent interruptions prevent others from having a chance to contribute?"

C. Redirect the individual and say, "Now let's hear what others have to say about this."

D. Restructure the task by selecting a group activity that requires sequential turn taking.

118. A COTA wants to alter the seating arrangement of a community skills group in order to facilitate communication amongst the members. The BEST arrangement would be to:

A. provide enough chairs around a rectangular table.

B. provide enough chairs around a round table.

C. provide enough pillows to sit on the floor.

D. use the couches and chairs that are already in the room.

119. "The patient has taken a more active role in the task group, as evidenced by the patient's willingness to contribute ideas and offer to assist in designing the unit mural." This statement would MOST appropriately be documented in which portion of a SOAP note?

A. Subjective
B. Objective
C. Assessment
D. Plan

120. Which of the following community activities provides an appropriate level of challenge for a client beginning assertiveness training?

A. Asking a department store salesperson for information about an item without buying it

B. In a restaurant, requesting that food be sent back to be rewarmed

C. Returning an item to a department store for cash, with the receipt

D. Questioning whether a restaurant bill is accurate and asking for an account

Physical Disabilities

121. Which of the following components is MOST essential to include when designing a work hardening program?

A. Pain management techniques
B. Achieving a balance between work and leisure
C. Energy conservation techniques
D. Vocational counseling

122. A COTA is performing a kitchen activity with an individual with limited shoulder range of motion the day before discharge. The individual demonstrates difficulty retrieving items from the higher shelves. Which of the following recommendations will BEST facilitate home management for this individual?

A. Store the most frequently used items on shelves just above or below the counter.

B. Use the largest joint available to move or lift items from high shelves.

C. Perform shoulder range-of-motion exercises 10 times each, twice a day.

D. Continue reaching for items on high shelves because it will help improve range of motion.

123. To improve written communication, a COTA would be MOST likely to recommend a large keyboard to enhance computer access when a client:

A. has limited UE range of motion but adequate fine coordination.

B. fatigues rapidly when reaching for the keys.

C. uses only one hand to access the keyboard.

D. has good UE range of motion but difficulty accessing small targets.

124. A fall prevention program is being implemented by a COTA who works in a life-care retirement community. The BEST way to implement this type of program at the primary level of prevention would be to:

A. develop a protocol for environmental modification to reduce fall risks in the life-care retirement community.

B. observe ADL performance to identify those residents at highest risk for falls.

C. make recommendations for wheelchair positioning for those who have had at least one fall.

D. provide intervention to improve balance with those residents who demonstrate the need.

125. What wheelchair feature would be MOST appropriate to recommend for an individual who will be traveling by car with the family to community outings and bringing his or her wheelchair?

A. A lightweight folding frame
B. A one-arm drive
C. An amputee frame
D. A reclining backrest

126. **A COTA is working with a group of individuals with Parkinson's disease in an aquatic exercise program. The three performance components MOST important for successfully walking across the pool are:**

    A. strength, fine motor coordination, and kinesthesia.
    B. visual motor integration, postural control, and gross motor coordination.
    C. vestibular processing, postural control, and muscle tone.
    D. range of motion, praxis, and crossing the midline.

127. **An elderly man was admitted to the hospital after a car accident. He sustained a right pelvic fracture and verbalizes extreme pain with ambulation. The orthopedic doctor has recommended that the patient perform "toe touch only" weight bearing on his right foot for 6 to 8 weeks. The COTA should instruct the patient to do which of the following?**

    A. Transfer on and off a commode seat while using a rolling walker.
    B. Work on bed mobility by rolling and pushing with both heels.
    C. Perform self-feeding in bed only.
    D. Work on distal lower extremity dressing without assistive devices.

128. **An OTR has asked a COTA to contribute information about a client's computer performance for a discharge summary. Which is the MOST appropriate statement of information for the objective section of the client's discharge summary?**

    A. Patient reports he can work at the computer much longer and more comfortably than he could initially.
    B. Patient's ability to work at the computer has increased from 10 minutes to 3 hours with stretch breaks every 30 minutes.
    C. Patient has improved significantly in his ability to work at the computer.
    D. Patient reports he is now able to work at the computer for 3 hours, where initially he was only able to tolerate 10 minutes.

129. **An individual diagnosed with Guillain-Barré syndrome exhibits good upper extremity strength. The activity that would be MOST appropriate for further strengthening and endurance building would be:**

    A. peeling potatoes.
    B. bedmaking.
    C. polishing furniture.
    D. washing windows.

130. **An individual with poor writing skills needs to produce large amounts of legible material upon returning to work. The MOST appropriate method of compensation the COTA could recommend would involve having the person:**

    A. learn to type.
    B. practice fine motor coordination exercises.
    C. practice letter or shape formations.
    D. strengthen the finger flexors and extensors.

131. **A COTA is addressing concerns about sexual activity with a person who has left-sided hemiplegia with spasticity. The BEST recommendation for positioning during sexual intercourse for this person would be:**

    A. lying on the left side, propped up with pillows.
    B. lying on the right side, propped up with pillows.
    C. lying in a supine position.
    D. lying in a prone position.

132. **A COTA employed by a senior center has been asked to develop a group to address the motor needs of people with Parkinson's disease. Which of the following activities would be MOST appropriate to include?**

    A. A game of rhythmic exercises performed to music
    B. Creating time capsules for their grandchildren
    C. Wheelchair races performed in pairs
    D. Taking turns reading out loud from the newspaper

133. **A COTA is working on lower extremity dressing with a young adult with a spinal cord injury. As the client attempts to put on his underwear, he notices an erection and asks the practitioner how this is possible, and if he will be able to have sexual intercourse. The COTA is uncomfortable with the question and unsure of the answer. The BEST action for her to take is to:**

    A. tell him she will find out the answers to his questions, and get back to him with an answer by the next morning.

B. answer his questions to the best of her ability, and quickly return to the lower extremity dressing program.

C. refer him to his psychiatrist.

D. refer him to her OTR supervisor who has attended a workshop on sexuality and spinal cord injury.

134. A COTA is planning intervention for a patient with limited shoulder abduction and external rotation. The craft activity that would provide the desired upper extremity movement at the lowest level of challenge is:

A. macramé with short cords.

B. macramé with long cords.

C. macramé with fine cords.

D. macramé with thick cords.

135. A COTA is working on keyboarding activities with a client with asymmetrical muscle tone who keeps falling to the side while sitting in a wheelchair. What is the MOST appropriate wheelchair adaptation the COTA can use to stabilize the upper body in a midline position?

A. Change to a reclining wheelchair.

B. Use an arm trough.

C. Provide lateral trunk support.

D. Provide lateral pelvic support.

136. A patient who has had surgery for a malignant tumor was seen once in OT and is being discharged home. The patient is weak and needs to continue receiving IV chemotherapy with a home health nurse. The MOST appropriate discharge recommendation for this patient to receive OT services would be:

A. from a home health OTR or COTA.

B. staying in the hospital a little longer.

C. going to a rehabilitation center.

D. coming back for outpatient OT.

137. A COTA is working with a client in a work program setting. What is the FIRST step to achieving the program objective of preventing reinjury within a work program?

A. Performing a prework screening

B. Learning proper body mechanics

C. Participating in work hardening

D. Engaging in vocational counseling

138. A person with a long history of Parkinson's disease is experiencing considerable fatigue during the day. The COTA's

MOST appropriate response to help the individual maintain his or her level of function is to teach them how to:

A. "work through" the fatigue.

B. perform desired activities in a simplified manner to conserve energy.

C. perform additional exercises to increase energy level.

D. eliminate activities or reduce activity level as much as possible.

139. A COTA is providing splint education to an outpatient who has received a resting hand splint. At the time of discharge, it is MOST important that the patient and caregivers understand the need to:

A. bend the splint if it doesn't fit comfortably.

B. discontinue use of the splint if it isn't cosmetically pleasing.

C. care for the splint with special washing directions.

D. observe for signs of pain, redness, and irritation.

140. A COTA has been asked to design a series of stress management sessions for individuals with multiple sclerosis. The COTA should include which of the following in the FIRST session?

A. Time management techniques

B. Self-assessment

C. Aerobic exercise

D. Progressive resistive exercise

141. A COTA is working with a patient with a high level spinal cord injury who has no functional movements to determine the best method of input access for a powered wheelchair. The MOST likely recommendation for this patient to activate the wheelchair would be to use a:

A. joystick.

B. sip and puff switch.

C. single-switch digital control.

D. mouth stick.

142. A COTA working with an individual to develop meal preparation skills, observes that the individual demonstrates minimal to moderate difficulty when asked to prepare a macaroni and cheese dish. Which cooking activity is MOST appropriate to use for the next OT session?

A. Making baked chicken and mashed potatoes

B. Making a peanut butter and jelly sandwich

C. Preparing a frozen dinner

D. Making instant pudding

143. An individual with a low back injury lives alone and must be able to do laundry independently. Which of the following recommendations will BEST protect his back from reinjury?

A. Place the clean laundry basket on the floor next to a chair and sit for folding.

B. Stop the activity when pain becomes severe.

C. Divide the laundry into several small loads for carrying.

D. Carry the laundry into one or two large loads.

144. A COTA is performing a functional ROM assessment on an elderly individual with arthritis. How should the COTA evaluate internal rotation?

A. Ask the individual to touch the back of his neck.

B. Use a goniometer to measure internal rotation in a supine position.

C. Observe the individual tucking a shirt in the back of his pants.

D. Interview the individual regarding areas of pain and stiffness.

145. A COTA is transferring a client from a wheelchair to a car. The BEST way for the COTA to perform a stand pivot transfer is to:

A. move slowly, twisting the body from the trunk.

B. keep feet a shoulder width apart, lifting with the arms.

C. keep knees bent and feet planted when moving.

D. maintain a normal curve of the back, slowly shifting feet as the turn is completed.

146. A COTA is assisting an individual with mild hemiparesis in transferring from the wheelchair to a mat table using a stand pivot transfer technique. The FIRST verbal cue the COTA gives to the individual is:

A. "stand up."

B. "scoot forward to the edge of the wheelchair."

C. "unfasten the wheelchair brakes."

D. "position the wheelchair so that it directly faces the mat table."

147. A local branch of the Arthritis Association has hired a COTA to develop pro- gramming to promote socialization, joint flexibility and overall physical fitness in individuals with rheumatoid arthritis. The intervention that would BEST satisfy these requirements is:

A. a weightlifting program.

B. providing adaptive equipment.

C. an aquatic therapy class.

D. educational programming in joint protection and energy conservation.

148. An individual reports that back pain during sexual activity is so severe that it prevents any enjoyment. The BEST strategy for the COTA to recommend is:

A. use a sidelying position.

B. time sexual activity for periods of high energy.

C. do not discuss pain with the sexual partner because it may be a "turn off."

D. identify alternative methods for meeting sexual needs that don't cause pain.

149. In establishing a wellness program for older adults, the OT practitioner is MOST likely to incorporate activities that:

A. improve weakness following a CVA.

B. increase physical activity and fitness.

C. improve social skills for depressed elders.

D. increase independent performance of transfers.

150. A COTA is ordering a wheelchair for an individual with MS. The MOST important consideration the COTA can make is the adaptability of the wheelchair in anticipation of:

A. gradual gains in strength.

B. growth of the individual

C. further decline.

D. improved wheelchair mobility.

151. To practice transfers using a transfer board with a patient, the COTA must have the patient use a wheelchair that has:

A. detachable footrests.

B. detachable armrests.

C. anti-tip bars.

D. brake handle extensions.

152. An individual with an upper extremity fracture has asked a COTA how to maintain strength in her arm until the cast is removed. The activities that would BEST

accomplish this goal are those which incorporate:

A. isometric muscle contractions.
B. isotonic muscle contractions.
C. progressive resistance.
D. passive movement.

153. An individual with paraplegia wishes to become independent in driving an automobile. The MOST appropriate piece of adaptive equipment for this individual is:

A. a palmar cuff for the steering wheel.
B. a spinner knob on the steering wheel.
C. pedal extensions for acceleration and braking.
D. hand controls for acceleration and braking.

154. An individual who previously worked as a cashier in a clothing store has been referred to a work-hardening program following knee surgery. Limitations are present in standing tolerance and balance. The activity that will BEST prepare this individual to return to work is:

A. moving piles of clothing from one end of the clinic to the other.
B. folding laundry and putting it in a basket while standing.
C. washing dishes while standing.
D. putting price tags on clothing while sitting.

155. Following a heart attack, an inpatient reports to the COTA that his wife overreacted and that there is really nothing wrong with him. The nurse reports poor compliance with cardiac precautions. Which of the following is the MOST important action for the COTA to take?

A. Monitor the individual's response to activities to prevent him from performing at activity levels that are too high and unsafe.
B. Instruct the individual in energy conservation techniques to minimize energy expenditure.
C. Emphasize the consequences of not observing cardiac precautions, and provide concrete proof of the myocardial infarction to the individual.
D. Refer the individual for psychological services.

156. An individual who is s/p total hip arthroplasty (posterolateral approach) is working on independence in lower extremity dressing. Which of the following instructions is MOST important to convey to this individual regarding safety?

A. Sit during dressing activities.
B. Avoid internal rotation and adduction of the involved hip.
C. Use a long-handled shoe horn and dressing stick.
D. Wear shoes with elastic laces.

157. An individual in the early stages of amyotrophic lateral sclerosis has been referred for OT in an outpatient setting. Which of the following interventions is MOST appropriate for this individual?

A. Work simplification and energy conservation
B. Progressive resistive exercises
C. Splinting
D. Active and passive range-of-motion exercises

158. An elderly patient who was hospitalized for a right cerebrovascular accident with left upper extremity flaccidity and decreased sensation, is beginning to experience sensory return in the left upper extremity. Intervention strategies should now include:

A. remedial treatment, such as rubbing or stroking the involved extremity.
B. remedial treatment, such as the use of hot mitts to avoid burns.
C. compensatory treatment, such as testing bathwater with the uninvolved extremity.
D. compensatory treatment, such as using a one-handed cutting board to avoid cutting the insensate hand.

159. A COTA is working on transfer training with a young client who underwent bilateral below the knee amputations 10 days ago. Which of the following should the COTA FIRST suggest for independent transfers from the wheelchair to the bathroom tub seat?

A. Stand pivot transfers
B. Sliding board transfers
C. Dependent lift transfer
D. Transfers should not be initiated until receiving prosthetics.

160. During a tub transfer training session, an individual requires cueing to lock his wheelchair brakes, and requires assistance to lift his legs from the wheelchair into and out of the tub. He is able to scoot himself from the wheelchair to the tub bench using a slicing board with occasional loss of balance. How should

the individual's performance be documented?

A. Dependent
B. Minimal assistance
C. Moderate assistance
D. Maximal assistance

161. **A COTA is educating a caregiver regarding manual wheelchair mobility. Which of the following is the BEST way for the COTA to teach the caregiver to propel a wheelchair down a steep ramp?**

A. Tip the wheelchair backward and guide it down the ramp backwards.
B. Tip the wheelchair backward and guide it down the ramp forwards.
C. Allow the patient to propel the wheelchair independently.
D. Obtain the assistance of a second individual.

162. **A homemaker is learning how to perform transfers into a bathtub after a total knee replacement. Despite having surgery 2 weeks ago, the client is still unable to extend or flex the knee greater than 20 degrees. Which of the following would MOST likely allow for safe tub transfers?**

A. Wait another 2 to 4 weeks, because tub transfers are contraindicated until 4 to 6 weeks after surgery.
B. Use a hand rail attached to the side of the tub.
C. Use a tub transfer bench and leg lifter.
D. Use a low kitchen stool with rubber tips.

163. **An COTA is fabricating a splint for an individual who has carpal tunnel syndrome. Which of the following splint fabrication techniques should be adhered to in order to allow for adequate digit motion?**

A. Trim lines of the splint should extend distal to the MCP crease.
B. Trim lines of the splint should extend proximal to the DIP joint.
C. Trim lines of the splint should extend proximal to the MCP crease.
D. Trim lines of the splint should extend distal to the ulnar fifth MCP crease.

164. **A COTA is working with a patient who has recently experienced a traumatic amputation of his right upper extremity at the short below-elbow level. Which of the following areas of patient education**

would the COTA work on FIRST in the OT intervention program?

A. Training to put on and take off the prosthesis
B. Training in residual limb wrapping
C. Activities to teach grasp and prehension functions
D. Training to resume vocational activities

165. **The OT staff in an outpatient facility are developing goals for a new work hardening program. Which of the following goals is MOST appropriate for this program?**

A. ADL retraining to increase the ability to perform household skills independently
B. Progressive resistive exercise to increase endurance for self-care skills
C. Work simulation to increase strength and endurance for necessary work-related skills
D. Vocational retraining to increase the ability to reenter the job market

166. **A newly referred patient complains of frequently dropping lightweight items and reports a numb feeling in both hands. Which of the following instruments is MOST important for evaluating this individual?**

A. Goniometer
B. Dynamometer
C. Pinch meter
D. Aesthesiometer

167. **A COTA/OTR team has been asked to perform an ergonomic evaluation and provide ergonomic interventions to a job site where the rate of cumulative trauma disorders is unusually high. Which of the following actions BEST addresses this request?**

A. Introduce relaxation seminars for employees to decrease stress while on the job.
B. Treat corporate clients for cumulative trauma disorders.
C. Provide work-simulation activities.
D. Suggest furniture and accessories that promote better positioning at work.

168. **An individual with hand weakness has difficulty holding a fork. Using a biomechanical frame of reference, which of the following interventions would be MOST appropriate for the COTA to recommend?**

A. Elicit functional grasp using reflex inhibiting postures.

B. Stimulate the hand flexors to promote a functional grasp.

C. Repeatedly squeeze with the hand against increasing amounts of resistance.

D. Build up utensil handles.

169. A young individual with MS is about to be discharged to home. The client is independent with bathtub transfers using a grab bar. The MOST important self-care recommendation the COTA can make regarding bathing is to:

A. use cool water.

B. use moderately heated water.

C. take showers and avoid bathing.

D. bathe at the sink with a basin.

170. A patient's weight has changed during the course of hospitalization, and the wheelchair seat is now 2.5 inches wider on each side of the patient's hips. Which is the BEST recommendation the COTA can make regarding proper wheelchair fit?

A. Obtain a wider wheelchair because this one is now too narrow.

B. The patient should be encouraged to lose weight.

C. The sides of the chair should be padded to improve the fit.

D. Obtain a narrower wheelchair because this one is now too wide.

171. A COTA is planning a self-feeding session with an individual with a C5 spinal cord injury. Which piece of feeding equipment would be MOST appropriate for the COTA to introduce to the client?

A. A wrist-driven flexor hinge splint

B. A mobile arm support

C. An electric self-feeder

D. Built-up utensils

172. An adult with MS has decreased sensation of the buttocks and bilateral lower extremities. When educating an individual with absent sensation, the COTA should:

A. teach how to inspect for pressure sores on bony prominences and affected areas.

B. give instructions pertaining to careful trimming of fingernails and toenails.

C. provide extra padding to areas of a splint that cause redness on the individual.

D. provide a program of systematic desensitization training.

173. A COTA is training an individual in the principles of joint protection. The principles that the COTA would MOST likely include would be:

A. using the strongest joint and avoiding positions of deformity.

B. preparing muscles and joints with massage before exercise.

C. practicing vivid imagery and relaxation exercises during difficult functional activities.

D. application of heat before treatment, and application of cold after range-of-motion treatment.

174. An OT practitioner is assessing the range of motion of an individual who actively demonstrates internal rotation of the shoulder to 70 degrees. The practitioner would MOST likely document this measurement as:

A. within normal limits.

B. within functional limits.

C. hypermobility that requires further treatment.

D. limited mobility that requires further treatment.

175. An individual who works as a nurse reports difficulty squeezing the bulb of the sphygmomanometer when taking blood pressures and difficulty opening pill bottles. Which of the following instruments would be MOST appropriate for assessing this individual?

A. Goniometer

B. Aesthesiometer

C. Volumeter

D. Dynamometer

176. A client with a history of chronic obstructive pulmonary disorder has limited endurance. The long-term goal for this client is to prepare three meals a week. The MOST relevant short-term goal for the COTA to focus on is:

A. the use of energy conservation.

B. work-hardening activities.

C. graded activities to increase strength.

D. safety in the kitchen.

177. An individual recovering from a peripheral nerve injury demonstrates weakness in thumb opposition. Which of the following instruments most effectively evaluates strength in the affected area?

A. Aesthesiometer

B. Pinch meter

C. Dynamometer

D. Volumeter

178. In the middle of a wheelchair to bed transfer, an obese patient begins to slip from the grasp of an average size COTA. The BEST action for the COTA to take is to:

A. ease the patient onto the floor, cushioning his fall.

B. reverse the transfer getting the patient back in the wheelchair.

C. continue the transfer getting the patient to the bed.

D. call next door for assistance.

179. A COTA is working with an individual with AIDS who has become too weak to turn himself in bed. After collaboration with the OTR, what is the MOST important modification to the treatment plan for the COTA to recommend?

A. Begin a strengthening program.

B. Begin a bed-mobility program.

C. Teach a caregiver how to lift and turn the client safely.

D. Provide an environmental control unit to the client

180. A COTA observes an individual having difficulty trying to find a white sock on a bed with white sheets. This behavior MOST likely indicates a deficit in the area of:

A. figure-ground discrimination.

B. unilateral neglect.

C. position in space.

D. cognitive mapping.

181. An individual begins therapy with a blood-thinning medication after surgery for an endarterectomy. Which would be the BEST grooming tool for the COTA to recommend for use in the hospital and after discharge?

A. An electric razor

B. A single-blade safety razor

C. A straight razor

D. A double-blade safety razor

182. Evaluation results for a person with arthritis will MOST accurately reflect true functional abilities if scheduled:

A. early morning (8 to 10 A.M.).

B. afternoon.

C. late morning (10 to 11 A.M.).

D. early morning and again in the afternoon.

183. When measuring elbow range of motion with a goniometer, the axis of the goniometer must be positioned:

A. at the lateral epicondyle of the humerus.

B. at the medial epicondyle of the humerus.

C. parallel to the longitudinal axis of the humerus on the lateral aspect.

D. parallel to the longitudinal axis of the radius on the lateral aspect.

184. An individual with Parkinson's disease exhibits a lack of facial expression, resulting in decreased communication. The BEST strategy to promote improved social interaction through facial expression is to:

A. teach caregivers to give the patient time to reply, and to ask questions that require short responses.

B. give a word chart or communication board to prevent frustration.

C. teach use of mirror feedback to make the person aware of his or her facial expression.

D. instruct in deep breathing, articulation, speech volume, and breaking up sentences into segments.

185. The COTA is participating in the evaluation of a high school teacher who recently experienced a right-hemisphere CVA. The individual is presented with letters of the alphabet typed in random order across a page. When instructed to cross out all of the "M's," the individual misses half of the "M's" in a random pattern. This behavior MOST likely indicates:

A. a left visual field cut.

B. a right visual field cut.

C. functional illiteracy.

D. decreased attention.

186. A COTA is treating a client who developed a severe PIP joint contracture in the third digit, 2 months after a burn injury. Which of the following static splinting techniques would BEST address the needs of this individual?

A. Plaster cylindrical splint

B. Dynamic outrigger splint

C. Blocking splint

D. PIP-DIP splint

Service Management and Professional Practice

187. The MOST important way for an entry level COTA to prepare for taking a level I fieldwork student is to:

A. initiate contact with the program director at an academic institution.

B. demonstrate competence as a fieldwork educator.

C. develop skills for providing feedback to the student.

D. develop learning objectives for the fieldwork experience.

188. A COTA decides to accept a position as activity director in an assisted living center. The role and job description are outside OT service delivery. Which one of the following statements BEST describes the necessary level of supervision by an OTR?

A. General supervision during program development and implementation in this work environment is appropriate.

B. OTR supervision is recommended only on a need basis, and may be less than monthly.

C. Minimal supervision on an as needed basis with the use of various communication methods is appropriate.

D. OTR supervision is not necessary.

189. An OT practitioner is supervising an OT aide. The MOST appropriate kinds of activities and level of supervision for the aide include:

A. selected tasks in which aides have been trained, with intense close supervision.

B. various intervention activities with routine supervision.

C. completing ADL training with a patient without supervision.

D. selecting adaptive equipment from a catalog with general supervision.

190. A client refuses to be treated by a level II OTA fieldwork student, stating he would only participate in OT "with someone who's qualified." What action should the supervising COTA take FIRST under these circumstances?

A. Attempt to persuade the client to participate with the student.

B. Cancel the session for that day and document that the client refused OT.

C. Consult with the supervising OTR.

D. Treat the client with the student observing the session.

191. An OT practitioner has been running a "beauty group" with a group of chronically mentally ill older women. Which of the following is the MOST important action to take with the makeup at the end of the session?

A. Put all supplies in a basket to be used next time.

B. Label any supplies used by individuals with communicable diseases with the individual's name, and put the rest in a basket.

C. Label lipstick with the individuals' names. Eye makeup and blush can be shared.

D. Label each item with the individuals' names. Cosmetics should never be shared.

192. The rehabilitation director asks a COTA to screen two clients who were admitted to the facility and do not have OT orders. What would be the MOST appropriate action for the OTA to take in this situation?

A. Complete the screens and report the findings to the rehabilitation director.

B. Contribute to the screening process in collaboration with the OTR.

C. Select the method appropriate to screen the clients, and then conduct the screens.

D. Complete the screens, meet with the OTR to discuss the screen results, then report findings to the rehabilitation director.

193. The OT staff in an inpatient psychiatric unit consists of an OTR and a COTA. Each works 4 days a week, overlapping only on Mondays. When a referral for a new patient is received by the COTA on a day the OTR is not present, the COTA should:

A. assess the patient's roles and interests.

B. include the new patient in group activities until the OTR returns.

C. begin the ADL evaluation.

D. wait for the OTR to return.

194. A COTA working in an outpatient setting would like to provide ultrasound as a treatment modality using skills and knowledge acquired in a previous work setting. However, the supervising OTR has had no training in the use of ultrasound. What is the best course of action for the COTA to take?

A. Use alternative modalities until the OTR can

establish competency with this treatment technique.

B. Ask the staff PT to supervise the COTA's performance.

C. Use ultrasound as a treatment modality only when the OTR is not on site.

D. Review basic ultrasound procedures with the OTR, then begin to use this modality for treatment.

195. An OT practitioner is supervising volunteers in an OT department. Which of the following tasks is MOST appropriate to delegate to a volunteer?

A. Help the patient with simple self-care tasks in the patient's room.

B. Independently work with a patient after the therapist has set up the activity.

C. Assist with stock and inventory control.

D. Complete chart reviews.

196. A COTA on an inpatient psychiatric unit calls in sick to work. The COTA's schedule for that day includes a task group and a coping skills group. The only other person available to lead groups on that day is the certified therapeutic recreation specialist. Which of the following options is MOST appropriate?

A. The CTRS could lead two task groups during the OT time and bill for OT.

B. A nurse could lead the coping skills groups during the OT time and bill for OT.

C. The CTRS could substitute recreational activities during the OT time, without billing for OT services.

D. A nurse could have patients work on tasks they were given by the COTA during OT group time; the COTA could then bill for OT services upon returning to work.

197. Which of the following is the BEST method for ensuring that all tools are accounted for at the beginning and end of a craft group?

A. Keep track of keys to storage cabinets and unit doors.

B. Have all materials and supplies ready before the group begins.

C. Allow only clients who have no behavioral risk precautions to attend groups.

D. Use a tool storage area, painted with tool shadows or outlines, that can be locked.

198. A client makes a bed with sheets and pillowcases to practice application of energy conservation techniques, then practices bed-to-wheelchair transfers. Which of the following actions must be taken upon completion of these activities?

A. Launder the linens if they are visibly dirty.

B. Reuse the linens until the end of the week, then launder them.

C. Wash any linens that came in contact with bodily fluids.

D. Launder the linens after the session.

199. A COTA working in an outpatient setting has completed ROM measurements on an individual who is s/p hand surgery. After bandaging the open wounds, what should the COTA do with the stainless steel goniometer?

A. Place it in a plastic bag and label it with the individual's name.

B. Sterilize it before using it again.

C. Store it with the other goniometers, and sterilize them all at the end of the day.

D. Wash it with hot, soapy water before using it again.

200. While practicing wheelchair to tub transfers, an individual's external catheter is dislodged and urine spills onto the floor. The COTA notes that the urine appears to have blood in it. Which one of the following responses is the MOST appropriate?

A. Clean up the area with paper towels and resume treatment as quickly as possible.

B. Close off the area until it can be disinfected and resume treatment as quickly as possible.

C. Clean up the spill with towels, place towels in the dirty laundry bin, and resume treatment as quickly as possible.

D. Put gloves on, clean up the spill with paper towels, put the soiled paper towels in an infectious waste container, disinfect the area, and finish the patient's session with whatever time is still left.

ANSWERS FOR SIMULATION EXAMINATION 4

1. (B) form constancy perception. Form constancy perception (answer B) is the ability to match similar shapes regardless of change in their orientation in space. Figure-ground perception (answer A) is the ability to distinguish the bead from the background. Position in space perception (answer C) is the ability to determine the spatial relationships of the beads to each other. Visual sequencing (answer D) is an activity that requires the ability to copy the same sequence of beads. Although these abilities are all required for this bead stringing task, the error described refers to a form constancy error. See reference: AOTA: Uniform Terminology for Occupational Therapy, ed 3.

2. (A) Arrhythmic and unexpected. Sensory integration treatment is complex and highly individualized, and must be monitored carefully to observe the effects of sensory input of varying types on the individual. The characteristics of facilitatory sensory input are an unexpected, arrhythmic, uneven, or rapid input. Answer B is not correct because, although arrhythmic input is excitatory, slow sensory input is inhibitory. Sustained and slow sensory input (answer C) is inhibitory, not facilitatory. Answer D is incorrect because, although facilitatory input is unexpected, rhythmic input is inhibitory. See reference: Bruce and Borg: Movement-centered frame of reference.

3. (D) Rubber-coated spoons. "Children who have a strong tonic bite reflex can use rubber coated, plastic, or rubber spoons" (p. 225). This will allow the parent and/or child to more easily remove the utensil from the child's mouth. Rubber coated spoons provide a smoother surface than that of a regular stainless steel utensil. Answers A, B, and C would not be recommended for a child with a strong tonic reflex, but for other limitations such as incoordination, tremors and apraxia. See reference: Solomon (ed): Jones, LMW and Machover, PZ: Occupational performance areas: Daily living and work and productive activities.

4. (A) Teach the child to dress in a sidelying position. The sidelying position eliminates the need for the child to maintain balance in order to dress the lower extremities. Answer B is not correct because the primary purpose of putting loops on waistbands is to help a child with limited grasp strength to pull on garments. Answer C is not correct because using Velcro in place of zippers is also an adaptation designed to help children with limited ability to grasp and pull, whereas answer D, teaching the child to dress in a standing position, is considered to be more difficult than dressing in a sitting position. See reference: Case-Smith (ed): Shepherd, J: Self-care and adaptations for independent living.

5. (A) exploratory play. Exploratory play provides children with experiences that develop body scheme, sensory integrative and motor skills, and concepts of sensory characteristics and actions on objects. Therefore, the obstacle course is an example of exploratory play. Symbolic play is associated with the development of language and concepts (e.g., use of "dress-up" materials). Creative play and interests are characterized by refinement of skills in activities that allow construction, social relationships, and dramatic play (e.g., finger painting). Recreational play is leisure experiences that allow the exploration of interests and roles such as arts and crafts or sports. See reference: Case-Smith (ed): Morrison, CD and Metzher, P: Play.

6. (B) a local wheelchair equipment vendor. Although any community resource may be helpful to a child and family with a severe physical disability, answer B is correct because of the possible breakdown of this already purchased piece of equipment. The OT practitioner needs to consider this possible problem and provide local support for a solution. Therefore, although answers A, C, and D may serve as resources for other needs of the child, only a specialist in wheelchair equipment would be able to solve mechanical problems that arise. See reference: Case-Smith (ed): Wright-Ott, C and Egilson, S: Mobility.

7. (C) Handle the child slowly and gently. Answer C is correct because the child with hypertonicity will be most relaxed and easier to handle if tone is inhibited by slow and gentle handling of the body. Answer A is incorrect because adaptive equipment is frequently needed to provide a child with a sense of security during bathing. Answer B is not correct because an explanation of the procedures also increases a parent and child's sense of security during bathing. Answer D is not correct because it provides the parent with a poor model of good body mechanics; the COTA should kneel by the tub or sit on a stool while bathing the child. See reference: Case-Smith (ed): Shepherd, J: Self-care and adaptations for independent living.

8. (B) flexion righting reaction. The flexion righting reaction (answer B) is correct because "the development of antigravity neck strength is first associated with the ability to maintain the head aligned with the body when pulled to a sitting position" (p. 273). Answer A is incorrect because protective reactions are elicited through displacement (such as falling forward), and these reactions protect infants from falls. Answer C is incorrect because the body righting on body reaction is represented by the rotation between trunk segments (also a rotational righting reaction). Answer D is incorrect because the optical righting reaction incorporates vision and allows the child to right the head against gravity (this is also referred to as a vertical righting reaction). See reference: Case-Smith (ed): Nichols, DS: Development of postural control.

9. (A) neck flexion. Answer A is correct because this method decreases the abnormal extension pattern that is influencing the oral motor patterns. Jaw and tongue thrust are part of an overall extension pattern. Answers B, C, and D would only increase the abnormal pattern in the mouth because they are part of an extension pattern. See reference: Case-Smith (ed): Case-Smith, J and Humphry, R: Feeding intervention.

10. (C) demonstrating typical development for a child with Down syndrome. Answer C is correct because exclusive "W" sitting is commonly seen in children with low muscle tone. The child is compensating for an inability to achieve stability in a variety of positions that require dynamic postural control, depending on skeletal rather than neuromuscular structures for stability. Answers A and D are not correct because exclusive "W" sitting would be considered both typical and age appropriate for a 5-year-old child with Down syndrome. Answer B is not correct because exclusive "W" sitting is considered to be a compensatory position. See reference: Kramer and Hinojosa (eds): Schoen, SA and Anderson, J: Neurodevelopmental treatment frame of reference.

11. (C) increase the management of texture by slowly increasing texture of food with a baby food grinder. This method offers a gradual increase in texture that encourages chewing. Answer A is not correct because scraping off food from a spoon with the child's teeth does not encourage any voluntary oral motor control. Answer B is incorrect because it combines liquid with pieces of food (soft and chewy), and this combination of textures will be too unpredictable for a child who is having difficulty organizing oral motor skills to manage food. Answer D is incorrect because a raisin is too large of a step from pureed food in terms of texture. See reference: Case-Smith (ed): Case-Smith, J and Humphry, R: Feeding intervention.

12. (C) follow administration instructions and note changes in behavior. Although the tester may not deviate from the protocol, changes in behavior represent important test data and should be recorded. The responses described in answers A, B, and D may make the test results invalid by altering the sequence of test items, the grouping of items, or the actual test item itself. These may not be changed unless it is specified in the test manual. See reference: Case-Smith (ed): Richardson, PK: Use of standardized tests in pediatric practice.

13. (A) Ballet. To promote the development of anticipatory control, movement should be slow, predictable, and controlled from a stable base. Participation in a dance class would involve controlled movement from a stable base. Answers B, C, and D are activities that feature faster moving objects whose speed and direction of movement cannot be controlled by the player, and require quick reactions to unpredictable stimuli. See reference: Case-Smith (ed): Nichols, DS: The development of postural control.

14. (C) Removing pants. Answer C is correct because, according to most developmental scales, children first learn to remove garments, especially socks. Answer A is not correct, because the ability to put garments on with the front and back correctly placed is a skill that is developed later. Buttoning and tying bows (answer D) is incorrect for the same reason. Answer B is incorrect because children are typically able to remove garments before they are able to put them on. See reference: Case-Smith (ed): Shepherd, J: Self-care and adaptations for independent living.

15. (C) Bring the seat in for reevaluation within 6 months. Fit and function of seating and mobility should be reassessed within 6 months to account for the child's growth, as well as any changes in posture. Parents should not make unsupervised adaptations (answer A), because improper positioning could harm the child. Weekly adjustment (answer B) are usually not necessary, and transporting the seat every week would be unnecessarily inconvenient. The end of the IEP (answer D) may be more than 6 months away and, therefore, too long to wait. See reference: Case-Smith (ed): Wright-Ott, C and Egilson, S: Mobility.

16. (B) playing clapping games. Answer B is the only one that requires bilateral movement and coordination. Finger painting (answer A), could require bilateral use if the child stabilized the paper with one hand as he painted with the other hand, but this is not required to perform the task. Turning pages in a book (answer C), and forming "Play Doh" "meatballs" (answer D) are activities that facilitate unilateral in-hand manipulation skills. See reference: Case-Smith (ed): Exner, CE: Development of hand skills.

17. (D) Removing a nut from a bolt. Answer D describes one type of in-hand manipulation called rotation. Rotation is the movement of an object around one or more of its axes, where objects may be turned horizontally or end over end, with the pads of the fingers, as when one would unscrew a nut from a bolt. Answers A, B, and C are incorrect because they describe activities with no in-hand manipulation that essentially keep an object in a certain position as it is grasped, released, or carried. See reference: Case-Smith (ed): Exner, CE: Development of hand skills.

18. (B) catching and bursting soap bubbles. This activity involves visually tracking a slow moving target and requires minimal fine motor precision to accomplish a successful "hit". Answers A, C and D also require visual tracking and eye-hand coordination, but they involve faster moving targets that require immediate, more precise movement. These activities can be used to promote advanced skills as the child's visual tracking ability improves. See reference: Case-Smith (ed): Dubois, SA: Preschool services.

19. (C) by tilting backward up to 60 degrees while rocking. By lowering the child backwards from the sitting position, the child is required to activate increasing degrees of antigravity control in the neck musculature. As the child's strength increases, the degree of incline can be increased. Answers A, B, and D do not address antigravity control using neck flexor musculature. See reference: Case-Smith (ed): Nichols, DS: Development of postural control.

20. (B) A noise machine producing white noise at bedtime. For a child who is easily aroused, a constant, monotonous auditory input can be calming enough to induce sleep. The other answers may actually increase arousal. Quick repetitive proprioceptive input, as experienced when jumping on a trampoline (answer A), and light touch provided by a fuzzy blanket (answer C), are types of sensory input that have direct arousing effect on the nervous system. Blocking out all light (answer D) may produce arousal as a result of fear generated by total darkness. See reference: Case-Smith (ed): Cronin, AF: Psychosocial and emotional domains of behavior.

21. (A) promote open-ended symbolic play, such as using action figures, puppets, and dolls. Toys that elicit feelings and expression can be used to promote beginning play skills, beginning interaction and communication skills. Inherent in open-ended play is the fact that there is no right or wrong way—that failure is not possible. Structured craft activities (answer B) do not provide sufficient opportunity for self-expression and carry the possibility of failure, because there is a right and wrong way to do them. As an initial activity, a game of tag (answer C), especially one that involves peers, may be perceived as threatening and overwhelming by the child. Activities that promote tension release (answer D) do not directly address play skills, rather, they focus on the powerful motor action only. See reference: Case-Smith (ed): Morrison, CD and Metzger, P: Play.

22. (D) Provide a therapy ball to sit on while the child is playing a game of checkers. Answer D is the most appropriate recommendation because it contributes to the development of postural background movements. This is done by requiring the client to continually adjust to the subtle movements of a usable surface. Answers A, B, and C provide additional external support (i.e., they provide adaptations using a compensatory approach, rather than facilitating the development of new skills). See reference: Case-Smith (ed): Nichols, DS: The development of postural control.

23. (B) observe him in his home during feeding time. "Considering the context of the child's environment is a critical process in occupational therapy assessments" (p. 167). The reason he does not feed himself may be environmental—for instance, his parents may have taught him not to touch food with his fingers or he may not have learned to feed himself because his grandmother always feeds him. In addition, the child may not be able to transfer skills learned at home to the clinic—that is, he may believe that "the place to eat is home, not the clinic." Although answers A and C provide useful information for treatment planning, they do not address feeding skills. Answer D does not put the skill to be assessed into an environmental context. See reference: Case-Smith (ed): Stewart, KB: Occupational therapy assessment in pediatrics.

24. (D) Visual perceptual. Running, hopping, using a tripod grasp, drawing a stick figure, and putting together a 10-piece puzzle are all developmentally appropriate skills for a 5-year-old child. Although the child cannot put together the 10-piece puzzle, the gross and fine motor skills that doing a puzzle require have been observed. No fine motor evaluation (answer A) is indicated because the child demonstrates a tripod grasp. No gross motor evaluation (answer B) is necessary because running and hopping skills are evident. Because the child's abilities appear developmentally appropriate, developmental evaluation (answer C) is not indicated. Because gross, fine, and developmental skills appear to be appropriate, visual perception should be evaluated. See reference: Case-Smith (ed): Case-Smith, J: Development of childhood occupations.

25. (C) Word prediction software. Word prediction software anticipates the word desired and increases the speed of input by decreasing the number of keystrokes required. A larger monitor (answer A) may be useful when a child has difficulty seeing a screen or details on the screen. Voice output systems (answer B), which read text and provide cues, can be useful for children with autism, learning disabilities, cognitive delays and visual impairments. Masking inappropriate keys (answer D) reduces the number of options, and can help children who have difficulty finding the correct key. See reference: Case-Smith (ed): Swinth, Y: Assistive technology: Computers and augmentative communication.

26. (C) Prone over a wedge. Considering the information given, answer C offers the best position because head control is isolated, with the trunk supported. The child does not have adequate control to stand in a standing frame (answer A). Answer B is not correct because, although the chest is supported by a sling, the child's shoulders, arms, and hips must be able to control the position. Sitting on a therapy ball (answer D) would require both head and trunk control. See reference: Case-Smith (ed): Nichols, DS: Development of postural control.

27. (B) Boy Scouts. While answers A, C, and D describe activities that may help build the boy's sense of competence, only participation in Boy Scouts includes the necessary interaction with peers. Noncompetitive activities, a uniform to signify belonging, predictable routines, and exposure to role models are all elements of the Boy Scouts that can help him develop social competence. See reference: Case-Smith (ed): Cronin, AF: Psychosocial and emotional domains.

28. (B) A corner chair with head support and padded abductor post. A corner chair provides hip, knee, and ankle flexion of 90 degrees, and the abductor post keeps the legs separated when or if extensor tone increases. The corner shape of the chair facilitates shoulder protraction or prevents shoulder retraction, which can prevent the child's hands from coming forward to assist with eating. The prone stander (answer A) would place the child in a standing or extended position, which would reinforce undesirable extensor tone. A supine position (answer C) is not appropriate for eating if other positions are available. The child would not be able to sit in a bolster chair without support (answer D), because of poor head control and extensor tone. See reference: Case-Smith (ed): Case-Smith, J and Humphry, R: Feeding intervention.

29. (A) Create a reliable route to the bathroom, encouraging the child to familiarize herself with the smells and sounds of the bathroom. A primary goal for the COTA working with a child with visual impairments is to address the development of self-care skills at an age appropriate level. By creating a reliable route to the bathroom, encouraging the child to focus on tactile and olfactory cues (answer A), the COTA can establish compensatory techniques for the visual deficit. Having the child practice with obstacle courses (answer B) would be appropriate for the development of movement in space and body image/awareness, but would not be considered part of a daily self care routine. Answer C, practicing handwriting and fine motor skills, would be more closely related to the development of hand manipulation skills. Introducing the child to other children with similar impairments would be an appropriate socialization activity for the child, but is not directly related to a self-care program. See reference: Case-Smith (ed): Snow-Russel, E: Services for children with visual or auditory impairments.

30. (A) Scribble on a piece of paper. The Bayley scales on infant development suggest that a child will be able to scribble on a piece of paper (answer A) between the ages of 10 to 12 months. Copying a triangle (answer B) is a task that is not anticipated until the age of 5 to 6 years. Copying a horizontal line (answer C) is typically not seen until the age of 2, while copying numerals (answer D) is typically not observed until the age of 5 to 6 years old. It is important to appreciate that despite these age/develop-

mental generalizations, each child's skill level can vary. See reference: Case-Smith (ed): Amundson, SJ: Prewriting and handwriting skills.

31. (B) Stability of the head and neck. Answer B is correct because the prone position allows the child to vertically right the head against gravity and develop the alternating flexion and extension control that provides head and neck stability. Answer A is not correct because the infant begins to protract, rather than retract, the shoulders, and hip extension develops during prone positioning in normal development. Answer C is not correct because the prone position provides the infant with the opportunity to develop trunk extension, rather than trunk flexion. Answer D is not correct because the prone position per se, during weight-bearing on the upper extremities, provides the opportunity to develop stability or cocontraction in the arms. See reference: Kramer and Hinojosa (eds): Colangeo, CA: Biomechanical frame of reference.

32. (B) Brushing her own hair. "The power grasp is often used to control tools or other objects. Oblique object placement in the hand, flexion of the ulnar fingers, less flexion with the radial fingers, and thumb extension and adduction facilitate precision handling with this grasp (e.g., for brushing hair)" (p. 295). Answer A, pegboard activities, would most likely be introduced to facilitate the pincer grasp or tip pinch, while answer C, carrying a briefcase, such as a child's art case, would encourage the hook grasp position. Lastly, the activity of ball throwing, would most likely be introduced to encourage a spherical grasp position. See reference: Case-Smith (ed): Exner, C: Development of hand skills.

33. (D) installation of a bidet with a spray wash and air drying mechanism. Use of a bidet for hygiene after use of the toilet eliminates any upper extremity reach requirement. Answers A, B, and C describe adaptations appropriate for a child with poor postural control in need of external stability devices. These devices would not reduce reach requirements. See reference: Case-Smith (ed): Shepherd, J: Self-care and adaptations for independent living.

34. (D) Create a comfortable foundation for fostering parent skills through parent-therapist collaboration. All four answers describe possible ways for a COTA to impact an infant's developmental outcome. However, the most permanent action would capitalize upon developing family centered mutual collaboration. With this approach, communication is the key to creating a relationship that will foster parental skill development and expertise. This then provides the parents with effective tools to best nurture and care for their infant at any time and in any environment, and has a permanent impact on the developmental outcome for the infant. See reference: Case-Smith (ed): Hunter, JG: Neonatal intensive care unit.

35. (A) whether the areas of concern to the OT interfere with the child's education. Related services are defined as services needed to help a student benefit from education. If the student's disability no longer interferes with education, OT as a related service can be discontinued. Functional skills (answer B) and independence in ADL (answer C) may be ongoing goals in therapy, as provided in a rehab setting or hospital, but would not be provided as a related service in schools. Accessibility of the learning environment (answer D) is an important concern, but it would be covered by consultation with the school or teacher, not through direct service provision. See reference: Case-Smith (ed): Case-Smith, J, Rogers, J, and Johnson, JH: School-based occupational therapy.

36. (A) a body-length prone scooter. Spastic diplegia is defined as abnormal tone affecting all four extremities, but with primary involvement of the lower extremities. Therefore, the child may use his upper extremities to propel himself through space while having his lower extremities positioned on a scooter (answer A). The airplane mobility device (answer B) is designed for children with good lower extremity function who need support in the upper body. A tricycle (answer C) requires good lower extremity control, including reciprocal movement. A power wheelchair (answer D) is designed for individuals with limited upper and lower extremity function. See reference: Case-Smith (ed): Wright-Ott, C and Egilson, S: Mobility.

37. (C) supervision. At this level, the child performs the task on his own, but cannot be safely left alone, or he may need verbal cueing or physical prompts for 1% to 24% of the task. At the independent level (answer A), the child performs the complete task, including the set-up. At the independent with setup level (answer B), the child performs the task after someone sets it up. Minimal assist (answer D) signifies that the child performs 50% to 75% of the task independently, but needs physical assistance, or other cueing, for the remainder of the task. See reference: Case-Smith (ed): Shepherd, J: Self-care and adaptations for independent living.

38. (D) applesauce. Foods with even consistency, uniform texture, and increased density such as applesauce, are the easiest to control and swallow. Foods with multiple textures like chicken noodle soup (answer A), sticky foods like peanut butter (answer B), and foods that are fibrous or break up in the mouth like carrot sticks (answer C), should be avoided. See reference: Case-Smith (ed): Case-Smith, J and Humphry, R: Feeding intervention.

39. (B) upright. For a child with increased tone, the upright position gives the best postural control. A forward (answer A) or backward tilt (answer C) increases the effect of gravity, and thus adds to the difficulty of maintaining posture. At all times, the child should sit squarely with even weight distribution on both buttocks, never tilted asymmetrically (answer D). See reference: Case-Smith (ed): Wright-Ott, C and Egilson, S: Mobility.

40. (B) Incorporate therapeutic activities into family routines. "Suggestions that the family can incorporate into the daily routine are the most successful" (p. 722). Separate "therapeutic activities" (answers A and D) can take up an excessive amount of time and energy, and may interfere with family life. Therefore long-term follow-through may not be as effective as when activities can be made to fit existing daily routines and develop into habits. Activities provided on an as-needed basis (answer C) will never become habits, and therefore follow-through is less effective. See reference: Case-Smith (ed): Stephens, LC and Tauber, SK: Early intervention.

41. (C) allow the child to self-apply tactile stimuli to maximize the child's tolerance. Tactile defensiveness is an overreaction or negative reaction to sensations of touch. Answer C is correct because "generally, tactile stimuli that are actively self-applied by the child are tolerated much better than stimuli that are passively received, as when being touched by another person" (p. 352). Answer A is incorrect because light touch sensations are particularly disturbing for children with tactile defensiveness, and may create overwhelming feelings of anxiety. Answer B is not correct because avoiding all forms of tactile sensation is virtually impossible, and such complete avoidance would not help the child to develop coping skills. Answer D is also incorrect because deep touch stimuli is often comfortable for children with tactile defensiveness, however, it may possibly provide "relief from irritating stimuli when deep pressure is applied over the involved skin areas" (p. 350). See reference: Case-Smith (ed): Parham, LD and Mailloux, Z: Sensory integration.

42. (A) poor postural responses. Poor postural responses, such as poor balance and postural control against gravity, are often symptoms of an underreactive vestibular system. Possible symptoms of an overreactive vestibular system are given in answers B, C, and D, which are problems of intolerance for motion, and gravitational insecurity. See reference: Fisher, Murray, and Bundy (eds): Fisher, AG: Vestibular-proprioceptive processing and bilateral integration and sequencing deficits.

43. (B) decreased muscle tone. Decreased muscle tone is usually characterized by joints that are lax and hyperextensible. Low muscle tone and joint hyperextensibility are also common characteristics of Down syndrome. Answer A is incorrect because loss of range of motion would be the joint characteristic of increased muscle tone. Answers C and D are incorrect because they are diagnoses that cannot be made on the basis of joint laxness, even though instability at the joint may occur with either of these conditions. The observation of joint hyperextensibility is merely an indication of below normal muscle tone and not necessarily the indication of a specific condition or disease process. See reference: Kramer and Hinojosa (eds): Colangelo, CA: Biomechanical frame of reference.

44. (C) cruising. The described pattern is cruising. Cruising occurs at approximately 12 months of age and directly precedes walking. Creeping (answer A) refers to four-point mobility in a prone position with only hands and knees on the floor, a pattern that occurs between the ages of 7 and 12 months. Crawling (answer B) is the term for the ability to move forward while in a prone position; this pattern occurs at about 7 months of age. Clawing (answer D), also called "fanning," is the ability to spread the toes to maintain balance in standing. See reference: Case-Smith (ed): Wright-Ott, C and Egilson, S: Mobility.

45. (B) Visual attention skills. According to Todd, answer B is correct because development of visual attention skills should be worked on first as they prepare and provide foundation skills for other aspects of visual perception. Answer A is incorrect because visual memory skills can only be developed after visual attention skills are established. Answers C and D are incorrect because general and specific visual perceptual skills develop after visual memory. See reference: Kramer and Hinojosa (eds): Todd, VR: Visual information analysis: Frame of reference for visual perception.

46. (C) the sidelying position. The sidelying position reduces the influence of reflexes, extensor tone, and gravity, all of which make protraction of the shoulders and forward reach difficult. Answer A is incorrect because the standing position will not reduce extensor tone. Moreover, it encourages shoulder retraction and makes forward reaching of both arms to midline more difficult. Answer B is also incorrect because in the prone position the upper extremities are involved in weight bearing. However, this position may help facilitate forward reach by developing shoulder protraction. Answer D is not correct because in the quadruped position, the upper extremities are involved in weight bearing. However, if the position is attainable, shoulder protraction and forward reach may be facilitated. See reference: Kramer and Hinojosa (eds): Colangelo, CA: Biomechanical frame of reference.

47. (B) play and self-care activities. "When providing OT care for children with terminal illness, the underlying principle is to add quality to their remaining days. There are two performance areas that occupational therapists should address in children with terminal illness: (1) play activities; and (2) activities of daily living" (p. 838). Educational activities (answer A) would not address the emphasis of adding quality of life. Play activities help the child to focus interest and express feelings, and may incorporate socializa-

tion and motor activities (answers C and D), but neither of these types of activities alone would be the primary goal. Self-care activities allow the child to maintain independence and purposefulness. See reference: Case-Smith (ed): Barnstorff, MJ: The dying child.

48. (B) Teach the child to sit in a chair and lift and place the affected foot up on a small stool. "For a child with hemiplegia or limited balance, sitting with back support may be the best starting position for putting on and removing socks. The child lifts the affected leg onto a box or step to bring the foot closer to the unaffected hand" (p. 235). Answer A, encourage the child to wear tight fitting socks, would make it more difficult for the child to put on and take off his or her socks. The child would benefit more from socks that have a wide opening. Answer C, encourage the child to lay on his back in bed when putting on socks, and answer D, placing the unaffected foot on a small stool, would not assist in dressing skills independence for this child. See reference: Solomon (ed): Jones, LMW and Machover, PZ: Occupational performance areas: Daily living and work and productive activities

49. (D) accommodation. Visual accommodation (answer D) is the ability to focus efficiently from near to far distance, and vice versa. Answer A, ocular motility, refers to the ability to pursue an object visually in an efficient and smooth manner. Answer B, binocular vision, is the ability to focus the eyes on an object at varying distances and on seeing a single object clearly. Answer C, convergence, is the ability to move the eyes inward or outward with continued focus on the object. See reference: Kramer and Hinojosa (eds): Todd, VR: Visual information analysis: Frames of reference for visual perception.

50. (D) the presence of self-stimulatory behavior. Self-stimulatory behavior is often seen in autistic children and frequently interferes with function. The other answers are less relevant in terms of essential data for intervention planning. An autistic child may be normal in terms of his or her ability to focus at close range (answer A), wrist flexibility (answer B), and hand preference (answer C), but show poor adaptive behavior. See reference: Neistadt and Crepeau (eds): Florey, L: Psychosocial dysfunction in childhood and adolescence.

51. (A) A large key ring. According to Solomon, "a large key ring or a piece of fishing line make inexpensive zipping aids for children with limited grasping ability, ROM, strength, or coordination" (p. 236). Answer B, oversized fasteners, would not address the child's need to become independent in zipping, unless all of the zippers were removed from the child's pants and replaced with fasteners. Colored zippers, answer C, would mostly be helpful for a child with visual discrimination problems. Velcro fasteners, answer D, is something the COTA may recommend if the more convenient and less expensive key ring adaptation does not assist the child in meeting his goals. See reference: Solomon (ed): Jones, LMW and Machover, PZ: Occupational performance areas: Daily living and work and productive activities.

52. (D) Playing on a trampoline. Postural control refers to the ability to maintain balance during functional movements. Activities that require a child to respond by changing body position to maintain balance encourage the use of postural reactions. Playing on a trampoline would be the best activity, because it requires a child to continuously change body position to adapt to changes in gravity while jumping. Answer A, sliding down a sliding board, would stimulate vestibular processing. Imitating gestures, as in answer B, playing "Simon Says," would facilitate perceptual processing. Swimming, answer C, would be a good activity to improve a child's endurance. See reference: Solomon (ed): O'Brien, JC: Play.

53. (C) Pencil gripper. These are all adaptive devices that can be used with a child who has JRA for various reasons. However, the correct answer is C because the pencil gripper will probably make grasping the pencil easier and reduce hand grasp fatigue. Because printing and handwriting are common tasks for children this age, it is important to reduce fatigue from hand weakness. The reacher (answer A) frequently requires grasp strength, and is more useful for children who have problems with extended reach. The jar opener (answer B) is a useful tool for individuals with hand weakness, but opening jars is not a task frequently performed by school-age children. The plate guard (answer D) is a useful device for those with incoordination or one-handedness, but is not particularly necessary when hand strength is decreased (adapting the utensil would be more reasonable). See reference: Case-Smith (ed): Rogers, SL, Gordon, CY, Schanzenbacher, KE and Case-Smith, J: Common diagnoses in pediatric occupational therapy practice.

54. (D) perform slow push-ups against the wall. Having the child perform push-ups against the wall is an activity which provides joint compression of the upper extremities with motor activity—a combination which will have a normalizing effect on the nervous system. Answers A and C are not correct because they emphasize additional tactile input. Answer B is not correct because it emphasizes slow vestibular input. See reference: Kramer and Hinojosa (eds): Kimball, JG: Sensory integration frame of reference: Theoretical base, function/dysfunction continua, and guide to evaluation.

55. (A) A small spoon. According to Solomon "by 24 months, children can hold a spoon and bring it to the mouth with the wrist supinated into the palm-up position...at 30-36 months children experiment with forks to stab at food" (p. 92), thus making answer D, a small fork incorrect. The COTA may allow the child

to eat with his fingers (answer B), however the child would most likely be developmentally ready to attempt to use a spoon. Answer C, a swivel spoon, would be indicated when a child is unable to deviate the wrist radially and/or supinate the forearm. See reference: Solomon (ed): O'Brien, JC, Koontz Lowman, D and Solomon, JW: Development of occupational performance areas.

56. (C) A phone with extra large buttons. "Phone companies offer adapted phone systems for children and adults who have various limitations...some phones have extra large buttons for those with incoordination or visual impairments" (p. 267). A phone with extra large buttons would most likely be the best solution for the child with mild visual impairments who desires to use the phone without assistance. Answers A, B, and C would assist individuals who are unable to hold the phone independently due to incoordination, weakness or loss of function in the hand or upper extremity. See reference: Solomon (ed): Jones, LMW and Machover, PZ: Occupational performance areas: Daily living and work and productive activities.

57. (C) Having the child roll around in a carpeted barrel. Tactile defensiveness is an area of sensory integration treatment that should be approached cautiously. Rolling on a textured surface is a child-controlled activity and, therefore, less intrusive to the nervous system than gentle brushing or rubbing (answers A and B). Brushing and rubbing lotion on sensitive areas such as the face, neck, and arms are powerful sensory techniques which can be overwhelming if the child does not have control of the tactile experience. Swinging activities (answer D) generally do not address the problem of tactile defensiveness. See reference: Solomon (ed): Graham, G, McCreedy, P, and Solomon, JW: Sensorimotor treatment approaches.

58. (A) Position the child's trunk, head, neck, and shoulders in proper alignment. Proper positioning is the first thing the COTA must address prior to feeding the child. "Proper positioning is vital for tongue control. The trunk, head, neck, and shoulders need to be stable and aligned" (p. 224). Answer B, hyperextend the child's head, would be contraindicated because "abnormal tongue movements tend to occur more frequently when the head is hyperextended" (p. 224). Answers C and D are techniques commonly utilized to facilitate proper feeding techniques, but they should not be initiated until after the child is appropriately positioned. See reference: Solomon (ed): Jones, LMW and Machover, PZ: Occupational performance areas: Daily living and work and productive activities

59. (D) Place Velcro fasteners in the child's clothing in place of zippers and buttons. After practicing for 2 months on dressing skills, this individual may benefit most from Velcro fasteners. "Velcro fasteners may make dressing and undressing easier and quicker; they can be sewn into clothing in place of buttons, snaps, zippers, or ties" (p. 236). In addition, using Velcro closures in the child's pants would require less time to fasten his pants after toileting. Answer A, encouraging the child to work with a dressing stick, would not address the issue of manipulating buttons and zippers, rather more gross motor removing or applying of clothing. While answer B, practicing with fastening boards, might eventually assist the child with buttons and zippers, Velcro fasteners would be the most appropriate intervention for this child. Finally, answer C, encouraging the child's mother to assist with buttons and zippers does not address the child's independence or feelings regarding his ability to fasten his pants efficiently after toileting while at school. See reference: Solomon (ed): Jones, LMW and Machover, PZ: Occupational performance areas: Daily living and work and productive activities.

60. (B) self-assessment. Self assessment of each individual's stressors and stress reactions is the first step in designing a stress management program. Time management techniques (answer A), which help individuals schedule, prioritize and develop appropriate attitudes about daily task requirements, may comprise one of the following sessions. Aerobic exercise (answer C) is an appropriate method for reducing stress in individuals with MS, but care should be taken in designing a program that will not lead to overheating. Progressive relaxation exercises (answer D) involve systematic tensing and relaxing of muscles and are not appropriate for individuals with hypertension, cardiac disease, upper motor neuron lesions, or spasticity. See reference: Neistadt and Crepeau (eds): Giles, GM and Neistadt, ME: Treatment for psychosocial components: stress management.

61. (A) Discharge recommendations. The COTA would contribute to the process of making discharge recommendations (answer A), but this section of the discharge evaluation is to be completed by the OTR. Answers B, C, and D may be completed independently by the COTA because these areas reflect factual data at the time of discharge. See reference: AOTA: Occupational therapy roles.

62. (A) Controlled stimulation with meaningful sensory cues. An environment that provides controlled stimulation with visual, tactile, and auditory cues that are meaningful to the resident, is preferable because it will best facilitate correct perception of the environment. Difficulty in perceiving or misunderstanding environmental cues can lead to behavioral problems or agitation. Environments that are too stimulating (answer B), or too unstimulating (answer C) can increase confusion. Answer D is incorrect because while dementia units should have a homelike atmosphere, and residents should have familiar objects near them to maintain links with me-

mories, the more important consideration in overall environmental design is to incorporate the special environmental adaptations that will enhance function. See reference: Larson, Stevens-Ratchford, Pedretti, and Crabtree (eds): Christenson, MA: Environmental design, modification, and adaptation.

63. (D) State strengths and limitations regarding performance in the activity. Self-concept is defined as the value of one's physical and emotional self. Stating one's strengths and limitations about one's own performance is a reflection of an individual's self-concept. Planning a healthy meal (answer A) addresses the goal of health maintenance. Developing a budget and shopping (answer B) address the goal of money management. Delegating tasks and preparing the meal address the goals of interpersonal skills and meal preparation skills, respectively. See reference: AOTA: Uniform Terminology for Occupational Therapy, ed 3.

64. (B) Develop awareness about what produces anger and how the clients respond to anger. All of the answers are steps in the cognitive-behavioral process. Treatment begins, however, with developing awareness of what produces anger and how individuals respond (answer B). Therapy should then move to changing behavior to achieve alternative, more healthy ways of responding to anger, and examining the benefits of responding in a more healthy fashion (answer A). Graded tasks are used to reinforce the new beliefs, behaviors, and responses, beginning with easier and progressing to more challenging tasks (answers C and D). See reference: Bruce and Borg: Cognitive-behavioral frame of reference.

65. (D) Conduct a group discussion about responsibilities people have when living in a group home. Discussion that heightens awareness in an attempt to modify behavior is one example of a cognitive intervention. Rewards and praise (answers A and B) are used when a behavioral approach is desired. Posting a schedule (answer C) is an example of an environmental adaptation that may facilitate compliance with chores, but does not represent a cognitive approach. See reference: Christiansen (ed): Self-care strategies in intervention for psychosocial conditions.

66. (D) Show a video about nutrition and keep a meal diary for a week. The psychoeducational model utilizes a teacher-student format as opposed to a learning by doing approach. It often includes a homework component. Answers A, B, and C can all be used to promote healthier eating, however, they all involve learning by doing. See reference: Cottrell (ed): Crist, PH: Community living skills: A psychoeducational community-based program.

67. (B) assembling packets that include a knife, fork, spoon, and napkin based on a sample. This individual is functioning at Allen's Cognitive Level 4. Individuals functioning at this level are able to copy demonstrated directions presented one step at a time. They find it easier to copy a sample than to follow directions or diagrams. Individuals functioning at cognitive level 3 are capable of using their hands for simple, repetitive tasks, but are unlikely to produce a consistent end product. They are also more successful performing a sorting task (answer A). The shoelace task (answer C) is more appropriate for those functioning at cognitive level 5. These individuals are interested in the relationships between objects and can generally perform a three-step task. Individuals functioning at cognitive level 6 can anticipate errors and plan ways to avoid them, and would be successful with tasks that are more complex and require attention to detail (answer D). See reference: Early: Some practice models for occupational therapy in mental health.

68. (D) Termination of activity. This individual demonstrated difficulty ending the task of brushing his teeth. Trying to put toothpaste on the toothbrush before taking off the cap would be an example of a deficit in sequencing (answer A). Difficulty following directions (answer B) could be evident if the individual attempted to brush his hair or shave rather than brush his teeth. An example of impaired problem solving ability (answer C) would be if the individual tried to squeeze the tube of toothpaste too softly so that nothing came out, and then gave up on the task. See reference: Early: Cognitive and sensorimotor activities.

69. (B) Set a time to meet with the individual after group and let him know that you will hear what he has to say at that time. Giving the individual a specific time to meet helps set boundaries, while reassuring him that you are available to him. Answers A and C might send the message that it is acceptable to interrupt the group, and may even reward his behavior. Refusing to listen (answer D) is likely to increase the individual's feelings of isolation, which is likely to increase his anxiety. See reference: Early: Responding to symptoms and behaviors.

70. (A) Social conduct. Appropriate social conduct requires individuals to use manners, observe personal space, make eye contact, and use body language appropriate to the environment. While poor eye contact may indicate low self-esteem (answer B), and grabbing may indicate poor self-control (answer C), the combination of behaviors described is most indicative of poor social conduct. By developing her interpersonal and coping skills (answer D), the individual may be able to demonstrate improved social conduct. See reference: Early: Psychosocial skills and psychological components.

71. (B) Administer a time-use assessment. Time use assessments (e.g., the Barth Time Construction) examine how individuals spend their time in work, leisure and self-care activities. The individual records all activities he engaged in each day on a chart, often for a full week. The OT practitioner may also want to obtain information on the individual's feelings about the various activities. As with all self-report assessments, the value of the assessment is dependent on the individual's ability and willingness to be honest and accurate. Interest checklists (answer A) typically assess the individual's level of interest and perceived skill in various leisure activities, but not how time is actually utilized. Actual skill in leisure activities would best be evaluated through direct observation (answers C and D), but this method would not provide useful information about how the individual actually spends his time. See reference: Early: Data collection and evaluation.

72. (D) stenciling project on poster board. Stenciling on poster board is the safest craft choice because it is free of sharp, toxic, and cordlike materials. A ceramic object (answer C) could be broken into sharp pieces that an individual could use to harm themself. Craft projects that contain rope or cordlike materials that can be used for hanging (answers A and B) should also be avoided. See reference: Early: Safety techniques.

73. (C) Relationships with others. The primary problem area for most individuals with a personality disorder is their inability to interact with others. Specific personality disorder categories indicate that there is some variation among the types of relationships that are impacted. For example, authority relationships seem particularly dysfunctional in those with antisocial personality disorders, and difficulty in establishing relationships is linked to avoidant personality disorders. Answers A and B (ADLs) are often problems for individuals with mood and thought disorders. Answer D is often a problem in those with schizophrenia. See reference: Early: Understanding psychiatric diagnosis: The DSM-IV.

74. (A) jogging. Forceful gross motor activities that involve no physical contact, such as exercising, wedging clay, and woodworking, can provide a physical outlet for sexual tension. Macramé (answer B) is predominantly a fine motor activity that would provide no such outlet. Reading a pornographic magazine (answer C) would only serve to increase sexual tension. This individual would not have the tolerance or self-control for ballroom dancing (answer D), which involves close physical contact with members of the opposite gender. See reference: Early: Responding to symptoms and behaviors.

75. (B) avoid use of power tools and sharp instruments. Individuals experiencing extrapyramidal syndrome, which may cause muscular rigidity, tremors, and/or sudden muscle spasms, should avoid using power tools or sharp instruments. Photosensitivity, an increased sensitivity to the sun, is another side effect often associated with neuroleptic medications that can be addressed by limiting sun exposure (answer A). Answer C is a strategy that can be used to avoid postural hypotension, a sudden drop in blood pressure resulting in feeling faint, or loss of consciousness when moving from lying or sitting to standing. Dry mouth is a common side effect of many drugs, and can be intensified by the dehydrating effects of caffeinated drinks and alcohol (answer D). Of all the above possible side effects of neuroleptic medications answer B is most important precaution because it relates to the only side effect the client has experienced. See reference: Early: Psychotropic medications and somatic treatments.

76. (D) Group members pass around and smell a basket of scented potpourri. Using sensory stimuli such as smell helps arouse an individual's attention and increase their level of participation. Individuals with severe depression tend to have difficulty initiating a physical activity such as throwing a ball (answer B), therefore, having a warm-up activity is useful. These individuals are also likely to have difficulty initiating conversations (answers A and C), and these activities are not consistent with a sensorimotor format. However, they may be effective activities for individuals functioning at a higher level. See reference: Early: Cognitive and sensorimotor activities.

77. (A) Perform a job analysis. A job analysis identifies essential functions of a particular job. Based on the results, the OT practitioner can then work with the individual to maximize performance or request reasonable accommodation (answer B). Activities that promote self-efficacy (answer C) are beneficial for individuals with depression, but should not be used at this stage of the individual's program. A weekly support group (answer D) may be an effective way for the individual to obtain support and can be recommended, but it is not the first action the OT practitioner would take. See reference: Early: Work, homemaking and childcare.

78. (D) Determine the individual's home environment and her need for meal preparation skills. It is important to include the context in which an individual performs, or will need to perform, work, self-care and leisure activities as part of the evaluation process, as well as the individual's needs, interests, strengths and weaknesses. It is possible that this individual has always lived in environments where others cooked for her and that she may never need to cook for herself. If indeed meal preparation skills are important to this individual, it may then be necessary to evaluate her cognitive level (answer A) in order to develop appropriate short- and long-term goals (answer B). After evaluation is complete and goals are established, the individual can be scheduled for an intervention such as a meal preparation group (answer C). See reference: Early: Data collection and evaluation.

79. (A) Wedging the clay. Individuals with tactile defensiveness often have an aversion to materials such as clay, paste, and fingerpaints. They react most strongly to stimulation of the hands, feet, and face. Answers B, C, and D involve stimuli that would not be perceived as noxious to an individual with tactile defensiveness. See reference: Early: Analyzing, adapting, and grading activities.

80. (B) are structured by the COTA to encourage self-reflection and feedback. For a graded program designed to develop an individual's self-awareness, the most essential element, is the opportunity to verbalize one's ideas and feelings, and to receive feedback from others in a safe setting (answer B). Therefore, it is not the activities that are graded, but the way the OT practitioner structures the activities to encourage self-reflection and feedback. See reference: Early: Analyzing, adapting, and grading activities.

81. (B) adult daycare. Adult daycare (answer B) is an environment that provides programming that is psychosocial in nature and focuses on vocational skills and social activities. Partial hospitalization (answer A) is a type of outpatient program that serves as a transition to community living. It offers most of the structure and services available on an inpatient unit, while allowing individuals to live in the community. Home health care (answer C) provides treatment services to individuals who have chronic or debilitating illnesses in their own homes in order to increase their functional independence. Although most individuals who receive home health services have disabilities that are primarily physical, secondary psychiatric disorders are quite common. Psychosocial rehabilitation centers (answer D) focus on the social rather than the medical aspects of mental illness. Psychosocial clubs and rehabilitation centers provide socialization programs, daily living skills counseling, prevocational rehabilitation, and transitional employment. See reference: Early: Treatment settings.

82. (D) Assist clients in the selection of simple, short-term tasks. The skills required at the parallel level are the "ability to work and play in the presence of others comfortably and with an awareness of their presence" (p. 295). At this level, the COTA must be available to provide support, encouragement and assistance when indicated. Parallel group members (answer D) typically work together on individual tasks. Therefore, it would not be expected that the COTA encourage experimentation (answer A), because this level would require the client to be working at the project group level. This level focuses on the client working with another group member while encouraging trust. Answer C, the COTA participating as an active member is also inappropriate. This level of assistance typically occurs during the mature group level, where individuals take on the roles necessary to achieve a balance between meeting the group task, and the emotional needs of the group.

Answer B would also be an incorrect selection because the COTA must act as an authority figure in the parallel group in order to set limits, encourage interaction and assist the patient in feeling safe. See reference: Early: Group concepts and techniques.

83. (B) vestibular stimulation and gross motor exercise. The sensory integration treatment approach, which aims to improve the reception and processing of sensory information within the central nervous system, uses both vestibular stimulation and gross motor exercises (answer B). Social skills training (answer A), role-playing activities (answer C), and discussion groups (answer D) might be used when an individual needs help in relating appropriately and effectively with others. Although these interventions may be a part of the overall treatment program, this type of individual must be able to receive and process sensory information before embarking on a higher level of social interaction. See reference: Early: Medical and psychological models of mental health and illness.

84. (A) provide each patient with an individual project and have him or her choose a tile color. The activity should begin with the most basic level of decision making. Each of the other choices provide increasingly more challenging decision making abilities. Choosing from an assortment of projects (answer B) requires a higher level decision making ability than only selecting a color. Answer C requires not only decisions on design, color, and size, but also involves decision making among group members. Answer D involves decision making on two separate aspects, pattern and colors, resulting in a higher level of complexity than answer A. See reference: Early: Analyzing, adapting, and grading activities.

85. (B) Ask the individual to try some lacing with distant supervision and praise her for what she has been able to do. All of the responses are increments of approaches used for decreasing dependency needs. Answer B is the best next step in this case because it allows the individual to attempt some lacing in the presence of the OT, who in turn offers reassurance that the individual is actually able to do the activity. The step in answer B would be followed by that in answer D. Here the individual is required to attempt some lacing without the benefit of the OT at her side. The OT is nearby, but working with another client. As the individual is able to do more of the activity independently, written instructions (answer A) replace the OT as the instructor. Finally, when the individual is feeling comfortable with self-instruction, asking her to work on the project without OT assistance (answer C) heightens the level of self-responsibility. See reference: Early: Analyzing, adapting, and grading activities.

86. (A) Dine as a group using a family style dining format. Goals for individual's with bulemia typically include restoration of normal eating patterns,

participation in appropriate exercise levels, and developing the ability to challenge distorted cultural values related to physical appearance. A client who is successful with eating individually sized portions should progress to family style dining, where portion size is not predetermined. Answers B, C, and D are all counterproductive for an individual with bulemia. See reference: Early: Understanding psychiatric diagnosis: the DSM-IV.

87. (C) Participate in writing a group rock song using "I" statements. Rock music is an important interest to most adolescent males and would probably be an engaging activity for this individual. The use of "I" statements in the song will allow group members to express themselves in a non-aggressive way. Telling his peers what makes him angry (answer A) is important, but is not activity based. Learning relaxation and karate techniques (answers B and D) are constructive ways to gain control of his aggressive drives, but are not geared toward emotional expression. See reference: Early: Psychosocial skills and psychological components.

88. (C) encourage the patient to describe what makes him fearful about going on this trip. Encouraging a person with anxiety to describe and identify exactly which aspects of an activity make them fearful, and to express their fearful feelings, is an important first step in helping them cope with their fears. Answer A, changing the topic or redirecting attention, is a strategy for distracting a person from certain thoughts, such as patients with psychotic disorders who express their delusions. Answer B, being firm about expectations, would be useful for establishing consistent limits, as with a patient who is manic. Answer D, stating why there is nothing to fear, is a useful for clarifying reality, such as when a person is experiencing hallucinations. But with an anxious person, this response might send the patient the message that their fears are not recognized or validated by the COTA. See reference: Early: Responding to symptoms and behaviors.

89. (A) Dismiss her from the group. It is important to prevent the client from doing something that she will be embarrassed about later. Since she did not respond to earlier attempts to get her to stop, dismissing her from the group is the only option. She would likely continue to draw attention to herself, even in the back of the room (answer C). Ending the activity (answer B) would deny treatment to the others in the group. Another medium (answer D) may indeed benefit the client; however. it does not provide the immediate solution required. See reference: Early: Responding to symptoms and behaviors.

90. (B) Require that she ride the bus according to a designated schedule. Getting to work on time is critical to successful job performance. Individuals with a history of substance abuse often have issues with time management. The introduction of a time management component is an appropriate way to upgrade this community mobility activity (answer B). Taking the bus to a second, different location is also an appropriate upgrade, and AA meetings are important (answer A). However, the question emphasizes skills needed for successful performance of the worker role. The ability to develop strategies for bad weather (answer C) is important, but is only an occasional need, whereas arriving on time is a daily need, therefore a higher priority. Because the individual has already ridden the bus independently, we may assume she can provide the correct fare (answer D) and there is nothing to indicate she is unable to count change accurately. See reference: Early: Understanding psychiatric diagnosis: The DSM IV.

91. (C) Acknowledge that he uses rituals to cope with anxiety. Individuals with obsessive compulsive disorder (OCD) perform unnecessary and meaningless actions repeatedly. The OT practitioner should "never criticize the patient's behavior. Instead, recognize that no matter how ridiculous the ritual may appear, it is one the patient uses to cope with anxiety" (p. 240). Telling him the behavior is unnecessary (answer A) will not help him to modify his behavior. Individuals with phobias should be encouraged to talk about their fears (answer B). Individual treatment (answer D) is indicated when an individual cannot tolerate a group environment. See reference: Early: Responding to symptoms and behaviors.

92. (A) Listen to what the individual says and reflect back to him. This individual is exhibiting signs of depression. Active listening allows depressed individuals to talk about what is bothering them and why, recognizing the importance of their feelings. Redirection, praise, predicting future girlfriends, and asking him to do something beyond his current abilities (answers B, C, and D) are all counterproductive. See reference: Early: Responding to symptoms and behaviors.

93. (D) sheltered work program. Sheltered work programs offer opportunities for severely disabled persons to perform simple, structured work tasks, such as assembling and packaging small items, in supervised, low stress settings. This would be the most appropriate choice for the client. Answer A, supported employment, is a work experience designed to help clients with psychiatric disabilities to get back into permanent employment. Answer B, volunteer work, would also be more appropriate as a trial work experience for a person with a psychiatric disorder. Answer C, transitional employment, is designed to allow temporary work placements for preparation of eventual permanent employment. See reference: Early: Work, homemaking, and child care.

94. (D) suggest a more realistic activity. Manic individuals are often unaware of their problem areas, and therefore tend to make grandiose or inappropriate choices. This lack of awareness may make it diffi-

cult for the individual to recognize or accept telling him that his attention span is too limited (answer B). Whereas a depressed individual may need support for his choices (answer A), a manic individual may need to be redirected. It is not the type of tool, however, that is problematic (answer C), but the qualities of building a clubhouse related to cost, space, time, complexity and possibly skill. See reference: Early: Responding to symptoms and behaviors.

95. (A) Have the individual contribute to a discussion identifying the "rules" for the group. This approach is most likely to elicit cooperation and to heighten the individual's awareness regarding his behavior. Rules such as showing respect for others, asking permission to borrow tools and supplies, and waiting for another person to finish speaking, are more likely to be respected when the individual contributes to the development of these rules. Ignoring his inappropriate behavior during group (answer C) disregards the needs of other group members. This individual may not have the skills or insight to treat others with respect at this time, and explaining that the behavior is unacceptable (answer D) may not be enough. Denying him access to groups (answer B) may be a last resort only after all other options have been exhausted. See reference: Early: Psychosocial skills and psychological components

96. (D) provide him with regular forceful gross motor activities. Forceful gross motor activity is one way of releasing sexual tension. Telling a psychotic individual to change a long-standing behavior (answer A), is usually not effective. Revoking cigarette privileges (answer C) is punitive, and would probably not be effective. Activities that involve close proximity to others (answer B), are not recommended for an individual who demonstrate inappropriate sexual behavior. See reference: Early: Responding to symptoms and behaviors.

97. (B) Collaboration with the OTR to change the short-term goal. In addition to implementing treatment, one of the roles of the COTA is to monitor the client's response to treatment, including achievement of goals. If the client can easily accomplish the intervention activity, or if the short-term goal appears to have been met, "the COTA should consult with the therapist about how to change the treatment plan" (p. 381). Continuing to follow the same treatment plan, answer A, would not reflect the changes in behavior that have been observed. Answer C, formally re-evaluate the client, is the responsibility of the OTR. The progress noted would be insufficient reason to revise the long-term goal, and doing so would be beyond the scope of the COTA. See reference: Early: Treatment planning.

98. (C) Pull her aside and ask her if she is upset. Mealtime for someone with an eating disorder is a source of high stress and conflict. Anorexia nervosa is characterized by abnormally low body weight with refusal to gain weight. Purging after a meal is one technique used to avoid weight gain. By taking the woman aside and allowing her to verbally express her current feelings, the COTA is providing her with an immediate emotional outlet and this may avoid an episode of purging. A common theme with clients with eating disorder is the need to control themselves and others through their food intake. Denying her request to go to the bathroom (answer A), would prove to be non-therapeutic and could challenge the trust that has been built between client and COTA. Allowing the request (answer B) is contraindicated because there is a good chance she will use the bathroom visit to purge the meal. The COTA cannot count on the nurse being readily available for advice or assistance (answer D). It would be important, however, after the group, to let her nurse know of the incident so it could be further processed on the unit. See reference: Early: Understanding psychiatric diagnosis: The DSM-IV.

99. (A) Involve the individual in a three-member task group. Adding an additional group member to the experience is the most appropriate way to upgrade this activity when addressing the goal of social interaction. Progressing from slip molds to coil pots (answer B) may be a way of providing an outlet for creativity or self-expression. Adding the responsibility of pouring the molds in addition to glazing them (answer C) may progress the individual toward more independent performance of ceramics activities. Decision making skills can be enhanced by providing opportunities for the individual to make choices about his project (answer D). See reference: Early: Analyzing, adapting and grading activities.

100. (C) Hand-over-hand assistance. In this method, the caregiver places one hand over the resident's hand and provides assistance while guiding the resident's hand through the steps of the task, in this case, guiding the resident's hand from the food into the mouth. This method provides maximum assistance while still allowing the resident to feel involved and connected to the task. Given the resident's attention span deficits, the use of demonstration (answer A), verbal feedback (answer B) and even chaining (answer C) would be insufficient to sustain the resident's active participation. See reference: Hellen: Daily life care activities.

101. (A) Limit the time available to answer each question. Individuals with OCD frequently experience time consuming compulsions having to do with thoughts and/or actions. Limiting the time available to answer questions (answer A) will help these individuals structure their time and be able to more effectively complete the evaluation process. Open-ended questions (answer C) are useful for eliciting more information, but are more difficult to time limit than closed ended questions. Instructing the individual to take as much time as necessary (answer B) may be beneficial for a highly anxious individual. Individuals

with attention deficits would most likely benefit from limiting environmental distractions (answer D). See reference: Neistadt and Crepeau (eds): Henry, AD: The interview process.

102. (D) gradual fading of cues. "Emphasis is on a specific task, rather than on the underlying skills needed to perform the task" (p. 429). This approach is for individuals who are not expected to be able to generalize learning (answer C). Other behavioral techniques that may be successfully employed include backward (not forward) chaining and positive (not negative) reinforcement (answers A and B). See reference: Neistadt and Crepeau (eds): Toglia, JP: Cognitive-perceptual retraining and rehabilitation.

103. (B) having the only red toothbrush. This is an environmental adaptation, and does not require new learning that may be beyond the individual's ability. The color red is easily recognizable, and if it is the only red one (answer B), he will not get it mixed up with others. Switching to an electric toothbrush (answer A) requires a new set of skills and this individual is likely to have difficulty with new learning. A built-up handle (answer C) is appropriate for individuals who have difficulty grasping the handle of a toothbrush. Having the individual's teeth brushed by a caregiver (answer D) is not desirable if the individual is able to do it himself. See reference: Neistadt and Crepeau (eds): Holm, MB, Rogers, JC, and James, AB: Treatment activities of daily living.

104. (C) Clothing care, cleaning, and volunteering. Doing laundry, cleaning, and volunteering are all examples of work and productive activities. Answers A and B are examples of ADLs. Reading, watching television, and doing small handicrafts (answer D) are examples of play and leisure activities. See reference: Neistadt and Crepeau (eds): Neistadt, ME: Introduction to evaluation and interviewing.

105. (C) Role playing of social situations. Social skills training is accomplished in four progressive steps: instruction, demonstration of desired behaviors by the group leader, guided practice and independent activities. The first step in this process, teaching about social skills and breaking down skills into smaller components, such as nonverbal behavior and listening skills, has been addressed in the group. The second step, directly demonstrating how the skills are performed has also been accomplished. The group members are now ready for guided practice, which "involves having the client perform an actual social skill under the watchful eye of the therapist and other members of the group." (p. 485). Role playing of social situations is a technique used in guided practice. Answers A and B would occur after guided practice. Answer D, providing feedback on hygiene and appearance, may have some impact on social functioning, but would relate more to ADL competence than social skill development.

See reference: Stein and Cutler: Leisure-time occupations, self-care, and social skills training.

106. (B) Eat well, exercise, and participate in meaningful occupations. Eating well and participating in exercise and meaningful occupations are essential for managing stress and developing good coping skills. Honestly expressing feelings of fear, sadness and loss (answer A), and identifying values and interests (answer D), are both appropriate methods for developing a healthy self-concept. Listing personal accomplishments (answer C) may help develop motivation. See reference: Neistadt and Crepeau (eds): Robertson, SC: Treatments for psychosocial components: Intervention for mental health.

107. (C) When the individual has worked to tolerance. "Intervention involves positively reinforcing (praising) the client's attempts at physical activity or exercise. Activity increases are done on a gradual basis with the client working to "tolerance" (gradual increase in task completion) as opposed to "pain" before a scheduled rest period" (p. 456). Working until the pain becomes intolerable (answer A) would be counterproductive, but allowing the individual to stop when he thinks the pain is about to begin (answer B) may reinforce pain behaviors. Although rest breaks should be scheduled, 30 minutes (answer D) is just an arbitrary number in this situation. See reference: Neistadt and Crepeau (eds): Engel, JM: Treatments for psychosocial components: Pain management.

108. (D) Information about the disease, its management, and communication strategies. Learning about the disease, its management and how to communicate with a family member who has schizophrenia can help the family cope with problems that may arise. Answer A, environmental adaptations, would be a relevant education topic for the family of persons with dementia. Answer B, encouraging attendance at a twelve-step self-help program, would be more relevant for clients with substance abuse problems. Answer C, monitoring of nutrition, physical activity and rest might relate to overall health, but would not provide strategies to deal with the specific issues of a person with schizophrenia. See reference: Neistadt and Crepeau (eds): Ward, JD: Psychosocial dysfunction in adults.

109. (C) applying grout to a tile trivet and waiting for it to dry. Activities provide a variety of opportunities for therapeutic gains. The process of grouting a tile trivet involves covering the individual's tile design with a grout mixture (which tends to be very liquid in consistency) before setting up the material to dry. Waiting for the grout to dry requires an individual to delay gratification. Working in a group (answer A) promotes cooperation. Selecting a tile design (answer B) involves decision making. Cleaning off the table (answer D) may promote the experience of success after a mess, but does not involve the

concept of delaying gratification. See reference: Neistadt and Crepeau (eds): Crepeau, EB: Activity analysis: A way of thinking about occupational performance.

110. (B) Awareness, minimal deficits, and learning potential. The client most likely to benefit from remedial activities would be one with minimal deficits, awareness of limitations, and learning potential. Answer A is incorrect because remedial approaches attempt to change skill levels, and this is less likely to be accomplished in a short time frame. Answer C, difficulty transferring skills to new situations, is incorrect because the rationale for using remedial techniques is that practice of the impaired skill will then result in improved performance in functional activities, requiring ability to transfer learning. A remedial approach for a client who has a long history of cognitive deficits, answer D, would not be warranted unless the client exhibited some potential for further improvement. See reference: Neistadt and Crepeau (eds): Toglia, JP: Cognitive-perceptual retraining and rehabilitation.

111. (D) Read the questions to the individual and check off his responses. It may be necessary to adapt the administration of some standardized tests to accommodate individuals with visual deficits. When this occurs, it is important to read the instructions and information to the individual exactly as it is written on the evaluation. It is also important to describe any modification to the assessment when documenting the evaluation results. In this case, it would be better to read the evaluation to the individual than to waste a day of inpatient hospitalization (answer A). It would not be appropriate to begin treatment (answer C) before the evaluation is complete, goals set, and a treatment plan developed. Administering an evaluation (answer B) is beyond the scope of what an aide may do. See reference: Neistadt and Crepeau (eds): Golisz, KM and Toglia, JP: Evaluation of perception and cognition.

112. (B) bringing about change among the members. Change is the overall purpose of therapeutic groups. Answers A and C are methods by which members may change. Answer D is an advantage of groups, but is not a primary purpose. See reference: Posthuma: The small group counseling and therapy.

113. (D) select appropriate evaluation procedures. An OT evaluation begins with the initial interview and chart review, which guide the OT practitioners in deciding on a frame of reference and the identification of specific evaluation procedures or assessments. Assessments are then performed (answer C) to gather information to identify problem areas and plan treatment. After the assessments are complete, the OTR uses clinical reasoning skills to analyze data (answer A) and to identify the person's strengths and weaknesses. The treatment plan (answer B) is developed after the individual's problems have been identified and evaluation data have been analyzed. Finally, specific interventions are selected. See reference: Pedretti and Early (eds): Pedretti, LW and Early, MB: Occupational therapy evaluation and assessment of physical dysfunction.

114. (B) Have the individual sit in a rocking chair. Activities that provide increased vestibular input (i.e. rocking) can help reorganize the way the central nervous system organizes and interprets sensory input, which can help decrease agitation. Lying down on a sofa (answer A) may make the individual more comfortable but would not necessarily decrease agitation. It would also be inappropriate to have an individual lie down during a group activity. Directing the individual to leave the room (answer C) without attempting to decrease his agitation first would limit the individual's ability to participate in and benefit from group activities thereby decreasing the chances of becoming an active member of the community. OT practitioners are not licensed to dispense prescribed medications (answer D). See reference: Pedretti and Early (eds): Royeen, CB, Duncan, M, and McCormack, G: The Rood approach: A reconstruction.

115. (D) Continuous reinforcement of correct responses. Continuous reinforcement is helpful with learning of new behaviors and should be provided every time the correct behavior occurs. Time-based and intermittent reinforcement (answers A, B, and C) are best for maintaining behaviors. See reference: Pedretti and Early (eds): Sabari, JS: Teacing activities in occupational therapy.

116. (B) Stress management. Many addicts use drugs and alcohol as a way to fill leisure time and to manage stress or boredom. When this individual experienced frustration with the birdhouse project, he was unable to manage this stress, became agitated, escaped the challenge, and sought out an addictive substance (the cigarette). Individuals with problems related to eye-hand coordination, visual perception, or fine motor performance (answers A, C, and D) may also have difficulty gluing pieces of a birdhouse together. However, the behaviors described above, in combination with the diagnosis of substance abuse, make B the most likely answer. See reference: Neistadt and Crepeau (eds): Ward, JD: Psychosocial dysfunction in adults.

117. (B) Confront the individual's behavior and ask, "Are you aware that your frequent interruptions prevent others from having a chance to contribute?" In general, the group leader should try answers A, C, or D before confronting the individual who is monopolizing the conversation. However, considering that these more conservative attempts have failed the practitioner, Answer B, confronting the behavior, would be the best approach for the COTA to take to modify the behavior. See reference: Posthuma: What to do if....

118. (B) provide enough chairs around a round table. Circular seating arrangements generally facilitate the most communication among members. Rectangular tables (answer A) can lead to unbalanced communications. Difficulties in maintaining comfort and attention are problems related to floor seating arrangements (answer C). Using available chairs and couches (answer D) frequently provides different seating heights and are often in rectangular or square seating arrangements. See reference: Posthuma: Group dimensions.

119. (B) Objective. The objective portion of the SOAP note (answer B) focuses on measurable or observable data obtained by the OT practitioner through specific evaluations, observations, or use of therapeutic activities. The subjective portion of a SOAP note (answer A) should feature relevant patient reports or comments. The assessment part of a SOAP note (answer C) addresses the effectiveness of treatment and changes needed, the status of the goals, and the justification for continuing OT treatment. The plan section of a SOAP note (answer D) includes statements related to continuing treatment; the frequency and duration of the treatment; suggestions for additional activities or treatment techniques; the need for further evaluations; and, when needed, recommendations for new goals. See reference: Sabonis-Chafee and Hussey: Treatment planning and implementation.

120. (A) Asking a department store salesperson for information about an item without buying it. Intervention to develop assertive behavior is a process of gradually empowering clients to make their own decisions, request assistance, avoid being taken advantage of, and provide constructive criticism when it is warranted in a variety of situations. Activities to assist in this process need to be graded for success by starting with situations that are less threatening to the client. Answer A, asking for information about an item without buying it, requires a request for information, but one which is well within the expectations of a department salesperson, making it a suitable exercise for beginning assertiveness training. Answers B, C, and D each require the client to make a special request, and question or criticize a service, which requires more skill and confidence. See reference: Stein and Cutler: Leisure-time occupations, self-care, and social skills training.

121. (A) Pain management techniques. Work-hardening programs focus on returning individuals to work in physically appropriate settings, as quickly as is feasible, through reconditioning. As part of that program, pain management techniques (answer A) are included to assist the person with managing and coping with pain during work-related activities. A work hardening program would teach proper body mechanics to prevent further injury rather than focus on energy conservation (answer C), which is emphasized with individuals who need to minimize or avoid fatigue. Vocational counseling (answer D) helps individuals enhance their vocational potential and addresses skills necessary for identify job seeking and job acquisition. While balancing work and leisure (answer B) is important for maintaining overall health, it is not the emphasis of a work-hardening program. See reference: Pedretti and Early (eds): Burt, CM: Work evaluation and work hardening.

122. (A) Store the most frequently used items on shelves just above or below the counter. When an individual experiences difficulty reaching because of limited range of motion, convenient placement of commonly used items will facilitate home management. Using the largest joint available (answer B) is an important principle of joint protection, and although it may be an appropriate suggestion if this individual has arthritis, it would not address the specific problem of reaching high shelves. Although it is possible that range of motion exercises, and reaching for high shelves (answers C and D), may eventually improve this individual's shoulder function, neither provides a home management solution. See reference: Pedretti and Early (eds): Foti, D: Activities of daily living.

123. (D) has good UE range of motion but difficulty accessing small targets. A large keyboard would be best for someone who has good range of motion, but difficulty accessing small targets (answer D). A person with limited range of motion, but adequate fine coordination (answer A) would benefit from a smaller or contracted keyboard. If someone fatigues rapidly when reaching for the keys (answer B), having to reach further on a large keyboard would cause more fatigue. A large keyboard would be more difficult for a person using one hand (answer C), because the hand would have to move farther to complete typing, adding more work to the process. See reference: Pedretti and Early (eds): Anson, D: Assistive technology.

124. (A) develop a protocol for environmental modification to reduce fall risks in the life-care retirement community. Developing a protocol for environmental modification of general hazards to reduce falls throughout the community is an example of a primary prevention strategy. Activities that focus on eliminating fall risk factors specific to individuals represents secondary prevention (answers B, C, and D). See reference: Larson, Stevens-Ratchford, Pedretti, and Crabtree (eds): Cook, M and Miller, PA: Prevention of falls in the elderly.

125. (A) A lightweight folding frame. A lightweight folding frame is needed when a wheelchair will be frequently lifted in and out of a car trunk or back seat, and folded to fit into the space. This is much easier on the individual or family member who will be lifting the wheelchair. Answers B, C, and D will add a great deal of weight and bulk, which makes the wheelchair much more difficult to lift. This in turn

may cause an individual or family member to be more reluctant to go on a community outing. See reference: Angelo and Lane (eds): Taylor, SJ: Evaluation for wheelchair seating.

126. (C) vestibular processing, postural control, and muscle tone. Vestibular processing and postural control are required for maintaining balance. Muscle tone that is too high or too low will limit an individual's ability to move the lower extremities for ambulation. Therefore, the three components given in answer C are important for successfully walking across the pool. Fine motor coordination (answer A) is not required to walk across the pool. In addition, although walking in water requires some strength, it can still be successfully performed with significantly decreased strength, because the body weighs significantly less when submerged. Answer B includes postural control and gross motor coordination, which are both important for walking in the pool, but it also includes visual motor integration, which is not important. Answer D includes range of motion and praxis, both of which are required to some degree for walking in the pool, but it also includes crossing the midline, which is not required. See reference: AOTA: Uniform Terminology for Occupational Therapy, ed 3.

127. (A) Transfer on and off a commode seat while using a rolling walker. The patient will most likely utilize a walker to transfer on and off a commode seat. In this case, the assistive device (the walker) will permit the patient to adhere to the mandated toe touch precautions, while providing balance, decreasing pain and encouraging safe transfers. Answer B, bed mobility, should not be performed by rolling and pushing with both heels, because this will most likely increase the patient's pelvic pain. In this case, the patient may benefit from the use of a trapeze attached to the bed to increase the use of both upper extremities, while performing bed mobility. Answer C, self-feeding, can be performed in bed, but the patient would most likely be encouraged to get out of bed to prevent immobility and risk of pneumonia. Answer D, distal lower extremity dressing, is actually facilitated with devices such as a long handled shoehorn, sock aid, dressing stick, elastic shoelaces and reacher, which help prevent pain and increase independence. See reference: Bernstein (ed): Bernstein, LC and Daleiden, S: Clinical implications of neurologic changes in the aging process.

128. (B) Patient's ability to work at the computer has increased from 10 minutes to 3 hours with stretch breaks every 30 minutes. The objective section of a discharge summary should summarize the patient's condition upon discharge from the facility and "summarize the patient's stay" (p. 49). Some facilities compare initial and final evaluations, while others only address progress from the time of the previous note. Answers A and D are subjective reports. Answer C is an example of a statement that belongs in the assessment section of a discharge summary. See reference: Borcherding: Writing the "O"-objective.

129. (D) washing windows. Washing windows (answer D) is a repetitive activity that involves resisted, elevated upper extremity activity. Rests can be taken as needed. Making the bed, peeling potatoes, and polishing furniture (answers A, B, and C) do not provide adequate resistance to achieve upper extremity strengthening. See reference: Dutton: Introduction to biomechanical frames of reference.

130. (A) learn to type. Typing would allow the individual to communicate legibly in writing, while circumventing the individual's poor handwriting skills. Answer B, fine motor coordination exercises, and answer C, practicing letter or shape formations, are both ways to improve control of writing utensils by improving coordination through exercises that will provide a greater smoothness to the writing. Answer D, exercises or activities for strengthening finger flexors and extensors, also allows improved use of the writing utensil by providing enough strength to properly position the writing tool. However, answers B, C, and D do not offer an alternative to the individual having to perform handwriting with a pen or pencil. See reference: Fisher, Murray, and Bundy (eds): Cermak, S: Somatodyspraxia.

131. (A) lying on the left side, propped up with pillows. This position allows the unaffected right extremities to remain free, and provides weight bearing to the affected side to assist with tone reduction. The pillows behind the individual allow support, and the individual may lean against the pillows to also provide pressure relief as needed to the affected side, because sensation may be reduced on that side along with movement. Sidelying on the right (answer B) would not provide any tone reduction, which is needed during a stressful activity such as sexual intercourse. This position also impairs the movement of the unaffected extremities, which would be needed for activities involving foreplay or applying contraceptive devices. Lying in a supine (answer C) or prone (answer D) position would not provide tone reduction to an individual with spasticity, and may be uncomfortable without many pillows to assist with positioning comfortably. Also, an individual lying prone has less mobility than when he or she is lying on the right side. See reference: Griffith and Lemberg: Neurological impairments relating to sexuality.

132. (A) A game of rhythmic exercises performed to music. Rhythmic activities facilitate motor performance in individuals with Parkinson's disease, especially when performed to music. Time capsules (answer B) are a meaningful activity for those who are approaching the end of life, but the description of the activity provides no rationale for why it would benefit the motor skills of those individu-

als with Parkinson's disease. Races (answer C) are generally not a good idea for this population because of the difficulty they often have stopping during ambulation. Reading out loud (answer D) is an effective intervention for addressing the communication, not motor deficits, frequently experienced by these individuals. Group activities are particularly beneficial because of the added advantage of social interaction. See reference: Sladyk, K and Ryan, SE (eds): Eberhardt, KM: A homemaker and volunteer with Parkinson's disease.

133. (D) refer him to her OTR supervisor who has attended a workshop on sexuality and spinal cord injury. Anyone providing sexuality counseling must not only be comfortable with his or her own sexuality, but must have certain competencies as well. These competencies include awareness of personal and societal attitudes concerning sexuality, knowledge of male and female reproductive systems and how different disabilities affect sexuality, and the interpersonal skills to communicate with patients about sensitive and personal issues concerned with sexuality. When an OT practitioner has developed these skills through continuing education and is available to the patient (answer D), it is not necessary to refer the patient to his psychiatrist (answer C). The COTA in this situation, who is unknowledgable and embarrassed by the patient's question (answers A and B), should not counsel him on these issues. See reference: Neistadt and Crepeau (eds): Freda, M: Treatment of activities of daily living: Sexuality and disability.

134. (A) macramé with short cords. Longer cords require more shoulder abduction with external rotation. Therefore, short cords (answer A) would be easiest for this type of individual. Fine cords (answer C) would be challenging for individuals with limited finger function. Thick cords (answer D) could be used to downgrade the activity for those individuals. The thickness of the cord, however, would have no bearing on shoulder range of motion requirements. See reference: Neistadt and Crepeau (eds): Crepeau, EB: Activity analysis: A way of thinking about occupational performance.

135. (C) Provide lateral trunk support. A lateral trunk support in the frontal plane stabilizes the side, helping to maintain correct alignment of the pelvis and trunk in the chair by counteracting the twisting effect of asymmetrical muscle tone. By providing upper extremity support, the lateral trunk support would also prevent improper loading onto an unstable shoulder joint. Using a reclining wheelchair (answer A) is incorrect because doing so would shift the client's weight to the posterior, but would not prevent the lateral shift of the trunk. An arm trough (answer B) may help maintain a more centered position of the trunk, but the weight of the affected extremity would result in instability and improper alignment of the shoulder, which could lead to shoulder pain. A lateral pelvic support (answer D) would provide stabilization of the pelvis to prevent it from shifting sideways, but this support would be too low to prevent the trunk from moving laterally. See reference: Neistadt and Crepeau (eds): Dutton, R: Treatment of performance components.

136. (A) from a home health OTR or COTA. Home health services, which may include nursing, OT, PT and speech therapy, are provided in the patient's home. Individuals who require continued care following discharge from the hospital may be appropriate for home health services if they are unable to travel to the hospital for outpatient services. If the decision to discharge the person has already been made, recommendations for a continued stay in the acute care hospital, or transfer to a rehabilitation center (answer B and C), are not appropriate. The patient's weakness and continuing requirement for IV drug therapy would make it extremely difficult for this patient to return to the hospital for outpatient therapy (answer D). See reference: Neistadt and Crepeau (eds): Griswold, LS: Community-based practice arenas.

137. (B) Learning proper body mechanics. Learning proper body mechanics (along with achieving a good fitness level) is one of the first steps to reducing the risk of reinjury in a work program. Answer C, work hardening, is appropriate to implement after the physical demands of the job's specific tasks are achieved. Answer D, engaging in vocational counseling, is appropriate after it is determined that a client cannot return to the same job or employer. Answer A, a prework screening, is typically completed by the practitioner before the employer offers the new employee a job. See reference: Neistadt and Crepeau (eds): Fenton, S and Gagnon, P: Treatment of work and productive activities: Functional restoration, an industrial approach.

138. (B) perform desired activities in a simplified manner to conserve energy. One method used to extend an individual's occupational performance as Parkinson's disease progresses is to introduce task simplification. This allows conservation of energy which can then be expended on desired activities. In a person with long-standing Parkinson's disease, encouragement to "work through" fatigue (answer A), and to perform additional exercises (answer B), would further deplete available energy. Recommendations to decrease activity level as much as possible (answer D), would also be detrimental to maintaining occupational performance levels. See reference: Neistadt and Crepeau (eds): Pulaski, KH: Adult neurological dysfunction.

139. (D) observe for signs of pain, redness, and irritation. Of the answers listed, the most important aspect of splint education is the need to monitor splinted skin areas for presence of problems, such as pain, redness, blisters or skin irritations, which

can lead to injury. If such signs exist, the next step is to discontinue use of the splint and report the problem to the therapist, who can then re-evaluate the splint. Answer A, teaching the client to bend or modify the splint themselves, would be inappropriate, could make the splint ineffective, or cause injury. Poor cosmesis (answer B) would be an inadequate reason to discontinue splint use. Splint care instructions (answer C) are important to maintain the splint, but are much less of a priority than informing the patient about precautions. See reference: Neistadt and Crepeau (eds): Wylett-Rendall, J: Treatment of performance components.

140. (B) Self-assessment. Self-assessment of each individual's stressors and stress reactions is the first step in designing a stress management program. Time management techniques (answer A), which help individuals schedule, prioritize, and develop appropriate attitudes about daily task requirements, may comprise one of the following sessions. Aerobic exercise (answer C) is an appropriate method for reducing stress in individuals with MS, but care should be taken in designing a program that will not lead to overheating. Progressive relaxation exercises (answer D) involve systematic tensing and relaxing of muscles, and are not appropriate for individuals with hypertension, cardiac disease, upper motor neuron lesions, or spasticity. See reference: Neistadt and Crepeau (eds): Giles, GM and Neistadt, ME: Treatment for psychosocial components: stress management.

141. (B) sip and puff switch. A sip and puff switch allows control through respiration (i.e.,: blowing air into and sucking air out of a straw positioned in front of the mouth activates the switch). This method would be particularly appropriate for a client with no functional movements. Answers A and C, joysticks and single digital switches, require mechanical activation through movement of some part of the body (e.g., hand, foot, head, chin). Mouth sticks, answer D, are usually used for direct access on keyboards or on ECU control panels. See reference: Neistadt and Crepeau (eds): Bain, BK: Assistive technology in occupational therapy.

142. (C) Preparing a frozen dinner. The Rehabilitation Institute of Chicago identified five levels of complexity for meal preparation ranging from easiest (level one) to hardest (level five). Preparing macaroni and cheese, a hot one dish meal, falls into the fourth level. Because the individual is unable to successfully perform at this level, the task must be downgraded to the next lowest level, i.e., level three, which includes preparation of hot beverages, soups, or frozen dinners. Having the individual prepare a multicourse meal, such as chicken and mashed potatoes (answer A), would be upgrading the activity to level five. Cold meals and foods such as instant pudding and peanut butter and jelly sandwiches (answers B and D), are at level two. Downgrading to this level would be appropriate if the individual had experienced significant difficulty not minimal to moderate as demonstrated here. See reference: Neistadt and Crepeau (eds): Culler, KH: Treatment for work and productive activities: Home and family management.

143. (C) Divide the laundry into several small loads for carrying. Dividing the laundry into several small loads will decrease low back strain as opposed to one or two large loads. Folding laundry from a basket on the floor next to the chair (answer A) would require bending and twisting, two movements that people with low back pain should avoid. Pain should be avoided when possible (answer D), and therefore preventive strategies should be urged to help the person avoid getting to the point of severe pain. See reference: Pedretti and Early (eds): Smithline, J and Dunlop, LE: Low back pain.

144. (C) Observe the individual tucking a shirt in the back of his pants. Tucking a shirt in the back requires shoulder abduction and internal rotation. Reaching the back of the neck (answer A) requires external rotation. Functional evaluations are best performed by observing movements during functional activities. A goniometer would be used when formal joint measurement is required (answer B). An interview (answer D) will provide useful information concerning pain, stiffness, and limitations in occupational performance, but is not a reliable method for assessing ROM. See reference: Neistadt and Crepeau (eds): Kohlmeyer, K: Evaluation of sensory and neuromuscular performance components.

145. (D) maintain a normal curve of the back, slowly shifting feet as the turn is completed. A correct transfer is performed slowly with the knees bent and the feet a shoulder width apart, while the normal curve of the back is maintained, and the lifting is performed with the legs. The body should not be twisted at the trunk (answer A), as this could cause back injury. Lifting with the arms (answer B), instead of the legs, could also injure the COTA's back. Another cause of back injury during a transfer is to keep the feet planted when moving (answer C), because this causes twisting of the back and may damage the knees. See reference: Palmer and Toms: Body mechanics and guarding techniques.

146. (B) "scoot forward to the edge of the wheelchair." When the COTA has the individual scoot forward to the edge of the wheelchair, this helps the individual position the body over the feet and causes the weight to shift forward during a transfer. The individual is much easier to transfer when the weight is shifted forward. If the person attempts to stand up (answer A) from a regular seated position, and the weight is shifted back during a transfer, it may require more than one person to assist with the transfer or it may be a total lift by one or more individuals. Answer C, unfasten the wheelchair

brakes, is incorrect because the wheelchair needs to be stabilized in a locked position before standing. Positioning the wheelchair facing the mat table (answer D) allows no room for the COTA to stand and assist with the pivot. See reference: Palmer and Toms: Body mechanics and guarding techniques.

147. (C) an aquatic therapy class. Many community centers offer aquatic therapy programs for individuals with physical disabilities. In a warm water environment, people with arthritis can perform AROM further, and with less pain, than on land. The group format also provides excellent opportunities for socialization and information sharing. A weightlifting program (answer A) would be contraindicated for individuals with RA. Providing and instructing in the use of adaptive equipment (answer B) is very important for this population, as is education in energy conservation and joint protection (answer D). However, these options do not address the physical fitness and socialization components required. See reference: Pedretti and Early (eds): Buckner, WS: Arthritis.

148. (D) identify alternative methods for meeting sexual needs that don't cause pain. Because the individual's pain cannot be seen or felt by the sexual partner, communication is particularly important. The couple can discuss alternate positions and methods for achieving sexual fulfillment that are acceptable to them and do not cause pain, such as alternate positions, masturbation, and fantasy. Good communication will ensure the needs of both partners are met and will prevent misunderstandings. Therefore, answer C is inappropriate. A pain-free position is important for successful sexual expression, but there is insufficient information to determine whether answer A, a sidelying position, is a pain-free position for this individual. Timing sex for periods of high energy (answer B) is an appropriate strategy for individuals with low endurance. However, timing sex for periods of lessened pain, such as after taking pain medication, may be a useful strategy for individuals with severe pain. See reference: Pedretti and Early (eds): Burton, GU: Sexuality and physical dysfunction.

149. (B) increase physical activity and fitness. Wellness programs focus on developing personal control of behaviors through educational approaches and active participation in activities that promote health, such as increasing levels of physical activity to improve physical fitness. Answers A, C, and D reflect traditional occupational therapy therapeutic interventions to improve performance in specific deficit areas, rather than promoting general good health. See reference: Cottrell (ed): Swarbrick, P: A wellness model for an acute psychiatric setting.

150. (C) further decline. Because MS is a degenerative disease, it is likely that the individual receiving a wheelchair will eventually decline further in functional performance. Improved wheelchair mobility and gains in strength (answers A and D) are not characteristic of progressive degenerative diseases. When ordering a wheelchair for a pediatric or adolescent client, it is important to anticipate growth of the individual (answer B). See reference: Neistadt and Crepeau (eds): Pulaski, KH: Adult neurological dysfunction.

151. (B) detachable armrests. Armrests need to be removed to allow the individual to move sideways out of the wheelchair. Footrests (answer A) may be swung away, but do not need to be detached to perform a transfer. Anti-tip bars (answer C) prevent a wheelchair from tipping over backwards (such as when performing a "wheelie" or when going up or down a step), but not when transferring. Brake handle extensions (answer D) allow the brakes to be locked more easily, but would be in the way of a board transfer. See reference: Pedretti and Early (eds): Adler, C and Tipton-Burton, M: Wheelchair assessment and transfers.

152. (A) isometric muscle contractions. Isometric muscle contraction involves contracting the muscle without joint movement or a change in muscle length. Isotonic contractions (answer B) shorten the muscle length with accompanying joint movement. Progressive resistance (answer C) is a type of isotonic exercise that uses an increase in weight during consecutive exercise repetitions. A person who has a cast obstructing movement would be unable to perform either type of isotonic exercise. Passive movements (answer D) are performed by an outside force to the arm and involve joint motion, but no muscle contraction. Passive movement could not be performed with a casted joint. See reference: Pedretti and Early (eds): Breines, E: Therapeutic occupations and modalities.

153. (D) hand controls for acceleration and braking. Hand controls use hand motions to control the accelerator and brake mechanisms, eliminating the need for any lower extremity function. The palmar cuff and spinner knob (answers A and B) are steering options for individuals who need to steer single-handed and allow constant contact with the steering wheel. Pedal extensions (answer C) can be installed on accelerator and brake pedal for individuals with limited lower extremity reach. See reference: Pedretti and Early (eds): Lillie, SM: Transportation, community mobility, and driving assessment.

154. (B) folding laundry and putting it in a basket while standing. Work-hardening programs prepare individuals to return to work by combining work simulation, strengthening, and behavioral components. A cashier stands during the job, removes clothing from a hanger, folds it, puts it in a bag, runs price tags through a scanner, operates a cash register, and makes change. Putting price tags on clothing while seated (answer D) does not include stand-

ing, a critical component of the job. Washing dishes while standing (answer C) incorporates the standing aspect of the client's job, but not the other aspects. Moving piles of clothing from one end of the clinic to the other (answer A) involves walking, not standing. The activity that incorporates the most components of the client's job is folding laundry and putting it in a basket while standing (answer B). See reference: Pedretti and Early (eds): Burt, CM: Work evaluation and work hardening.

155. (A) Monitor the individual's response to activities to prevent him from performing at activity levels that are too high and unsafe. "Denial is common among patients with cardiac disease. Patients in denial must be closely monitored during the acute phase of recovery. Persons in denial may ignore all precautions and could stress and further damage their cardiovascular systems" (p. 970). This individual, because of his denial, is unlikely to be willing to learn or apply energy conservation techniques (answer B), which can benefit him. The COTA should attempt to understand and modify the individual's behavior through collaborative goal setting. The COTA and supervising OTR, along with the patient and his family should engage in educational sessions prior to referring for psychological services. See reference: Pedretti and Early (eds): Matthews, MM: Cardiac and pulmonary diseases.

156. (B) Avoid internal rotation and adduction of the involved hip. Following hip arthroplasty, positions such as flexion of the hip past a prescribed range (usually 60 to 90 degrees), internal rotation, and adduction can result in dislocation of the hip. Therefore, answer B, avoid internal rotation and adduction of the involved hip, is the priority set of instructions to convey. OT practitioners instruct patients in hip precautions and provide them with adaptive equipment so they can safely perform self-care, work, and leisure activities. Answers C and D may help an individual comply more easily with hip precautions. Sitting during LE dressing (answer A) is also recommended. See reference: Pedretti and Early (eds): Coleman, S: Hip fractures and lower extremity joint replacement.

157. (A) Work simplification and energy conservation. In the first stage of ALS, mild limitations in function and endurance begin to develop. The individual becomes easily fatigued, so work simplification and energy conservation techniques are the most beneficial. Progressive resistive exercises (answer B) may cause cramping and fatigue, and are therefore not recommended for individuals with ALS. Splinting (answer C) will be required in later stages to prevent contractures, support weak muscles, and assist with function. Active range of motion and PROM activities will also be required later as the disease progresses, to prevent contractures and maintain strength. See reference: Pedretti and Early (eds): Schultz-Krohn, W, Foti, D, and Glogoski, C:

Degenerative diseases of the central nervous system.

158. (A) remedial treatment, such as rubbing or stroking the involved extremity. When sensation begins to return, it is appropriate to initiate remedial activities for sensory retraining. Stimulating the involved extremity by rubbing or stroking (to provide tactile input), or through weight-bearing activities (to provide proprioceptive input), are examples of remedial activities. Compensatory activities, which are essential for individuals with decreased or absent sensation, would have been part of the original treatment plan. Answers B, C, and D are all examples of compensatory strategies. See reference: Pedretti and Early (eds): Iyer, MB and Pedretti, LW: Evaluation of sensation and treatment of sensory dysfunction.

159. (B) Sliding board transfers. Sliding board transfers, or push-up-and-over transfer techniques, would be the safest and most efficient technique when transferring to a tub seat for this client. Answer A, stand pivot transfers, would only be effective with unilateral amputations protheses or crutches. Answers C and D would not address independent transfer training with the client. See reference: Pedretti and Early (eds): Adler, C and Tipton-Burton, M: Wheelchair assessment and transfers.

160. (C) Moderate assistance. Moderate assistance is defined as having the ability to complete the task with supervision and cueing, while requiring physical assistance for 20% to 50% of the task. The individual who requires minimal assistance (answer B) is able to complete a task with supervision and cueing, while requiring physical assistance for less than 20% of the task. An individual who needs supervision, cueing, and physical assistance for 50% to 80% of the task is performing at the maximal assistance level (answer D). An individual is rated dependent (answer A) when he or she is able to perform less than 20%, or a few steps, of the activity independently. This individual may require elaborate equipment, may perform the activity extremely slowly, and may fatigue easily. See reference: Pedretti and Early (eds): Foti, D: Activities of daily living.

161. (B) Tip the wheelchair backward and guide it down the ramp forward. This is the recommended technique for going down a steep ramp. The individual sitting in the wheelchair can also help to control the wheels, if capable of doing so, by grasping the hand rims. It would be difficult for the person guiding a wheelchair backwards down a ramp (answer A) to see where he or she is going. Only extremely strong individuals can propel themselves independently down a steep ramp (answer C). Using two people to move a wheelchair down a steep ramp could be awkward and dangerous (answer D). See reference: Pedretti and Early (eds): Adler, C and Tipton-Burton, M: Wheelchair assessment and transfers.

162. (C) Use a tub transfer bench and leg lifter. The use of a tub transfer bench would allow the client to back up to the tub bench, sit, and manually lift the knee over the side of the tub, either by using her own hands or a leg lifter. Answer A, the postponing of bathing, is not considered to be a standard course of treatment. Answer B, use of a hand rail, would assist with transfers, but would not address the limitation of knee motion. Answer D, use of a low kitchen stool in the tub, even one with rubber tips, would not be considered a safe or stable selection for transfer training. See reference: Pedretti and Early (eds): Coleman, S: Hip fractures and lower extremity joint replacement.

163. (C) Trim lines of the splint should extend proximal to the MCP crease. Trim lines of a splint that extend proximal to the MCP crease allow for adequate MCP digit extension and flexion. Answers A, B, and D fall distal to the MCP crease, thus restricting full extension and flexion of the digits at the metacarpal heads. See reference: Pedretti and Early (eds): Bekin, J and Yasuda, L: Orthotics.

164. (B) Training in residual limb wrapping. Residual limb wrapping would help prepare the residual limb by shrinking and shaping it to fit in the prosthesis. Training in how to put on and take off the prosthesis (answer A), and activities to improve grasp and prehension (answer C), come later in the intervention process when the prosthesis has been selected, prescribed, and fitted. Training to resume vocational activities (answer D) would also normally occur later in rehabilitation process, after the patient has mastered the basics of prosthetic use. See reference: Pedretti and Early (eds): Keenan, DD and Morris, PA: General considerations of upper and lower extremity amputations.

165. (C) Work simulation to increase strength and endurance for necessary work-related skills. Work simulation is considered to be a primary goal of work hardening, in addition to increasing productivity and feasibility through work-simulated activities. Answers A and B, ADL retraining and progressive resistive exercises, are not typical goals associated with the description of a work hardening program. Answer D, vocational retraining, is incorrect. It is vital that a work hardening program be viewed as an adjunct to vocational retraining, not as a vocational training program in and of itself. OT practitioners typically measure and assess a client's overall physical ability to perform the requirements of a particular job. See reference: Pedretti and Early (eds): Burt, CM: Work evluation and work hardening.

166. (D) Aesthesiometer. People with sensory loss in the hand often drop things because they are not receiving adequate sensory input. An aesthesiometer measures two-point discrimination with a moveable point attached to a ruler that has a stationary point at one end. The dynamometer (answer B) and pinch meter (answer C) are both used to measure strength. An individual with a loss of strength would drop heavy, not lightweight items. A goniometer (answer A) is a tool with two arms used to measure movement at a joint. One arm is held stationary while the other arm moves around an axis of 360 degrees. See reference: Pedretti and Early (eds): Kasch, MC and Nickerson, E: Hand and upper extremity injuries.

167. (D) Suggest furniture and accessories that promote better positioning at work. The best recommendation is for ergonomically correct furniture and accessories (answer D). Additional adaptations may include tool modification and the training of workers in appropriate positioning. Answers A and C, setting up stress management and work simulation activities, are not considered to be ergonomic interventions. Answer B is not an example of an ergonomic intervention, but is a treatment intervention. See reference: Sladyk, K and Ryan, SE (eds): Larson, B: Work injury activities.

168. (C) Repeatedly squeeze with the hand against increasing amounts of resistance. The biomechanical approach is a treatment approach used when a person has a deficit in strength, endurance, or range of motion, but has voluntary muscle control during performance of activities. The biomechanical approach focuses on decreasing the deficit area to improve the person's performance of daily activities. Eliciting functional grasp using reflex inhibiting postures (answer A) is a neurophysiological approach, which emphasizes an understanding of the nervous system in a person with brain damage, and how to elicit a desired response from that person. Muscles can be stimulated through a variety of neurodevelopmental techniques (answer B), using an understanding of the nervous system to elicit a response in a developmental sequence. Building up utensils (answer D) is an example of the rehabilitative approach, which teaches a person how to compensate for a deficit on either a temporary or permanent basis. See reference: Trombly (ed): Zemke, R: Remediating biomechanical and physiological impairments of motor performance.

169. (B) use moderately heated water. Hot water may contribute to fatigue in individuals with MS, and should therefore, be avoided. Moderate water temperature is recommended (answer B). Bathing in cool water (answer A) is unnecessary and may cause chilling and increase spasticity. Bathing rather than showering (answer C) is recommended for individuals with poor balance or standing tolerance, such as those with MS or COPD. Bathing at the sink (answer D) may be recommended for individuals who experience difficulty bending, such as those with hip or knee replacements or back pain. However, dura-

ble medical equipment is typically available for all of these diagnoses, so bathing in the tub would be possible through the use of a tub bench and hand held shower. See reference: Sladyk, K and Ryan, SE (eds): Kornblau, BL: A mother and a caterer with Multiple Sclerosis.

170. (D) Obtain a narrower wheelchair because this one is now too wide. The recommended wheelchair seat width is 2 inches wider than the widest point across the hips and thighs of the seated individual. If the seat is 2.5 inches wider than the patient, it is too wide, not too narrow (answer A). In addition, "wheelchairs should be as narrow as possible while allowing for comfort, ease of repositioning, and transfers" (p. 605). The narrower the wheelchair, the easier it is to maneuver. Because a narrower wheelchair would be better, padding the sides (answer C) is a less desirable option. The need to lose or gain weight (answer B) should be discussed first with a patient's physician. See reference: Trombly (ed): Deitz, J and Dudgeon, B: Wheelchair selection process.

171. (B) A mobile arm support. A C5 quadriplegic with fair shoulder flexors and abductors, and at least poor minus biceps, upper trapezius, and external rotators, will be able to operate a mobile arm support for self-feeding and facial hygiene activities. A wrist-driven flexor hinge splint (answer A), would be used for a lower level spinal cord injury (C6-C8), in which the individual had functional use of the shoulder and arm muscles, and has fair plus or better wrist extension strength. This splint is indicated for individuals who lack prehension power. An electric self-feeder is indicated for individuals with a higher level of involvement (C4), and who demonstrate poor plus, or weaker, shoulder strength. Built-up utensils may be indicated for individuals with C8 or T1 injuries, because they may lack the strength to tightly grasp regular utensils. See reference: Trombly (ed): Hollar, LD: Spinal cord injury.

172. (A) teach how to inspect for pressure sores on bony prominences and affected areas. Visual inspection of an area is important to prevent pressure sores, which may develop because there are no sensory cues for skin breakdown. It is recommended that an individual with absent sensation not trim his or her own nails (answer B) because of safety issues. Another person may be able to assist by trimming the nails or the individual could file his or her own nails, which may be difficult and time consuming. Extra padding on a splint (answer C) would cause increased pressure and redness to an area, which would lead to skin breakdown. Desensitization training (answer D) is performed with hypersensitivity or exaggerated sensation, not absent sensation. See reference: Trombly (ed): Bentzel, K: Remediating sensory impairment.

173. (A) using the strongest joint and avoiding positions of deformity. The significance of using these principles for individuals with preexisting joint conditions and adverse musculoskeletal changes may help to restore function as well as prevent further impairments. Answers B, C, and D involve common muscle relaxation and stress management techniques not related to joint protection techniques. See reference: Trombly (ed): Bear-Lehman, J: Orthopaedic conditions.

174. (A) within normal limits. Normal range of motion for internal rotation is 70 degrees (answer A). Rotation can be assessed with the humerus adducted against the trunk or with the shoulder abducted to 90 degrees. If the humeral movements for internal or external rotation are observed during the performance of activities and found to be adequate for performance of functional activities, range of motion may be noted as WFL (answer B). The OT practitioner may choose not to perform a formal joint measurement if the joint is WFL, even though the end of the range may be lacking a few degrees, because the loss of movement may not be significant to the individual. Hypermobility (answer C) at a joint is motion past the average range of motion, which at the shoulder would be past 70 degrees of internal rotation. If hypermobility is caused by an unstable joint as might occur after a surgical repair or a disease process, then splinting or another form of stabilization or immobilization can be used to correct the problem. If the practitioner observes hypermobility during range of motion, they should compare the range of motion to that on the individual's opposite side in order to assess normal range. A limitation of internal rotation (answer D) at the shoulder would be less than 70 degrees of motion. If a limitation is apparent, the rehabilitation team may choose not to treat it unless it interferes with the function of the upper extremity. See reference: Trombly (ed): Trombly, CA: Evaluation of biomechanical and physiological aspects of motor performance.

175. (D) Dynamometer. This individual exhibits difficulty in the area of strength. A dynamometer measures grip strength through gross hand grasp. A volumeter (answer C) is a container used to measure edema in the hand by measuring the amount of water displaced when the hand is placed into the container. A goniometer (answer A) is a tool with two arms used to measure movement at a joint. One arm is held stationary while the other arm moves around an axis of 360 degrees. An aesthesiometer (answer B) measures two-point discrimination with a moveable point attached to a ruler that has a stationary point at one end. See reference: Trombly (ed): Trombly, CA: Evaluation of biomechanical and physiological aspects of motor performance.

176. (A) the use of energy conservation. Energy conservation techniques reduce the amount of energy expenditure an individual requires to perform various activities. For a client with COPD and limited endurance, energy conservation techniques should be taught early so they can be implemented and reinforced while performing other activities, such as preparing meals. Work hardening (answer B) and graded activities to increase strength (answer C) would not address the need to perform meal preparation in the most energy efficient manner. Safety in the kitchen (answer D) would be more relevant to individuals with sensory or balance loss rather than limited endurance. See reference: Trombly (ed): Atchison, B: Cardiopulmonary diseases.

177. (B) Pinch meter. A pinch meter is used to measure the strength of a three-jaw chuck grasp pattern (also known as palmar pinch), as well as key (lateral) pinch and tip pinch. All of these pinch patterns require thumb opposition. For each of these tests, the individual performs three trials, which the tester averages together; the result is compared to a standardized norm. An aesthesiometer (answer A) measures two-point discrimination. A dynamometer (answer C) measures grip strength, but is not particularly sensitive to thumb opposition. A volumeter (answer D) measures edema in the hand. See reference: Trombly (ed): Trombly, CA: Evaluation of biomechanical and physiological aspects of motor performance.

178. (A) ease the patient onto the floor, cushioning his fall. Proper body mechanics must be used when transferring patients. No one should "attempt a transfer that seems unmanageable because of the discrepancy between the patient's size and her own or because of the patient's level of dependency" (p. 294). Attempting to continue or reverse the transfer of an obese patient who has already begun to slip (answers B and C), is likely to result in injury to the COTA and perhaps to the patient as well. Once the patient has started to slip, the COTA should immediately begin easing him to the floor. Although calling for assistance is an appropriate action, the higher priority action is to begin easing the patient to the floor to prevent injury to the individuals involved. See reference: Trombly (ed): Trombly, CA: Retraining basic and instrumental activities of daily living.

179. (C) Teach a caregiver how to lift and turn the client safely. Individuals unable to move themselves, especially those with sensory loss, are susceptible to the development of decubiti. Skin damage results from pressure on the skin over a prolonged period of time. The skin over bony prominences is particularly prone to the development of decubitus ulcers. Frequent position changes are essential for these individuals to prevent skin breakdown and the risk of serious infection. If the patient were already involved in a strengthening program (answer A), it may be appropriate to change it to a maintenance program at this point. A bed-mobility program (answer B) and an environmental control unit (answer

D) would be appropriate if the individual has potential in these areas, but instructing a caregiver in how to reposition the patient is the most important modification. See reference: Trombly (ed): Bentzel, K: Remediating sensory impairment.

180. (A) figure-ground discrimination. Figure-ground discrimination is the ability to distinguish an object from the background. A person with impaired figure-ground discrimination would have difficulty finding the sock despite its position on the bed (answer A). Other deficits that may be demonstrated by the person would be an inability to see the sock on one side of the bed (unilateral neglect), to find it in relation to the bed (position in space), and to know how to get back to the bed to look for the sock (cognitive mapping). See reference: Trombly (ed): Quintana, LA: Evaluation of perception and cognition.

181. (A) An electric razor. An electric razor (answer A) is the safest for shaving because a rotary head or foil, instead of a blade, is in contact with the skin. Any shaving over the incision area or near it would not be recommended until the incision area is healed. The other razors have blades that could nick or cut the skin, which should be avoided until the patient is no longer treated with blood thinners and normal blood coagulation can occur. See reference: Trombly (ed): Trombly, CA: Retraining basic and instrumental activities of daily living.

182. (D) early morning and again in the afternoon. Individuals with arthritis should be evaluated in the morning and afternoon to assess the functional abilities of the individual during and after morning stiffness. Evaluating the individual only in the morning (answers A and C) or only in the afternoon (answer B) accurately reveals the individual's functional level at only one time of day. Individuals with arthritis have many changes in functional status after morning stiffness has disappeared. See reference: Trombly (ed): Feinberg, JR and Trombly, CA: Arthritis.

183. (A) at the lateral epicondyle of the humerus. The lateral epicondyle of the humerus is the bony prominence on the lateral side of the elbow. The medial epicondyle (answer B) is the bony prominence on the medial side of the elbow. The stationary arm of the goniometer should be positioned parallel to the longitudinal axis of the humerus on the lateral aspect (answer C). The movable arm of the goniometer should be positioned parallel to the longitudinal axis of the radius on the lateral aspect (answer D). See reference: Trombly (ed): Trombly, CA: Evaluation of biomechanical and physiological aspects of motor performance.

184. (C) teach use of mirror feedback to make the person aware of his or her facial expression. Using mirror feedback can make an individual aware of his or her facial expressions and help them understand how they appear to others. It can also help the Parkinsons' patient learn to smile and use more facial expression, which can be accomplished with concentration. Answers A, B, and D are useful strategies for improving communication, rather than facial expression. See reference: Trombly (ed): Newman, EM, Echevarria, ME, and Digman, G: Degenerative diseases.

185. (D) decreased attention. An attention deficit (answer D) is indicated if the individual recognizes a letter and marks it accurately on both the right and left sides of the page but misses letters in a random pattern. A visual field cut (answers A and B) is evidenced by missed letters appearing close together in one area, on either the left or right side of the page. Illiteracy (answer C) is unlikely because the individual is a high school teacher. See reference: Trombly (ed): Quintana, LA: Remediating perceptual impairments.

186. (A) Plaster cylindrical splint. A plaster cylindrical splint would encourage a static stretch of the PIP joint contracture. Answer B is a form of PIP extension and is considered to be a dynamic splint. Answer C is used to isolate tendon and joint range of motion. Answer D is also a form of dynamic splinting. See reference: Pedretti and Early (eds): Belkin, J and Yasuda, L: Orthotics.

187. (C) develop skills for providing feedback to the student. One of the most important jobs of a fieldwork educator is to provide constructive and positive feedback as the student progresses through the experience. Other responsibilities include communicating with the academic program, facilitating the student's clinical reasoning and evaluating the student, to name just a few. The academic fieldwork coordinator, not the program director (answer A) is responsible for coordinating student fieldwork experiences. Competence in student supervision (answer B) is developed over time, and there is no one method for determining competence as a fieldwork educator, although AOTA has developed a self-assessment to facilitate development in this area. Learning objectives for level I fieldwork (answer D) are typically developed by the academic program, and level II objectives are typically developed by the fieldwork site. See reference: AOTA: Occupational therapy roles.

188. (D) OTR supervision is not necessary. When a COTA is functioning in a role outside of OT service delivery, supervision by an OTR is not required, according to the AOTA document *Guide For Supervision of Occupational Therapy Personnel in the Delivery of Occupational Therapy Services*. In this situation, the COTA does not use OT credentials. See reference: AOTA: Guide for supervision of occupational therapy personnel in the delivery of occupational therapy services.

189. (A) selected tasks in which aides have been trained, with intense close supervision. To maximize efficiency and cost-effectiveness of therapy services, there has been an increased use OT aides. Such aides must be very closely supervised, and are expected to receive site specific training in selected activities determined by the supervising OT practitioner, and must be utilized in accordance with state regulations. Activities and levels of supervision in answers B, C, and D are all beyond the scope of the OT aide. See reference: Neistadt and Crepeau (eds): Cohn, ES: Interdisciplinary communication and supervision of personnel.

190. (D) Treat the client with the student observing the session. Occupational therapy practitioners should always respect the recipients of their services. According to the *Occupational Therapy Code of Ethics*, under Principle 3d, "occupational therapy personnel shall respect the individual's right to refuse professional services or involvement in research or educational activities"; attempts to persuade the client (answer A) would conflict with this principle. Canceling the session (answer B) would be punitive. Consulting with other fieldwork educators (answer C) may help the COTA develop strategies for facilitating student involvement. See reference: AOTA: Occupational therapy code of ethics.

191. (D) Label each item with the individuals' names. Cosmetics should never be shared. Federal regulations prohibit the sharing of cosmetics if there is any likelihood of the cosmetics coming in contact with bodily fluids. This likelihood would be high in a geropsychiatric population. See reference: Early: Safety techniques.

192. (B) Contribute to the screening process in collaboration with the OTR. The COTA works under the supervision of an OTR. When a formal OT screen referral is received, the COTA can contribute to the screening process under the supervision of an OTR, therefore answers A and D are incorrect. According to the *Occupational Therapy Personnel Skill Mix Resources* developed by the AOTA Practice Department, it is important that service competency with the screening process be established by the supervising OTR. It is the OTR's responsibility to select the most appropriate screening method(s) (answer C). A COTA reports to the supervising OTR; reporting to the OTR and the rehabilitation director (answer D) would be redundant. See reference: AOTA Practice Department: Guide to role performance: OT, OTA, Aide.

193. (D) wait for the OTR to return. Referrals must be received by the OTR before a COTA can begin evaluating or treating the patient. Answers A and C are part of the evaluation process, and cannot be initiated without the OTR's involvement. Involving the patient in group activities (answer B) constitutes treatment, which cannot be initiated without the involvement of the OTR. In some facilities, the COTA may be able to screen individuals and collect data

the OTR will use for evaluation purposes, prior to the OTR taking action on the referral. See reference: Sladyk, K and Ryan, SE (eds): Ryan, SE: Therapeutic intervention process.

194. (A) Use alternative modalities until the OTR can establish competency with this treatment technique. COTAs providing services reimbursable under OT must be supervised by an OTR, therefore answers B and C are incorrect. The OTR must be able to determine COTA competency for specific interventions and must be able to monitor patient response to interventions and modalities. In this case, the OTR must establish competency in using ultrasound prior to considering its use in treatment by either the OTR or COTA; a simple review of the procedures (answer D) does not establish competency. See reference: AOTA Practice Department: Guide to role performance: OT, OTA, Aide.

195. (C) Assist with stock and inventory control. Volunteer interaction within an OT department must be limited, so that it is in the direct line of vision of an OT practitioner. Answer A, helping the patient with self-care in the room, would take the volunteer out of the direct line of vision. In addition, it is not appropriate for a volunteer to treat a patient, because he or she lacks the skill and expertise of an OT practitioner, so answer B is also incorrect. Answer D is incorrect because it violates the confidentiality of the patient. See reference: Sladyk, K and Ryan, SE (eds): Ryan, SE: The role of the OTA as an activities director.

196. (C) The CTRS could substitute recreational activities during the OT time, without billing for OT services. Answers A, B, and D are incorrect because they all involve billing for occupational therapy services when services were not actually provided by an OT practitioner. Therefore, the only correct answer is not billing for occupational therapy. See reference: AOTA: Occupational therapy code of ethics.

197. (D) Use a tool storage area, painted with tool shadows or outlines, that can be locked. Painting a lockable tool cabinet with shadows or outlines to indicate where tools are to be kept, is a very effective method that allows simple, rapid and accurate identification of missing items. This method also makes it easy to hold clients responsible for returning tools at the end of group sessions. Keeping track of keys (answer A) is an overall safety strategy that is not specific to the use of tools. Advance preparation (answer B) is a strategy to reduce the OT practitioner's distractions. Many clients treated for psychosocial problems would be excluded from OT treatment if they had to wait until all of their behavioral risks were being managed (answer C). Clients with severe suicidal or impulsive behaviors should rarely be involved with activities requiring tools that have potential to harm. See reference: Early: Safety techniques.

198. (D) Launder the linens after the session. "Linens....should be replaced or laundered after each use" (p. 272). The Occupational Safety and Health Administration has set out strategies to protect individuals from potential exposure to infectious diseases. Contamination by bodily fluids is not always visible or apparent (answers A and C). Waiting until the end of the week (answer B) may result in exposure to others. See reference: Early: Safety techniques.

199. (B) Sterilize it before using it again. OSHA has set out strategies to protect individuals from potential exposure to HIV and hepatitis B virus. This situation would be an example of an engineering control. These controls are to modify the work environment to reduce risk of exposure. Other examples are using sharps containers, eyewash stations, and biohazard waste containers. Answers A, C, and D would not meet guidelines set forth by OSHA regarding equipment that has come into contact with open wounds. See reference: Pedretti and Early (eds): Buckner, WS: Infection control and safety issues in the clinic.

200. (D) Put gloves on, clean up the spill with paper towels, put the soiled paper towels in an infectious waste container, disinfect the area, and finish the patient's session with whatever time is still left. The Occupational Safety and Health Administration (OSHA) has identified materials that require universal precautions to include blood, semen, vaginal secretions, cerebrospinal fluid, synovial fluid, pleural fluid, any body fluid with visible blood, any unidentifiable body fluid, and saliva from dental procedures. Items OSHA has identified as not needing universal precautions include feces, nasal secretions, sputum, sweat, tears, urine, and vomitus. Because the urine had blood in it, in this case it would be considered an exposure. Hospitals have policies regarding response to exposures such as this. Answer A is incorrect because it does not address disposal of the paper towels or disinfecting the area afterward. Leaving the area unavailable for other therapists and their patients who might need to use it (answer B) would be inconsiderate. Contaminated linens and towels (answer C) need to be placed in a specially designated laundry area. See reference: Pedretti and Early (eds): Buckner, WS: Infection control and safety issues in the clinic.

SIMULATION EXAMINATION 5

Directions: Circle the correct answer to the following questions. When you have completed this examination, check your answers against the answer key that follows. As you will see, an explanation is given for each answer along with a reference for further study. The book author is listed as well as the chapter author. See the bibliography for complete references.

1. An OT practitioner is providing accessibility consultation services to a local library. In the back of the library there is a reference room with a doorway that has a threshold height of 1 inch. Concerning the threshold and accessibility according to the ADA guidelines, which of the following recommendations would be best?
   A. Keep the threshold as is, and place a sign near the door alerting people to the threshold.
   B. Provide a throw rug that covers the threshold.
   C. Remove the threshold altogether.
   D. Ramp the threshold.

2. What wheelchair feature would be MOST appropriate to recommend for an individual who will be traveling by car with the family to community outings and bringing his or her wheelchair?
   A. A lightweight folding frame
   B. A one-arm drive
   C. An amputee frame
   D. A reclining backrest

3. A COTA working in an outpatient setting would like to provide ultrasound as a treatment modality using skills and knowledge acquired in a previous work setting. However, the supervising OTR has had no training in the use of ultrasound. What is the best course of action for the COTA to take?
   A. Use alternative modalities until the OTR can establish competency with this treatment technique.

   B. Ask the staff PT to supervise the COTA's performance.
   C. Use ultrasound as a treatment modality only when the OTR is not on site.
   D. Review basic ultrasound procedures with the OTR, then begin to use this modality for treatment.

4. An entry-level COTA has joined the staff of a rehabilitation facility and requires "close supervision" for the first few months. As specified by AOTA, the COTA should have contact with the supervising OTR:
   A. once a day.
   B. once a week.
   C. once a month.
   D. as needed.

5. A referral for a woman who has had a hip replacement is received in the OT department on a day when the only OTR is on vacation. The COTA observes that the patient is scheduled to be discharged before the OTR's return. The ONLY acceptable action for the COTA to take is to:
   A. obtain collaboration with supervision from an OTR to screen the individual before beginning treatment.
   B. perform an ADL evaluation.
   C. provide the individual with the adaptive equipment she will need.
   D. begin instruction in hip precautions.

6. Working with a preschooler in the home, the COTA observes the child climb into a highchair and jump up and down on a toy trampoline. When presented with a new rocking horse as a birthday present,

however, the child is unable to determine how to mount the horse. This **MOST** likely indicates a problem in the area of:

A. fine motor skills.
B. gross motor skills.
C. reflex integration.
D. motor planning.

7. **A COTA is putting together an inpatient group for individuals with schizophrenia. Which of the following would the COTA MOST likely attempt to facilitate amongst group members?**

A. Self-disclosure
B. Development of insight regarding a person's feelings
C. Appropriate social and life skills
D. Strategies used for dealing with anger

8. **A COTA is running a group for individuals who have difficulty managing anger. Based on a cognitive-behavioral frame of reference, which of the following steps would the COTA BEGIN with?**

A. Discuss the benefits of alternative beliefs about anger and alternative responses to anger.
B. Develop awareness about what produces anger and how the clients respond to anger.
C. Role-play a situation that presents minimal difficulty to group participants.
D. Role-play a situation that presents significant difficulty to group participants.

9. **A child with active juvenile rheumatoid arthritis has been fitted with hand splints. The COTA is explaining the purpose of the splints to the child's parents. Which is the MOST accurate description of how splinting will benefit the child?**

A. The splints will inhibit hypertonus.
B. The splints will increase range of motion.
C. The splints will prevent deformity.
D. The splints will correct deformity.

10. **A COTA learns that a young child receiving OT is easily aroused because of a sensory-modulation disorder. Which of the following describes the MOST effective environmental adaptation for assisting the child to fall asleep?**

A. A mini trampoline in the bedroom to tire the child out before going to bed
B. A noise machine producing white noise at bedtime
C. A lightweight, fuzzy blanket providing light touch
D. Shutters on the windows to produce total darkness

11. **A COTA and an OTR are working on discharge plans for a child with paraplegic spina bifida who has just started using a powered wheelchair. The community resource that would be recommended as MOST critical for this child is:**

A. the local social service agency.
B. a local wheelchair equipment vendor.
C. the family physician.
D. an early intervention program.

12. **A COTA needs to report the results of an ADL evaluation to the supervising OTR. The OTR, who is on her way to the cafeteria for lunch, states she has to leave immediately after lunch to go to another facility. Which is the BEST method for the COTA to use to communicate the evaluation results to the OTR?**

A. With a phone call
B. In a written report
C. During discussion at lunch in the cafeteria
D. During discussion in the OT office

13. **A COTA working with an infant observes the presence of the first stage of voluntary grasp. Which of the following would be the MOST appropriate statement for documenting this behavior?**

A. The infant is exhibiting radial palmar grasp.
B. The infant is exhibiting pincer grasp.
C. The infant is exhibiting ulnar palmar grasp.
D. The infant is exhibiting palmar grasp.

14. **A COTA has recommendations concerning adaptations for a child's artificial limb. This would require that the COTA consult the:**

A. physiatrist.
B. orthotist.
C. prosthetist.
D. physical therapist.

15. **A child who has difficulty with visual perception of "position in space" will soon be discharged from an outpatient OT program. Of the following, which would be the BEST activity to recommend to the child's classroom teacher and parents?**

A. Identifying letters on a distracting page
B. Finding geometric shapes scattered in a box
C. Following directions about objects located in front, in back, and to the side
D. Making judgments about moving through space

16. During a time-management group, an individual with severe anxiety begins to provide a description of the physical symptoms she experienced when on a community outing the previous day. The COTA should:
A. report this to the individual's supervising OTR.
B. report this to the individual's physician.
C. encourage the individual to elaborate on her concerns.
D. redirect the individual to a more neutral topic.

17. A 1-year-old child is working on increasing neck flexor strength. At this time, the child can maintain head alignment when tilted backward from an upright supported sitting position, to a 45-degree incline, but loses control when tilted further back. The COTA recommends that the NEXT important step in the intervention is to work on head and neck alignment:
A. in a sidelying position while batting a toy.
B. in a prone position while watching a peek-a-boo game.
C. by tilting backwards up to 60 degrees while rocking.
D. in a supine position while watching an overhead mobile.

18. A young child has been wearing a left upper extremity prosthesis for 3 weeks. The MOST important activity recommendation that the COTA gives to the child's preschool teacher is to:
A. offer toys that the child can manipulate with one hand.
B. stress bilateral play and school activities incorporating the prosthesis.
C. teach the child one-handed manipulation techniques.
D. involve the child in activities that do not require manipulation.

19. A COTA is scheduled to interview an individual with a head injury about her home environment, and family and child care

responsibilities. Knowing the individual has an attention span of 10 to 15 minutes, which of the following should the COTA do FIRST?
A. Schedule a 30-minute treatment session.
B. Obtain as much information as possible from the chart.
C. Interview the individual using appropriate verbal and nonverbal communication.
D. Perform the interview in an environment where distractions can be minimized.

20. The MOST appropriate device a COTA can recommend to a child's parents to promote the development of upper lip control while feeding is a:
A. straw.
B. "spork."
C. deep spoon.
D. shallow spoon.

21. A COTA/OTR team receives a consult for an infant in the NICU whose mother has a history of drug abuse during pregnancy. Using a sensory integrative approach, what is the FIRST action the COTA/OT team should take?
A. Determine the mother's current medical status, parental involvement, and support systems.
B. Recommend a social work referral to address social concerns, provide emotional support and community program information, and make a referral to the Department of Human Services.
C. Modify the environment to protect the infant from excessive and/or inappropriate sensory stimulation prior to direct intervention.
D. Assess motor and behavioral skills to identify areas of developmental delay in order to educate family and medical staff of necessary positional and environmental strategies for skill acquisition.

22. A COTA needs to document the following statement, "patient states she is frightened by the anger she feels when doing ceramics." In which portion of a SOAP note would the COTA place this information?
A. Subjective section
B. Objective section
C. Assessment section
D. Plan section

23. **A COTA is working with a group of 4 to 5-year-old children who have mild cerebral palsy. The goal of the group is to encourage the children to participate in some form of physical or "rough and tumble" play. Which of the following is the COTA MOST likely to recommend?**
   A. Drawing and puzzle activities.
   B. Constructing towers and buildings with blocks.
   C. Role-playing with stories the children make up.
   D. Playing "Simon Says."

24. **Which of the following describes the BEST treatment activity for improving coordination?**
   A. Walking sideways on a balance beam
   B. Crawling over and along a rope taped to the floor
   C. Kicking a ball with alternating feet when sitting on a T-stool
   D. Tossing a balloon with alternating hands

25. **A COTA is conducting an ongoing assertiveness training group. Which of the following strategies would be MOST helpful in the development of group cohesion?**
   A. Define assertiveness, passivity, and aggression for the group members.
   B. Allow and encourage all group members to release their aggressive feelings physically and verbally toward inanimate objects.
   C. Demonstrate commonly used assertiveness techniques to the group members.
   D. Encourage group members to share similar experiences and reactions with each other.

26. **A child has mastered brushing her teeth with the COTA giving verbal and physical cues. What would be the NEXT step in the process of reducing the intrusiveness of cues?**
   A. Verbal cues
   B. Verbal and gestural cues
   C. Physical cues
   D. Verbal and physical cues

27. **Which of the following devices will be required by an individual with C7-C8 quadriplegia when performing oral hygiene activities?**
   A. Mobile arm support with utensil holder
   B. Universal cuff
   C. Toothbrush with built-up handle
   D. Wrist support with utensil holder

28. **An individual about to be discharged from an inpatient psychiatric unit asks, "when I apply for jobs, what should I put down when the application asks if you have been hospitalized in the past 6 months?" The therapist's response should include strategies that address:**
   A. developing assertiveness.
   B. improving self-esteem.
   C. anger management.
   D. managing stigma.

29. **An OTR/COTA team is performing an assistive technology intervention with a client who has severe limitations of motor function resulting from CP. The FIRST function of the OTR/COTA team in this process is to:**
   A. identify the most appropriate commercially available forms of assistive technology.
   B. identify the abilities, needs, and life goals of the client.
   C. select the appropriate method of accessing the technology.
   D. modify the assistive technology device to meet the needs of the client.

30. **A COTA is working in a day program with older adults with severe mental illness who have been institutionalized for many years. The COTA is developing ideas for a work and productive activities program. However, because of their age and severely impaired performance, these individuals will never move into paid employment. Which of the following is the MOST important concept for the COTA to integrate?**
   A. Incorporate activities such as wiping the tables after lunch, which are concrete, consistent, and predictable.
   B. Train clients to sort objects, like nuts and bolts, to prepare them for piece-work employment.
   C. Teach clients jobs they can then generalize to their home environments, such as dusting furniture.
   D. When available, involve clients in stuffing envelopes for non-profit agencies, to develop a sense of community membership.

31. **While performing endurance training activities, an individual on a cardiac rehabilitation unit begins to slow down, using progressively smaller movements to perform the activity. Which of the following**

is the MOST appropriate action for the COTA to take?

A. Stop the activity.
B. Upgrade the activity for the next session.
C. Modify the activity to make it less challenging.
D. Replace the activity with isometric exercises.

32. **An individual with complete C7 quadriplegia demonstrates fair plus (3+) strength in the wrist extensors. Which of the following interventions would the COTA introduce to MOST effectively increase strength in the wrist extensors?**

A. A craft activity using increasingly heavy hand tools
B. Mildly resistive activities that are halted as soon as the individual begins to fatigue
C. Electric stimulation to the wrist extensors
D. Moderate resistance during AROM to the wrist

33. **A COTA is interviewing an individual diagnosed with Alzheimer's disease to obtain information about his level of independence in ADL's and IADL's. Halfway through the interview, the COTA realizes the client is confabulating. Which of the following options is MOST appropriate?**

A. Complete the interview using closed-ended questions.
B. Stop the interview and complete it the next day.
C. Interview a reliable informant instead of the individual.
D. Administer a written questionnaire using a checklist format.

34. **When teaching children with moderate mental retardation to feed, groom, and dress themselves, the COTA is MOST likely to use which technique?**

A. Chaining
B. Practice and repetition
C. Demonstration
D. Role modeling

35. **An 8-year-old boy with conduct disorder is disruptive, uncooperative and occasionally combative during therapy. From a behavioral point of view, the MOST appropriate strategy to use to address the child's conduct would be to:**

A. allow the child to express his anger without restraint for a short period to vent his frustration.

B. ignore the behavior and continue with therapy with or without the child's cooperation.
C. attempt to reason with the child to get his cooperation.
D. set clear expectations for behavior and enforce consequences, such as a time-out, if the child loses control.

36. **A COTA is working in a psychosocial setting with clients who are classified as being at risk for suicide. In selecting craft media, the activity that would MOST likely be the safest is a:**

A. leather checkbook cover with single cordovan lacing.
B. macramé plant hanger.
C. ceramic ashtray.
D. stenciling project on poster board.

37. **Which of the following is MOST important when using a remotivation approach with a group of elderly individuals?**

A. Use pictures, music, and discussion to encourage discussion of memories.
B. Discuss an upcoming holiday and base an activity on that holiday.
C. Adapt the environment to maximize independent functioning.
D. Focus on group activities designed to enhance interpersonal skills.

38. **An OT practitioner wishes to identify how a patient spends his leisure time, which leisure activities he especially enjoys, and which others he has participated in that he would be interested in renewing. The MOST appropriate tool for this purpose is a(n):**

A. evaluation of living skills.
B. interest checklist.
C. activity configuration.
D. self-care evaluation.

39. **The COTA is selecting activities for an 8-year-old child with Duchenne's muscular dystrophy. Which of the following developmental issues is MOST important to consider when identifying activities for this child?**

A. Establishment of basic trust
B. Freedom to use his initiative
C. Development of self-identity
D. Reinforcement of competence

40. **A COTA and OTR each carry out part of the initial evaluation of a newly admitted**

patient. Upon completion of the evaluation, each will write part of the initial note. The most appropriate part of the note for the COTA to write is the:

A. treatment plan.
B. source of the referral, the reason for the referral, and the date the referral was received.
C. summary and analysis of the patient's assets and deficits.
D. projected outcome of treatment.

41. **A COTA is collaborating with a new teacher to plan classroom activities for a 6-year-old child with developmental dyspraxia. Which would be the MOST accurate description for the COTA to provide to the teacher to explain this problem?**

A. A problem with learning new motor skills
B. A sensory integration problem
C. A lack of development of higher order reflex reactions
D. A problem of poor balance

42. **A sixth grader with a diagnosis of athetoid cerebral palsy needs an adapted computer for communication. Her upper extremity control is poor because of fluctuating muscle tone. The COTA suggests that the BEST way for her to operate her computer is to use a:**

A. single pressure switch, firmly mounted within easy reach.
B. lightweight keyboard placed at midline.
C. low-resistance mouse and pad.
D. mercury switch headband set to respond to minimal movement.

43. **A COTA is working with a group of children in an early intervention program. All of the children in the group are able to sit independently on the floor except for one child with cerebral palsy. The child has told the COTA that he wishes to sit on the floor like his peers and not in his wheelchair. The COTA would MOST likely recommend that the child use a(n):**

A. hammock.
B. floor sitter.
C. adapted wheelchair insert.
D. prone stander.

44. **An 18-year-old adolescent diagnosed with schizophrenia, takes a neuroleptic drug that has caused him to experience extreme thirst, but he must continue**

taking the drug. At the time of discharge, it is MOST important to remind him to:

A. limit sun exposure as much as possible.
B. drink coffee and caffeinated sodas whenever possible.
C. get up slowly from a standing, sitting, or lying position.
D. drink juices and caffeine-free colas when thirsty.

45. **The goal of an arts and crafts group for chronically mentally ill individuals is to improve their decision making abilities. The MOST appropriate approach to initiating a mosaic tile activity would be to:**

A. provide each patient with an individual project and have him or her choose a tile color.
B. have the patients choose from a variety of projects.
C. have the patients decide on a design, size, shape, and color for a group mosaics project.
D. have each patient decide on a pattern and two tile colors to use in his or her mosaic project.

46. **OT practitioners employed by a school district provide consultation to a vocational instructor in a high school program for students with moderate mental disabilities. Which of the following activities would be MOST appropriately provided by the OT practitioners?**

A. Developing an in-house prevocational work program
B. Bringing in outside speakers from different job settings
C. Teaching the vocational instructor different assessment tools and scoring procedures
D. Meeting the vocational instructor weekly to discuss adaptations to work tasks

47. **A COTA has been working on laundry skills with an adult with developmental disabilities who lives at home with her aging parents. Although the client is able to use the washer and dryer successfully with only verbal cues, her mother continues to do her laundry. The COTA should:**

A. explain to the mother that it is critical to allow the client to do her own laundry in order to achieve independence.
B. discuss the meaning and value of the

client's doing her own laundry with the mother and client.

C. ask the father to intercede to stop the mother from doing the client's laundry for her.

D. acknowledge that independence in laundry skills may not be an appropriate goal for this client.

48. An individual with borderline personality disorder has been referred to occupational therapy. Which of the following would be MOST important to evaluate?

A. Activities of daily living

B. Instrumental ADL's

C. Relationships with others

D. Sensorimotor skills

49. An OTR/COTA team begins to provide occupational therapy services through a Medicare-certified home health agency. What is the MOST critical component for establishing a successful collaborative relationship in this treatment setting?

A. Determining reimbursement when completing joint visits

B. Establishing a system for the OTR to countersign the COTA's documentation

C. Creating a written and specific supervisory plan based on competency levels for both practitioners

D. Developing a handout to educate future clients regarding how the OTR/COTA team will provide services

50. A COTA is discussing skills that can help a client with substance abuse problems to develop an alcohol-free lifestyle. The area that the COTA is MOST likely to address first with the client is:

A. work or job performance.

B. self-care skills.

C. time management and use of leisure time.

D. medication management.

51. A COTA is ready to introduce decision-making opportunities to an individual in a craft group. Which choice should the COTA begin with?

A. Which type of project is the client interested in: leather, wood, macramé or weaving?

B. Does the client want to paint the project blue or white?

C. Would the client like to give the finished project to a friend or relative?

D. Would the client like to work alone or in a group?

52. A lead guitar player in a band has been admitted to an inpatient psychiatric facility following a suicide attempt. At present, he is withdrawn and rarely participates during group activities. What would be the MOST effective method to use for increasing the individual's engagement in group activities?

A. Give him a guitar to play during break under the supervision of the COTA.

B. Give him a guitar to practice with in his room.

C. Have him compose music for the group.

D. Allow him to play the guitar in a separate room during group.

53. An OT practitioner is working to reduce the application of restraints for the population of a long-term care facility. The MOST appropriate form of intervention for the OT practitioner to provide is:

A. identifying legal issues related to restraint reduction.

B. providing staff education, recommendations, and support for restraint alternatives.

C. investigating incidents of resident abuse related to restraint reduction.

D. assessing the level of risk and liability involved with restraint use.

54. A COTA is positioning a child with low muscle tone and postural instability into a prone stander to develop head righting. The child rapidly shows fatigue and associated reactions. How can the COTA BEST adjust the stander to decrease these reactions while continuing to address the goal of head righting?

A. Place the child in prone on the floor.

B. Position the stander at 45 degrees from the floor.

C. Position the stander at 75 to 90 degrees from the floor.

D. Position the child upright in a prone or supine stander.

55. A child has considerable difficulty with problem solving when playing with Lego blocks and becomes frustrated and gives up easily. This MOST likely indicates a problem in which area of play?

A. Sensorimotor

B. Imaginary

C. Constructional

D. Game

56. **A COTA is planning to discharge an individual who recently had a stroke. Plans are to discharge the client home to live independently. The practitioner has worked with other individuals in similar situations, and has developed a keen sense for many of the issues that may arise and need to be problem solved. The form of clinical reasoning that this practitioner is MOST likely to use based on past experience will be:**

A. procedural reasoning.

B. conditional reasoning.

C. interactive reasoning.

D. narrative reasoning.

57. **A COTA working in a geropsychiatric day program runs a craft group after lunch. Many of the clients doze off during the group, which prevents them from benefiting from the activity. The COTA should recognize this as a problem with:**

A. motivation.

B. interest.

C. level of arousal.

D. attention span.

58. **A COTA is planning a simple meal preparation activity that will result in success for a patient with cognitive deficits. The SIMPLEST activity would be preparing:**

A. a can of soup.

B. a casserole.

C. brownies from a box mix.

D. a meal with two side dishes and an entrée.

59. **A patient who has had surgery for a malignant tumor was seen once in OT and is being discharged home. The patient is weak and needs to continue receiving IV chemotherapy with a home health nurse. The MOST appropriate discharge recommendation for this patient to receive OT services would be:**

A. from a home health OTR or COTA.

B. staying in the hospital a little longer.

C. going to a rehabilitation center.

D. coming back for outpatient OT.

60. **A COTA is working with a client who had a TBI and demonstrates deficits in sequencing and problem solving. The client has successfully prepared a cold meal in today's treatment session. The next**

meal preparation activity the COTA should have the client prepare is:

A. brownies.

B. a cheese sandwich.

C. a casserole.

D. a spaghetti dinner with salad and garlic bread.

61. **An individual diagnosed with borderline personality disorder tells a COTA that she is the only one she can trust. The next day she accuses the COTA of lying to her. The best way for the COTA to respond is to:**

A. tell the individual her feelings have been hurt.

B. remain matter of fact and consistent in approach.

C. ask the individual how she has felt when lied to in the past.

D. apologize and try to determine how the misunderstanding occurred.

62. **During a craft group comprised of individuals diagnosed with substance abuse, a COTA observes one individual having difficulty gluing two pieces of a birdhouse together. The individual becomes increasingly agitated. As the COTA approaches him, he storms out of the room and heads to the smoking area for a cigarette. This behavior MOST likely indicates a problem in which of the following?**

A. Eye-hand coordination

B. Stress management

C. Visual perception

D. Fine motor skills

63. **Which of the following is the MOST important precaution to emphasize to parents when discharging a child with lower extremity paralysis as a result of myelomeningocele?**

A. Practice regular skin inspection.

B. Avoid feeding the child chewy foods that may cause choking.

C. Monitor apnea episodes.

D. Avoid situations that can stimulate tactile defensiveness.

64. **A COTA provided information about adaptations that will assist in resuming sexual activity to a patient with a spinal cord injury. Afterward, the patient confides to the COTA that there are serious personal issues affecting his sexual rela-**

tionship with his wife. What is the BEST action for the COTA to take?

A. Encourage the patient to explain further about the problems he is having with his wife.
B. Explain that this is normal, and that divorce rates are actually higher after serious injuries.
C. Direct the patient to speak with his physiatrist about his concerns.
D. Encourage the patient to speak with the rehabilitation psychologist to discuss his concerns.

65. When working with an individual who is severely depressed and demonstrates psychomotor retardation, it is MOST important to:

A. encourage more rapid responses.
B. provide extensive visual and auditory sensory stimulation.
C. give simple directions and patiently wait for responses.
D. provide activities involving large groups.

66. A COTA is working with a client in a work program setting. What is the FIRST step to achieving the program objective of preventing reinjury within a work program?

A. Performing a prework screening
B. Learning proper body mechanics
C. Participating in work hardening
D. Engaging in vocational counseling

67. A young patient with neurological deficits has been unable to carry over skills learned previously in therapy, and has exhibited the inability to learn new information. The MOST appropriate strategy the COTA can suggest to the patient's mother to improve ADL functioning would be to recommend:

A. repetitive practice of simple ADL under the COTA's guidance.
B. environmental adaptations and assistance for ADL.
C. ADL training in the familiar home environment.
D. forward or backward chaining techniques.

68. A client with cognitive deficits exhibits little transfer of skills from one activity to the next. Which intervention would be BEST to assist this client in performing the steps of doing his laundry?

A. Performing memory drills of the steps involved in doing in a laundry activity
B. Placing serial pictures of a laundry activity in sequence
C. Making a checklist of steps in the process, then consulting the list while doing laundry in the actual setting
D. Reading a story about a person doing laundry with the client, then discussing the story

69. An individual who uses a wheelchair is being discharged from a rehabilitation facility to home. In determining accessibility of the interior home environment, the area the COTA should be MOST concerned with is:

A. location of telephones and appliances.
B. arrangement of furniture in bedrooms.
C. steps, width of doorways, and threshold heights.
D. presence of clutter in the environment.

70. A flight attendant with a back injury is participating in a work hardening program. The client can successfully simulate distributing magazines to all passengers in a plane using proper body mechanics. To upgrade the program gradually, the COTA should NEXT request that the client simulate:

A. putting blankets in the overhead compartments.
B. distributing full meal trays to the passengers.
C. distributing magazines to half of the passengers in the plane.
D. putting luggage in the overhead compartments.

71. A COTA is fabricating a resting pan splint for a client with extremely fragile skin. Which of the following areas will the COTA have to inspect most carefully for signs of skin breakdown?

A. Metacarpal heads, pisiform, and, trapezium
B. Volar PIP joints, medial fifth digit, and thumb MP joint
C. Ulnar styloid, distal head of radius, and thumb CMC joint
D. Thumb PIP joint, pisiform, and hamate

72. An OT practitioner is planning to provide a program to address the needs of persons with Alzheimer's disease, and their families, as part of a hospital outreach

program. One of the areas of intervention which would be **MOST** beneficial to maintaining safety and supporting function at home in the advanced stages of Alzheimer's is:

A. strength and endurance activities.
B. cognitive rehabilitation techniques.
C. environmental modification.
D. assertiveness skills.

73. **An individual has sustained a large, full-thickness burn to both upper extremities during a fireworks display. The client is in the acute care phase of treatment. Which of the following BEST represents an acute care rehabilitation goal?**

A. Prevent loss of joint and skin mobility.
B. Provide adaptive equipment.
C. Provide compression and vascular support garments.
D. Prevent scar hypertrophy through scar management techniques.

74. **The goal for an elderly client with lower extremity weakness is to be independent with bathing, but this requires the tub to be more accessible to the client who uses a walker. Which environmental adaptation would the COTA MOST likely recommend to achieve this?**

A. Place the light switch outside the door so the bathroom is lit before entering.
B. Provide long-handled adaptive devices to facilitate lower extremity dressing.
C. Provide a transfer tub bench and install grab bars.
D. Place nonskid decals in the tub and mats on the floor to prevent slipping on the wet floor.

75. **An individual is about to be discharged to home following a hip arthroplasty. He is able to ambulate with a quad cane, but his balance remains slightly impaired. During the home evaluation, which is the MOST important safety recommendation for the COTA to make?**

A. Remove all throw or scatter rugs.
B. Place lever handles on faucets.
C. Install a ramp if steps exist.
D. Install a handheld shower.

76. **Which of the following would the COTA recommend to a 12-year-old child with mild visual impairments who desires**

independent use of the telephone within his home?

A. A speaker phone
B. A hands free phone
C. A phone with extra large buttons
D. A phone with a receiver holder

77. **An COTA is fabricating a splint for an individual who has carpal tunnel syndrome. Which of the following splint fabrication techniques should be adhered to in order to allow for adequate digit motion?**

A. Trim lines of the splint should extend distal to the MCP crease.
B. Trim lines of the splint should extend proximal to the DIP joint.
C. Trim lines of the splint should extend proximal to the MCP crease.
D. Trim lines of the splint should extend distal to the ulnar fifth MCP crease.

78. **Which of the following is the MOST important adaptation to recommend to an individual returning home following a total hip replacement?**

A. Move items from high cabinets to lower locations.
B. Obtain a raised toilet seat.
C. Place high contrast tape at the edge of each step.
D. Install a handheld shower head.

79. **A patient diagnosed with Parkinson's disease is being seen by a COTA to develop a routine for performing self-care activities. The COTA is MOST likely to begin this process by instructing the patient that self-care activities:**

A. are more easily performed if coordinated with consistent timing of medications.
B. should be performed before medications are taken.
C. should be attempted only with the assistance of others.
D. should be performed at intervals throughout the day until completed.

80. **The COTA is working on dressing skills with a 7-year-old girl with limited balance. Which of the following would the COTA MOST likely recommend regarding socks?**

A. Use socks with a wide opening.
B. Attempt to use a sock aid.
C. Purchase nylon tights because they slip on more easily than socks.

D. Use socks with a narrow opening.

81. **A family would like to place grab bars around the toilets in the house for easy access during transfers by the mother, who uses a wheelchair and is of average height. The grab bars should be placed at a height range of:**
    A. 28 to 32 inches.
    B. 33 to 36 inches.
    C. 38 to 41 inches.
    D. 43 to 46 inches.

82. **An individual with left upper extremity flaccidity is observed sitting in a wheelchair with his left arm dangling over the side. The FIRST positioning device the COTA should introduce to the client is a(n):**
    A. lap tray.
    B. wheelchair armrest.
    C. arm sling.
    D. arm trough.

83. **During a cooking evaluation, an individual with a history of traumatic brain injury exhibits moderate upper extremity incoordination. Which of the following recommendations would be MOST beneficial for this individual?**
    A. Use built-up utensil handles.
    B. Use heavy utensils, pots, and pans.
    C. Use a high stool to work at counter height.
    D. Place the most commonly used items on shelves just above and below the counter.

84. **The COTA is attempting to increase playfulness with a 7-year-old girl with sensory integrative dysfunction. The child experiences difficulties with motor tasks and often complains that no one likes her. After establishing rapport with the child, the COTA would MOST likely introduce which of the following?**
    A. Playing a game of "Go Fish"
    B. Playing a game of checkers
    C. Jumping rope
    D. Role playing a tea party with "Barbie" dolls

85. **An instructor from a local nursing school has asked a COTA to speak about OT to a class of first year nursing students. The COTA feels uncertain about doing the lecture because of a lack of resources. The MOST appropriate action for the COTA to take is to:**
    A. recommend that the nursing course instructor call AOTA and obtain public relations information to share with the nursing students.
    B. decline to do the in-service, but send information to the instructor.
    C. decline to do the in-service and find an OTR to do the lecture.
    D. use brochures, posters, videotapes, and films available from the AOTA to enhance the presentation.

86. **While running a discussion group, the COTA encounters a group member who frequently monopolizes the discussion and interrupts other members. The COTA has unsuccessfully attempted various subtle and indirect methods to decrease the client's behavior. Which direct intervention should the COTA implement NEXT to modify the client's behavior?**
    A. Sit beside the person who is monopolizing the discussion and touch his or her hand or arm as a reminder not to interrupt others who are talking.
    B. Confront the individual's behavior and ask, "Are you aware that your frequent interruptions prevent others from having a chance to contribute?"
    C. Redirect the individual and say, "Now let's hear what others have to say about this."
    D. Restructure the task by selecting a group activity that requires sequential turn taking.

87. **A COTA is working with an elderly client who has diabetes, poor vision, and peripheral neuropathies. The client has difficulty discriminating between medications. The BEST adaptation for the COTA to provide is:**
    A. Braille labels.
    B. labels with white print on a black background.
    C. a pill organizer box.
    D. brightly colored pills with each type of medication a different color.

88. **A child with cerebral palsy has tongue thrust. Prior to feeding, the COTA should do which of the following FIRST?**
    A. Position the child's trunk, head, neck, and shoulders in proper alignment.
    B. Hyperextend the child's head.
    C. Place his digits directly under the child's chin, facilitating tongue retraction.
    D. Provide upward pressure under the child's lower jaw prior to chewing.

89. **A COTA working in an outpatient setting has completed ROM measurements on an individual who is s/p hand surgery. After bandaging the open wounds, what should the COTA do with the stainless steel goniometer?**
    A. Place it in a plastic bag and label it with the individual's name.
    B. Sterilize it before using it again.
    C. Store it with the other goniometers, and sterilize them all at the end of the day.
    D. Wash it with hot, soapy water before using it again.

90. **A COTA is instructing the parent's of a newborn infant regarding the facilitation of the suck-swallow reflex. Prior to feeding the infant a bottle the COTA encourages the parent's to perform which of the following?**
    A. Stroke the infant's cheek before feeding her a bottle.
    B. Gently touch the infant's lips to encourage her to open her mouth and begin sucking motions.
    C. Softly stimulate the infant's gums before bottle feeding.
    D. Gently rub the infant's gums and cheek simultaneously before feeding the baby her bottle.

91. **The COTA is setting up a feeding session with a normally developing 24-month-old boy. The COTA should encourage the child to eat a bowl of peas and carrots with which of the following?**
    A. A small spoon
    B. His fingers
    C. A swivel spoon
    D. A small fork

92. **An individual who had a stroke is copying a picture of a clock. The drawing appears as a lopsided circle with a flat side on the left. The numbers one through eight are written in numerical order around the right side of the clock. The hands are correctly drawn on the clock to represent three o'clock. The individual's performance appears to demonstrate:**
    A. right hemianopsia.
    B. left unilateral neglect.
    C. cataracts in the left eye.
    D. bitemporal hemianopia.

93. **An individual with a high level spinal cord injury is returning home. Which type of**

adaptive technology would the client MOST likely require to ensure safety in the home?
    A. An environmental control unit
    B. A call system for emergency and nonemergency use
    C. A remote control power door opener
    D. An electric page turner

94. **A client requests assistance with his ongoing memory problems. The MOST effective external compensation method of intervention the COTA can introduce is to:**
    A. teach the client to retrace steps mentally to stimulate memory.
    B. teach the client to use a diary or log.
    C. train the client to repeat important pieces of information aloud until memorized.
    D. work with a memory training computer program.

95. **An individual who had a myocardial infarction has been transferred from the acute care unit to a rehabilitation unit. During the initial interview, he displays good memory of information processed before the MI, but poor recall of the period spent in the acute care facility. He is able to recall information since the transfer. The OT practitioner would MOST likely document these behaviors as:**
    A. orientation problems.
    B. long-term memory deficits.
    C. anterograde amnesia.
    D. retrograde amnesia.

96. **An individual with joint changes that limit finger flexion would be MOST comfortable using utensils with:**
    A. regular handles.
    B. weighted handles.
    C. a universal cuff attachment.
    D. built-up handles.

97. **The COTA is participating in the evaluation of a high school teacher who recently experienced a right-hemisphere CVA. The individual is presented with letters of the alphabet typed in random order across a page. When instructed to cross out all of the "M's," the individual misses half of the "M's" in a random pattern. This behavior MOST likely indicates:**
    A. a left visual field cut.
    B. a right visual field cut.

C. functional illiteracy.

D. decreased attention.

98. **The COTA is working on handwriting skills with a school-age child with decreased proprioception in the hand and wrist. Which of the following would the COTA recommend the child use to increase proprioception while writing?**

    A. A wide pen

    B. Attach rubber bands to the eraser and the child's wrist

    C. A soft triangle grip

    D. A pediatric weighted utensil holder

99. **A COTA applies weights to the wrists of a woman who is making a macramé planter to improve strength in her shoulders. The COTA is MOST likely implementing which of the following treatment approaches?**

    A. Neurophysiological

    B. Neurodevelopmental

    C. Biomechanical

    D. Rehabilitative

100. **While assessing dressing skills with a patient who recently had a stroke, the OT practitioner notes that the individual is unable to see buttons on a printed fabric. This MOST likely indicates that the individual may be having difficulty with:**

    A. spatial relations.

    B. figure-ground perception.

    C. body image.

    D. visual closure.

101. **Each morning, a COTA performs ADL training with a teenage client who has quadriplegia. On the first day, the practitioner works with arranging the shirt on the client's lap. When the client masters that particular skill, they work on sliding both arms into the sleeves and pushing the shirt up past the elbows. When this skill is mastered, they will work on gathering the shirt up at the collar and pulling it on over the client's head. The COTA is MOST likely using which of the following techniques?**

    A. Repetition

    B. Cueing

    C. Rehearsal

    D. Chaining

102. **A COTA is treating a child with a standard above-elbow amputation who is ex-** periencing hypersensitivity of the residual limb. **The COTA would MOST likely perform which of the following interventions in the preprosthetic phase of treatment?**

    A. Play activities to strengthen the residual limb

    B. Activities to increase the range of motion of the residual limb

    C. Play activities which incorporate tapping, application of textures, and weight bearing to the residual limb

    D. Dressing activities for practicing putting on and taking off the UE prosthesis

103. **An OT practitioner is making a home visit to an elderly client who lives alone. The client exhibits severe hand weakness. When addressing safety in the home, the MOST important area to assess is the individual's ability to:**

    A. work locks and latches on doors and windows.

    B. use built-up utensils while eating.

    C. use energy conservation techniques.

    D. manipulate fasteners on clothing.

104. **An OT practitioner is assessing the range of motion of an individual who actively demonstrates internal rotation of the shoulder to 70 degrees. The practitioner would MOST likely document this measurement as:**

    A. within normal limits.

    B. within functional limits.

    C. hypermobility that requires further treatment.

    D. limited mobility that requires further treatment.

105. **A 60-year-old automobile mechanic with diabetes has been referred to OT following an above-knee amputation. The patient has impaired sensation in the remaining lower extremity and will be using a wheelchair for the foreseeable future. The FIRST patient education subject the COTA should cover is:**

    A. skin inspection.

    B. grooming techniques (shaving, trimming toenails, etc.).

    C. retirement planning.

    D. returning to work.

106. **A child running in the playground trips and falls forward, landing on out-**

stretched arms. This behavior is BEST described as a(n):

A. primitive reflex.
B. righting reaction.
C. equilibrium reaction.
D. protective extension response.

107. A patient is beginning to demonstrate return in the right upper extremity following a CVA, but has mildly impaired proprioception in the right hand, which results in uneven letter formation during writing activities. Which would be the BEST method to help improve letter formation?

A. The COTA verbally describes how to make a letter as the individual writes.
B. The individual watches her grip on a felt tip pen while writing.
C. The individual works with "theraputty" to strengthen her hand.
D. The individual traces letters through a pan of rice with her fingers.

108. A COTA has completed patient education with an individual who has just received a splint for carpal tunnel syndrome. When documenting this session, the COTA will indicate that the patient was instructed in precautions, splint wearing schedule, and care of a:

A. wrist cock-up splint.
B. thermoplastic splint.
C. resting hand splint.
D. dynamic MP flexion splint.

109. A young boy with hemiplegia has difficulty putting on his socks each morning before school. Which of the following should the COTA recommend?

A. Encourage the child to wear tight fitting socks.
B. Teach the child to sit in a chair and lift and place the affected foot up on a small stool.
C. Encourage the child to lay on his back in bed when putting on socks.
D. Teach the child to sit in a chair and lift and place the unaffected foot up on a small stool.

110. A COTA enters the room of a patient who recently had a RCVA with flaccidity to the left upper extremity. The COTA begins to perform upper extremity passive range of motion to the left arm when marked pitting edema of the left hand is

noted. Which of the following should the COTA do FIRST?

A. Continue to perform PROM and then position and elevate the affected extremity.
B. Fabricate a resting splint for the affected extremity.
C. Take no action and wait for the edema to subside.
D. Have the individual attempt to squeeze a ball.

111. When administering an evaluation of upper extremity function to a newly admitted patient with Guillain-Barré syndrome, it is MOST important to:

A. test proximal muscle strength first.
B. perform the evaluation over several sessions.
C. include sensory testing.
D. evaluate range of motion.

112. A COTA employed by a senior center has been asked to develop a group to address the motor needs of people with Parkinson's disease. Which of the following activities would be MOST appropriate to include?

A. A game of rhythmic exercises performed to music
B. Creating time capsules for their grandchildren
C. Wheelchair races performed in pairs
D. Taking turns reading out loud from the newspaper

113. An OTR and COTA, along with the assistive technology team, has made specific recommendations for electronic assistive technology for an adult with muscular dystrophy. After the devices are ordered, and modified as necessary, the NEXT step in the process of implementation is for the OT practitioners to:

A. evaluate how well the whole system works.
B. evaluate if the assistive technology devices match the needs of the client.
C. train the client in the operation of the AT system and in strategies for its use.
D. determine if funding is available for the recommended assistive technology.

114. The COTA is working with a child with low muscle tone who has difficulty engaging in activities against gravity. The COTA also wants to encourage the child to play. To best address these issues,

the COTA would MOST likely position the child:

A. long sitting along a wall.
B. side-lying on a mat.
C. supine on a large wedge.
D. prone over a bolster.

115. **A COTA making a bedside visit finds her patient poorly positioned with an edematous upper extremity caught between the mattress and the bed rail. The MOST appropriate intervention to address the edema in the upper extremity is to:**

A. elevate the arm on pillows so it rests higher than the heart.
B. massage the arm gently, stroking toward the fingers.
C. instruct the patient to avoid active range of motion.
D. instruct the patient to avoid PROM.

116. **"The patient has taken a more active role in the task group, as evidenced by the patient's willingness to contribute ideas and offer to assist in designing the unit mural." This statement would MOST appropriately be documented in which portion of a SOAP note?**

A. Subjective
B. Objective
C. Assessment
D. Plan

117. **A 5-year-old child has sustained burns to his bilateral upper extremities, hands, and trunk. The child is reluctant to perform any active range of motion despite encouragement from the OTR. The OTR has requested that the COTA attempt to engage the child in therapy since they seemed to have developed a good rapport together. Which of the following activities should the COTA attempt FIRST?**

A. Inform the child that if he does not participate in therapy he may have terrible scarring and limited range of motion.
B. Introduce active range of motion exercises through gentle swaying/dancing with the child's favorite music.
C. Introduce passive range of motion exercises while the child watches his favorite cartoon.
D. Attempt to position the child over a prone bolster while encouraging the child to reach for toys.

118. **A mother of four teenaged children who was diagnosed with a right CVA is receiving home care OT services. The treatment plan includes "activities to improve left upper extremity function" and "activities to improve balance in sitting and standing." The MOST appropriate activity for the COTA to recommend would be:**

A. stacking cones.
B. door pulley.
C. folding laundry.
D. throwing a ball.

119. **A COTA is preparing to lead a cooking group. He is new to the facility, and not certain of the facility's policies and procedures relating to food storage and handling. Which of the following actions would be MOST appropriate for the COTA to take?**

A. Read the facility's infection control plan.
B. Contact the dietary department for clarification.
C. Read the facility's risk management plan.
D. Use only canned food for the group activity this time.

120. **An individual with ALS and mild dysphagia becomes extremely fatigued at breakfast, lunch, and dinner. Which is the FIRST intervention the COTA should consider recommending?**

A. Speak with the physician about tube feedings.
B. Sit in a semireclined position during meals.
C. Eat six small meals a day.
D. Substitute pureed foods for liquids.

121. **An unmarried patient with a spinal cord injury is on a rehab unit and constantly flirts with a COTA. The MOST appropriate action for the COTA to take would be:**

A. firmly reject the patient's advances.
B. acknowledge the patient's actions and mildly flirt back in order to protect the patient's self-esteem.
C. request the supervising OTR discuss the effects of SCI and sexual functioning with the patient.
D. set personal boundaries appropriate to the therapist–patient relationship.

122. **An elderly client was hospitalized for an episode of acute depression after the death of his spouse. The client is preparing for discharge and would like to**

return to his home, but is fearful of spending his days alone. The **BEST** environment for the client to continue socialization and participation in meaningful occupation would be:

A. partial hospitalization.
B. adult day care.
C. home health care.
D. psychosocial rehabilitation center.

123. **A client who is s/p traumatic brain injury exhibits good strength with ataxia in both upper extremities. The writing adaptation that would be MOST appropriate in compensating for the patient's deficit areas would be:**

A. using a keyboard.
B. a universal cuff with pencil holder attachment.
C. using a balanced forearm orthosis with built-up felt-tip pen.
D. a weighted pen and weighted wrists.

124. **An individual with Guillain-Barré syndrome was recently admitted to a rehabilitation unit and is expected to remain for 3 to 4 weeks. At what point in the rehabilitative process should the COTA recommend adaptive equipment for this individual?**

A. After the patient and family have accepted the individual's disability
B. As soon as the insurance provider approves it
C. Within the first week of therapy
D. Just before discharge

125. **An OT practitioner is about to begin hand rehabilitation activities with a client who has open dorsal hand wounds. The MOST appropriate way for the practitioner to protect himself from bloodborne pathogens is to:**

A. wear a mask.
B. wear gloves.
C. refuse to work with the patient.
D. wash hands before and after treating the patient.

126. **A person with peripheral neuropathy exhibits loss of pinprick, light touch, pressure, and temperature sensation resulting in an absence of protective sensation. The COTA explains to the client that the most appropriate form of intervention to address this type of sensory loss would be a program of:**

A. sensory re-education.
B. sensory desensitization.
C. sensory bombardment.
D. sensory compensation.

127. **An elderly patient who was hospitalized for a right cerebrovascular accident with left upper extremity flaccidity and decreased sensation, is beginning to experience sensory return in the left upper extremity. Intervention strategies should now include:**

A. remedial treatment, such as rubbing or stroking the involved extremity.
B. remedial treatment, such as the use of hot mitts to avoid burns.
C. compensatory treatment, such as testing bathwater with the uninvolved extremity.
D. compensatory treatment, such as using a one-handed cutting board to avoid cutting the insensate hand.

128. **When treating individuals in the acute phase of cardiac rehabilitation, it is important for the COTA to FIRST select activities that:**

A. can be accomplished without causing fatigue.
B. decrease the effects of prolonged inactivity.
C. promote strength, ROM, and endurance.
D. can be carried out independently after discharge.

129. **A depressed client has completed a mosaic tray project. The end product that the client shows the COTA looks messy and poorly put together. Which type of feedback would be MOST appropriate?**

A. "You did a fine job, this looks very good."
B. "This could be much better, let me show you how you could fix this."
C. "I see you've finished the project, is there anything else you'd like to do with it?"
D. "It's understandable that you did a poor job, don't worry about it."

130. **Which of the following interventions is MOST appropriate for an individual who has recently been diagnosed with rheumatoid arthritis and is in the acute stage of the disease?**

A. Strengthening with resistive exercises
B. Positioning, adaptive equipment, and patient education
C. Discharge planning
D. Preparing the patient for surgical intervention

131. An individual with a C6 spinal cord injury has been referred to OT 2 days post-injury. Immobilized with a halo brace, the individual demonstrates fair plus wrist extension and poor minus finger flexion. Which of the following interventions should be implemented FIRST?

A. Volar resting pan splints to prevent flexion contractures

B. Wrist support with universal cuff to promote independence

C. Wrist splints to promote development of tenodesis

D. Instruction in bed mobility techniques to prevent decubiti

132. An OT practitioner is performing a home management evaluation of an ambulatory individual with cerebral palsy who is cognitively intact, but exhibits an ataxic gait pattern. The PRIMARY focus of the evaluation should be:

A. safety and stability.

B. the individual's ability to reach and bend.

C. whether the individual has adequate strength to perform homemaking tasks.

D. fatigue and endurance levels.

133. An individual with severe cognitive limitations frequently chokes while drinking liquids. Which of the following is the MOST appropriate course of action?

A. Use a straw for drinking liquids.

B. Use a "sippy cup" for drinking liquids.

C. Monitor fluid intake.

D. Add a thickening agent to liquids.

134. A patient with poor visual acuity is about to be discharged after completing a rehabilitation program following a total hip replacement. The MOST appropriate environmental adaptation to ensure that the client can go up and down stairs safely is:

A. installing a stair glide.

B. installing handrails on both sides of the steps.

C. marking the end of each step with high contrast tape.

D. instructing the patient to take only one step at a time when going up or down.

135. While observing a child for the first time, the COTA notes that the child responds to a loud noise by abducting and extending the arms. The reflex, or reaction,

observed in this child is documented by the COTA as a:

A. rooting reflex.

B. Moro reflex.

C. flexor withdrawal reflex.

D. neck righting reaction.

136. An individual with mental retardation insists on wearing the same outfit day after day, regardless of whether it is clean or dirty. What is the BEST approach for the COTA to use?

A. Force alternate clothing choices by limiting outfits available in the closet.

B. Encourage the caregiver to wash the outfit each night.

C. Tell the client the outfit is in the laundry and she will need to wear a different one.

D. Provide the client with several outfits similar to the preferred one.

137. A COTA/OTR team is considering the use of classical sensory integration therapy for a child with a learning disability. Which of the following techniques would be MOST consistent with this approach?

A. Include the child in a group of children using a program of sensory stimulation activities.

B. Encourage the child to participate in activities that are passive and do not require adaptive responses.

C. Design an individualized program directed at the underlying neurologic deficit.

D. Promote the development of specific motor skills, such as balance and coordination.

138. When planning treatment for individuals diagnosed with eating disorders, the COTA's initial OT treatment goals would MOST likely address:

A. increasing self-awareness through expressive activities.

B. increasing awareness of nutritional issues.

C. improving school performance skills.

D. making recommendations or referrals for family therapy.

139. After wearing a new splint for 20 minutes, an individual develops a reddened area along the ulnar styloid process. The FIRST modification the COTA should make to correct the splint is to:

A. line the splint with moleskin.

B. line the splint with adhesive backed foam.

C. flange the area around the ulnar styloid.

D. reheat and refabricate the entire splint.

140. **An individual has demonstrated competence in heating canned soup. The COTA recommends modifying the treatment plan and upgrading the cooking activity to:**
    A. baking brownies.
    B. making an apple pie.
    C. making toast.
    D. making a fresh fruit salad.

141. **An OT practitioner providing services to a community mental health program has been asked to examine the effectiveness of the OT groups that have been provided over the past 6 months. Which of the following procedures should be used to accomplish this goal?**
    A. Quality assurance
    B. Peer review
    C. Utilization review
    D. Program evaluation

142. **A COTA instructs a client with chronic neck pain to use psychosocial pain management techniques. Which of the following strategies should the COTA implement to assist in the management of this individual's chronic pain?**
    A. Biofeedback, distraction, and relaxation techniques
    B. Specific skill training
    C. Strength and endurance building techniques
    D. Cognitive retraining techniques

143. **A COTA is working with an individual who was admitted to an inpatient psychiatric program for major depression. This individual is also diagnosed with stage 4 AIDS. The BEST general focus of treatment at this point would be to:**
    A. restore and maintain performance of self-chosen occupations that support performance of valued occupational roles.
    B. increase physical endurance and maintain desired self-care tasks.
    C. facilitate resolution of current and anticipated losses through the grieving process.
    D. restore and maintain functional performance of the individual's primary work role.

144. **An OT practitioner is supervising an OT aide. The MOST appropriate kinds of activities and level of supervision for the aide include:**
    A. selected tasks in which aides have been trained, with intense close supervision.

B. various intervention activities with routine supervision.
    C. completing ADL training with a patient without supervision.
    D. selecting adaptive equipment from a catalog with general supervision.

145. **Which of the following activities would MOST effectively evaluate group interaction skills during a 45-minute OT session?**
    A. The clients make individual collages, sharing a set of magazines to complete the activity.
    B. All group members construct one tower that incorporates all of the pieces provided in a set of constructional materials (e.g., Lego blocks, Tinkertoys, or Erector set).
    C. All group members work together to make pizza and salad for their lunch that day.
    D. Each client selects a short-term craft activity from four available samples.

146. **A COTA is working with an elderly patient with early stage dementia who was admitted to the hospital after accidentally setting fire to his kitchen. The MOST appropriate follow-up services to identify relative to this patient's meal planning needs after discharge would be:**
    A. OT services to teach the patient to cook safely.
    B. volunteer companion services to supervise cooking at home.
    C. transportation services to bring the person to a community meal site.
    D. home-delivered meal services.

147. **A fifth-grade child with significantly low muscle tone caused by Duchenne's muscular dystrophy is losing trunk control when sitting. Which of the following frames of reference should the COTA consider when planning the treatment program?**
    A. Neurodevelopmental treatment
    B. Sensory integration
    C. Biomechanical
    D. Visual perceptual

148. **Results of an OT evaluation show that a young child has many tactile defensive behaviors. The MOST appropriate beginning activity for intervention to normalize sensory processing would require that:**

A. the therapist has the child play "sandwich" between heavy mats.

B. the therapist applies a feather brush lightly to the child's arms and legs.

C. the child is blindfolded and must guess where he or she is touched on the body.

D. the therapist has the child play the "duck, duck, goose" circle game.

149. A COTA in a long-term care facility is working with several residents who seem very isolated and disengaged from the other residents. The COTA has identified a need to provide these residents with a group activity that would enhance self-esteem, provide opportunities for social skills and assist residents in integrating past experiences with present life. The COTA should FIRST introduce a:

A. reminiscence group.

B. meditation group.

C. grooming activities group.

D. movement activities and games group.

150. A day camp for children with special needs offers a variety of indoor and outdoor activities emphasizing development of interpersonal and social skills. Which of the following activities provides the most appropriate opportunity for campers to BEGIN experiencing responsibility for others?

A. Having a buddy during a field trip to an amusement park

B. Roasting marshmallows over a fire

C. Feeding the camp pets

D. Lifeguarding at the kiddie pool

151. Which of the following is BEST to use when assessing three-jaw chuck strength?

A. An aesthesiometer

B. A pinch meter

C. A dynamometer

D. A volumeter

152. Which of the following is MOST important to include in the initial intervention for an individual with complete paralysis as a result of Guillain-Barré syndrome?

A. ADL training

B. Balance and stabilization activities

C. Passive ROM, positioning, and splinting

D. Resistive activities for the intrinsic hand muscles

153. A COTA is planning a community living program for clients who are to be discharged after an average of 25 to 30 years of hospitalization. One of the goals of this program is to train the clients to effectively manage their money. Which of the following activities should be used FIRST?

A. Provide each client with $25 to spend during a group trip to the local shopping center.

B. Provide samples of coins and paper money.

C. Use a board game to introduce the concept of receiving and spending money.

D. Establish a hospital-based community store where the clients can buy clothing.

154. A COTA is working with an elderly woman with a diagnosis of depression and dementia during the clean-up portion of a cooking activity. The patient begins to dry the plates and utensils she has already dried. The COTA should:

A. tell the client that the same dishes and utensils are being redried.

B. put the dried dishes away and begin to hand her wet dishes.

C. ask the client to stop the activity because it seems too difficult.

D. ask the client to describe what she is doing.

155. An individual with mental illness has been homeless for the past 4 years and recently began coming to a shelter. It has taken 3 weeks for the COTA to establish rapport, and the COTA believes attending a group is the next step. Which type of group is MOST likely to engage this individual?

A. Highly structured craft group

B. Volunteer activity group, such as stuffing envelopes

C. Simple meal preparation group

D. Social skills group

156. A COTA is working on prewriting skills with an 11-month-old child. Which of the following activities would be MOST appropriate for the COTA to instruct the child to perform?

A. Scribble on a piece of paper.

B. Copy a triangle.

C. Copy a horizontal line on a chalkboard.

D. Copy numerals on a sheet of paper.

157. While preparing a client with an anxiety disorder for discharge from OT, the

COTA is reviewing the client's plans for healthful activities. The BEST recommendation for activities to reduce the physical symptoms of muscle tension associated with anxiety disorder would be:

A. sewing and handcrafts.
B. aerobic exercise.
C. line dancing.
D. woodworking projects.

158. An adolescent with a history of shoplifting and gang violence has been hospitalized with a diagnosis of conduct disorder. During a craft group, the COTA should pay particular attention to the individual's:

A. perceptual-motor performance.
B. leisure and vocational interests.
C. attention span and social interaction skills.
D. interest in, and ability to, perform multiple roles.

159. A COTA is running a parallel group. What level of assistance should the COTA offer to address the needs of this particular group?

A. Encourage experimentation among group members.
B. Observe from the sidelines and not act as an authority figure.
C. Participate as an active member.
D. Assist clients in the selection of simple, short-term tasks.

160. A child displays poor postural stability because of low muscle tone. To promote beginning antigravity control, the FIRST activity that should be performed is:

A. pull-to-sit, leaning back against a therapy ball.
B. prone scooter obstacle course.
C. hippity-hop races.
D. batting a balloon, while the child is suspended in net.

161. A client with severe depression and suicidal ideation stops the COTA as she is about to leave the inpatient unit at the end of the day and asks her to accept her favorite necklace as a gift of thanks. Which of the following responses is MOST important?

A. Explain that the "Code of Ethics" prevents her from accepting gifts.
B. Accept the gift so as not to imply rejection.
C. Report the incident to the client's physician.

D. Ask the client about her reasons for wanting to give her a gift.

162. A COTA working with a person experiencing a manic episode would be MOST likely to select which type of activity?

A. Detailed needlepoint project requiring fine stitches
B. Using clay to mold an object of one's choice
C. A watercolor painting project
D. Finishing a prefabricated wood birdhouse from a kit

163. One week after a COTA begins a new job, half of the OT department is out with the flu, including the COTA's supervisor. The COTA observes an aide carrying out an ADL training session with a patient who is scheduled for discharge the next day. Which of the following actions should the COTA take?

A. Allow the aide to finish so the patient will be prepared for discharge.
B. Take over the session and terminate the aide.
C. Bring the issue to the attention of the faculty administrator.
D. Discuss the observations with an OTR who is present.

164. A COTA is working with a man diagnosed with schizophrenia. He states that his main goal is to have a girlfriend. Which of the following statements would then be the MOST appropriate short-term OT goal?

A. The client will develop a friendship with a female within 6 months.
B. After each group session, the client will identify the ways in which his disability has interfered with his thinking processes.
C. The client will initiate appropriate, casual greetings when beginning casual conversations with female staff.
D. During conversations with female group members, the client will make eye contact for 8 to 10 seconds, two times in each half-hour group.

165. A supermarket employee with obsessive-compulsive disorder takes an hour to stock 24 soup cans on the shelf. He reports that once he has placed all the cans on the shelf, he removes them all and starts over because "all the labels were not lined up exactly in the same direction." Which of the following methods

would **MOST** effectively evaluate this individual's work performance?

A. Functional assessment of work-related skills, such as carrying and opening cartons and shelving items
B. Cognitive assessment using the Allen's Cognitive Levels evaluation
C. Verbal interview focusing on the requirements of the individual's job
D. Task evaluation using a "clean" medium like a puzzle

166. **The OT practitioner has just completed observation of a child eating lunch. Which of the following statements BEST describes an objective observation?**

A. The child did not appear to like the food presented.
B. The child demonstrated tongue thrust.
C. The child was uncooperative and kept pushing the food out of her mouth.
D. The child was obviously not hungry at the time.

167. **A young man with a history of depression constantly makes negative statements about himself. The goal set for him in the task group is to increase self-esteem. After several sessions, he is showing more self-confidence and asks the COTA for her phone number because "you're so nice to me." The MOST appropriate response is for the COTA to:**

A. give him her phone number and tell him to call when he is feeling depressed.
B. ignore the request, but remind him he's doing a good job.
C. tell him she has a boyfriend.
D. in private, explain the nature of the client-therapist relationship.

168. **An individual with ALS swims three times a week to maximize strength and endurance. Initially able to swim for only 10 minutes, the individual is now able to swim 20 minutes without becoming fatigued. The NEXT step is:**

A. continue the program of swimming 20 minutes three times a week.
B. decrease swimming frequency to two times a week.
C. increase swimming time to 25 minutes or to tolerance.
D. provide adaptive equipment that will enable the individual to swim using less energy.

169. **While participating in activities to improve strength, an individual with multiple sclerosis who was recently admitted to the hospital complains of fatigue. Which of the following actions is the MOST appropriate for the COTA to take?**

A. Instruct the individual to work through the fatigue to complete the session.
B. Instruct the individual to work through the fatigue for another 5 to 10 minutes.
C. Discontinue strengthening activities.
D. Give the individual a rest break.

170. **A COTA has been hired to develop social skills training programs for persons with long-term mental illness in a community mental health facility. The COTA needs to select a behavior to assess as an outcome measure. Which would BEST indicate that the program was successful in achieving goals for this population?**

A. Improved ability to balance rest, work, play, and leisure
B. Improved verbal and nonverbal communication skills
C. Improved ability to identify areas for vocational exploration
D. Improved ability to perform daily self-care and home management activities

171. **The COTA is observing a 3-year-old child during tooth brushing. The child demonstrates good bilateral upper extremity/hand strength, but decreased dexterity. Which piece of equipment would the COTA MOST likely encourage the child to use during brushing?**

A. A small soft bristle toothbrush
B. A velcro strap attached to a toothbrush
C. An electric toothbrush
D. A soft sponge-tipped toothette

172. **A COTA working in a group home with individuals with serious mental illness is developing a program to promote healthier eating habits. Which of the following activities BEST represents a psychoeducational approach?**

A. Each client makes a healthy food collage.
B. Plan and shop for a meal as a group.
C. Designate 1 day a week for the residents to be responsible for cooking dinner.
D. Show a video about nutrition and keep a meal diary for a week.

173. **An individual with C4 quadriplegia is able to independently use a mouth stick to strike keys on a computer keyboard for 15 minutes. To upgrade this activity, the COTA should:**
    A. provide a heavier mouth stick.
    B. have the individual work at the keyboard for 30 minutes.
    C. progress the individual to a typing device that inserts into a wrist support.
    D. teach the individual how to correctly instruct a caregiver in use of the keyboard.

174. **An individual with a history of substance abuse lives in a group home. The residential manager has asked the COTA to work with the individual to develop house cleaning skills. Which of the following interventions is MOST appropriate when a cognitive approach is desired?**
    A. Reward the individual with a snack bar token when chores have been successfully completed.
    B. Praise the individual when chores have been successfully completed.
    C. Post a schedule of each individual's chore responsibilities in a highly visible location.
    D. Conduct a group discussion about responsibilities people have when living in a group home.

175. **Which of the following assessment methods would an OT practitioner MOST likely choose in order to learn about a family's values and priorities?**
    A. Interview
    B. Skilled observation
    C. Inventory
    D. Standardized test

176. **In a preschool setting, the COTA is providing information to the OTR concerning readiness for discharge of a 5-year-old preschooler with mild developmental delay. The MOST important information for the COTA to focus on is:**
    A. achievement of dressing independence.
    B. improved socialization and impulse control.
    C. attainment of kindergarten readiness skills.
    D. independence in toileting.

177. **An OTR and COTA are collaborating on a discharge summary. Which of the following is the MOST appropriate contribution for the COTA to make?**
    A. Describe the treatment received.
    B. Make the referral for community-based services.
    C. Compare the initial and final status.
    D. Formulate the OT follow-up plans.

178. **A COTA is working with a child whose poor visual attention is affecting his ability to perform school work. An adaptation of the sensory environment that would BEST improve attention during a visual task is to have the child:**
    A. work with lively background music to increase competing sensory input.
    B. work against a patterned background to increase competing visual input.
    C. use headphones during work to reduce competing sensory input.
    D. use dim lighting to reduce the visual input.

179. **A child with athetoid CP is working in OT to develop self-feeding skills. The COTA observes that when the child attempts to pick up food, it slides off the plate. Which adaptation does the COTA provide to solve this problem?**
    A. A swivel spoon
    B. A nonslip mat
    C. A mobile arm support
    D. A scoop dish

180. **In assessing the dressing skills of a 5-year-old child, the COTA observes that the child is able to put on a jacket, zip the zipper, and tie a knot in the draw string, but needs verbal cueing to tie a bow. The COTA would MOST likely determine that the child's dressing skills are:**
    A. age appropriate.
    B. delayed.
    C. advanced.
    D. limited.

181. **A COTA is planning a collage activity task group for several clients with depression. The PRIMARY purpose of using an OT task group with these clients is to:**
    A. provide opportunities to evaluate areas of function.
    B. focus the group on a topic that is common to all of the members and can be discussed by the members.
    C. encourage here-and-now explorations of member behaviors and issues, while promoting learning through doing.
    D. encourage the members to develop se-

quentially organized social interaction skills with the other members.

182. A young child exhibits tactile defensiveness with all dressing tasks. Which of the following would the COTA recommend as the MOST effective handling method for this child?
A. Tickle him prior to dressing and undressing.
B. Play loud music when undressing him.
C. Lightly stroke the child's arms and legs while dressing him.
D. Hold him firmly when picking him up and dressing him.

183. An OT practitioner is administering a standardized test to a young client who suddenly becomes uncooperative and complains that the test is "too hard." The MOST appropriate response would be to:
A. switch to easier items to improve the child's self-esteem.
B. terminate the session and schedule another session to administer the remainder of the test.
C. follow administration instructions and note changes in behavior.
D. adapt the remaining test items to ensure success.

184. A COTA is working with a 17-year-old with impaired mobility, dexterity and communication skills. The teenager is within function limits cognitively. Which of the following would the COTA MOST likely recommend to the family regarding emergency alert systems in the event of a fire?
A. Position a wireless cell phone within the child's reach.
B. Establish an exit routine in order to get out of the house quickly in the event of a fire.
C. Review "fire prevention within the home" literature.
D. Recommend that the child wear an emergency alert system pendant around her neck.

185. The occupational therapist is a member of the interdisciplinary team providing transition services for a 17-year-old male with moderate learning disabilities. The goal is to help the student engage in part-time work at a local stationery

store. **Which of the following interventions is MOST appropriate?**
A. Have the student practice work tasks in the classroom with peers.
B. Observe performance at the job site and make recommendations to increase productivity.
C. Teach math and money management skills to help the student handle his pay check.
D. Teach the student interviewing skills to increase the likelihood of eventually obtaining full-time employment.

186. When providing occupational therapy for children who have been diagnosed with a terminal illness, the PRIMARY focus for OT intervention would be:
A. educational activities.
B. play and self-care activities.
C. socialization activities.
D. motor activities.

187. A child has poor sitting balance, which interferes with seated tabletop activities. Which of the following should the COTA suggest to the child's teacher for the promotion of ongoing postural adjustments in sitting?
A. Use a sturdy chair with lateral trunk supports while the child is doing homework.
B. Use a corner floor seat with built in desk surface while the child is self-feeding.
C. Provide a bolster for back support while the child is coloring.
D. Provide a therapy ball to sit on while the child is playing a game of checkers.

188. When working with a child who exhibits tactile defensiveness, which of the following areas should be evaluated FIRST?
A. Reading skills
B. Dressing habits
C. Social skills
D. Leisure interests

189. A COTA is using leather stamping as part of a group activity but feels the need to increase the problem solving processes within the group. The BEST approach for encouraging problem solving in a craft media group is to:
A. begin with activities that have obvious solutions and high probabilities of success, and then gradually increase the complexity.
B. begin with activities that require gross motor responses and progress to activities that require fine motor responses.

C. structure the number and kinds of choices available.

D. gradually increase the time used in the activity by 15-minute increments.

190. While standing and holding onto furniture, a 3-year-old boy with delayed motor development shifts his weight onto one leg and steps to the side with the other. This movement pattern is BEST described as:

A. creeping.

B. crawling.

C. cruising.

D. clawing.

191. A school-age child demonstrates aggressive and disruptive behavior in school as a result of a low sensory threshold. Which of the following suggestions would be MOST useful to discuss with the teacher regarding an upcoming class bus trip to the zoo?

A. Review the bus rules with the child and apply consequences consistently.

B. Let the child sit at the front of the bus and use a tape player with earphones.

C. Give the child the responsibility of monitoring classmates as "bus patrol."

D. Let the child set the criteria for a successful trip, and provide a reward if the criteria are met.

192. Using the Model of Human Occupation as a frame of reference, evaluation of an individual should focus PRIMARILY on which of the following?

A. Identification of problem behaviors that need to be extinguished

B. Clarification of thoughts, feelings, and experiences that influence behavior

C. Cognitive function, including assets and limitations

D. The effect of personal traits and the environment on role performance

193. A COTA provides a leather-working activity to an individual with C7 quadriplegia in order to increase grip strength. Which component of this activity would be MOST effective in promoting this goal?

A. Holding the hammer

B. Holding the stamping tools

C. Squeezing the sponge to wet the leather

D. Lacing with the needle

194. A hospital's public relations department plans to take some pictures of the OT staff working with patients. Before proceeding, which of the following MUST be obtained?

A. The correct spelling of the patients' names for the photograph caption

B. The patients' written consents to take the photographs and use them for publicity

C. The department head's written consent to take the photographs and use them for hospital purposes

D. The correct spelling of the patients' diagnoses and names for the photographs' captions

195. Which aspects of psychosocial performance are MOST important to emphasize in developing a client's work potential in a prevocational program?

A. Punctuality, accepting directions from a supervisor, and interacting with coworkers

B. Memory, sequencing of work tasks, attending to work tasks, and making decisions

C. Standing tolerance, eye–hand coordination, and endurance

D. Maintaining personal cleanliness and adhering to safety precautions

196. An OT practitioner working for the school system has identified a general need to enhance the fine coordination skills of elementary school students to facilitate better writing skills. The BEST intervention to treat this population would be to:

A. screen students for writing problems, and provide in-depth assessment of those identified.

B. provide remedial activities for those students identified as having fine coordination deficits.

C. recommend activities to develop fine coordination that teachers can incorporate into classroom programming.

D. recommend additional OT staff to provide direct services for students.

197. A long-term goal for an individual with progressive weakness is for the family to carry out his feeding program. They have achieved the short-term goal of understanding how the individual's disability affects his ability to feed himself. Which statement is the BEST revised short-term goal?

A. Patient will participate in feeding program.

B. Patient will feed himself with moderate assistance.

C. Family will feed patient safely and independently 100% of the time.

D. Family will demonstrate independence in current positioning and feeding techniques.

198. A COTA is explaining to a teacher the kind of high technology aid that can be used to help a multiple handicapped student with speech and writing deficits function in the classroom. The COTA would MOST likely recommend which of the following for a child with speech and writing limitations?

A. Environmental control unit

B. Wanchik writer

C. Head pointer

D. Electronic augmentative communication device

199. An OT practitioner who is a member of an assistive technology team evaluating

an adult with severe motor limitations is MOST likely to:

A. make recommendations for ways of operating the technology.

B. recommend communication strategies.

C. seek funding sources for the technology.

D. solve mechanical or software problems.

200. A patient in an acute care facility with severe depression is withdrawn and exhibiting a low energy level. Of the following, which would be the MOST appropriate type of intervention activities for the COTA to present in the initial stages of treatment for this patient?

A. Selecting a leisure activity of interest and identifying materials needed

B. Performing a clerical task such as sorting papers

C. Practicing meditation

D. Writing suggestions for coping with daily life stresses

ANSWERS FOR SIMULATION EXAMINATION 5

1. (C) Remove the threshold altogether. Removing the threshold altogether would be the simplest and safest solution. Door thresholds may have a maximum height of half an inch and these must be beveled; keeping it as it is (answer A) would provide a barrier to wheelchair accessibility and a safety hazard for people with visual deficits. Placing a throw rug to cover the threshold (answer B) would not improve accessibility and would present a slipping hazard. Because the threshold height is over half an inch, placing a ramp over the threshold (answer D) would be required if the threshold could not be removed. The best solution would still be to remove the threshold altogether to provide the most accessible surface. See reference: Americans with Disabilities Act: ADA Accessibility Guidelines.

2. (A) A lightweight folding frame. A lightweight folding frame is needed when a wheelchair will be frequently lifted in and out of a car trunk or back seat, and folded to fit into the space. This is much easier on the individual or family member who will be lifting the wheelchair. Answers B, C, and D will add a great deal of weight and bulk, which makes the wheelchair much more difficult to lift. This in turn may cause an individual or family member to be more reluctant to go on a community outing. See reference: Angelo and Lane (eds): Taylor, SJ: Evaluation for wheelchair seating.

3. (A) Use alternative modalities until the OTR can establish competency with this treatment technique. COTAs providing services reimbursable

under OT must be supervised by an OTR, therefore answers B and C are incorrect. The OTR must be able to determine COTA competency for specific interventions and must be able to monitor patient response to interventions and modalities. In this case, the OTR must establish competency in using ultrasound prior to considering its use in treatment by either the OTR or COTA; a simple review of the procedures (answer D) does not establish competency. See reference: AOTA Practice Department: Guide to role performance: OT, OTA, Aide.

4. (A) once a day. The *Guide for Supervision of Occupational Therapy Personnel* provides definitions for levels of supervision. Close supervision is defined as "daily, direct contact at the site of work" (p. 592). Other levels of supervision are routine, general, and minimal. Routine supervision is provided when direct contact is made every 2 weeks with "interim supervision occurring by other methods such as telephone or written communication." Under general supervision, contact is made monthly (answer C). Minimal supervision is provided on an "as needed" basis as in answer D. It is possible that this may be less than once a month. Requirements for supervision are often specified in state licensure laws, and supercede AOTA guidelines. See reference: AOTA: Guide for supervision of occupational therapy personnel in the delivery of occupational therapy services.

5. (A) obtain collaboration with supervision from an OTR before beginning treatment. According to the *AOTA Statement of Occupational Therapy Refer-*

ral, a COTA may identify or screen individuals for potential referral, but may not accept or enter a case without the supervision or collaboration of an OTR. Answers B, C, and D are all actions the COTA would take after accepting the case. See reference: AOTA: Statement of occupational therapy referral.

6. (D) motor planning. Motor planning or praxis problems are often seen in young children when they are dealing with novel equipment. Motor planning requires an adequate body concept and the ability to cognitively plan movements. Fine motor skills (answer A) are required for dexterity and manipulation and are not required for mounting a rocking horse. In order to climb into the highchair and jump on a trampoline, the child must have integrated reflexes (answer C) and adequate gross motor skills (answer B). See reference: AOTA: Uniform Terminology for Occupational Therapy, ed 3.

7. (C) Appropriate social and life skills. Answer C is correct because practicing life skills is essential for learning, and has been found to be helpful in improving functional performance. Answers A, B, and D reflect verbally focused, rather than activity focused group environments that include insight development, self-disclosure, confrontation, and the open expression of anger. Intense treatment milieus that focus on these group environments have been found to be contraindicated in the inpatient treatment of individuals with schizophrenia. Structured, supportive milieus with an emphasis on enhancing positive social and life skills have been found to be helpful. See reference: Bonder: Schizophrenia and other psychotic disorders.

8. (B) Develop awareness about what produces anger and how the clients respond to anger. All of the answers are steps in the cognitive-behavioral process. Treatment begins, however, with developing awareness of what produces anger and how individuals respond (answer B). Therapy should then move to changing behavior to achieve alternative, more healthy ways of responding to anger, and examining the benefits of responding in a more healthy fashion (answer A). Graded tasks are used to reinforce the new beliefs, behaviors, and responses, beginning with easier and progressing to more challenging tasks (answers C and D). See reference: Bruce and Borg: Cognitive-behavioral frame of reference.

9. (C) The splints will prevent deformity. A child with juvenile rheumatoid arthritis will need splinting to prevent deformity and maintain range of motion. Hypertonus (answer A) is not a characteristic of this condition. Due to the active nature of the child's condition, increasing range of motion (answer B) may be contraindicated. The correction of deformity (answer D) may also be contraindicated with this child due to the active nature of the disease. See reference: Case-Smith (ed): Rogers, SL, Gordon, CY,

Schanzenbacher, KE, and Case-Smith, J: Common diagnoses in pediatric occupational therapy practice.

10. (B) A noise machine producing white noise at bedtime. For a child who is easily aroused, a constant, monotonous auditory input can be calming enough to induce sleep. The other answers may actually increase arousal. Quick repetitive proprioceptive input, as experienced when jumping on a trampoline (answer A), and light touch provided by a fuzzy blanket (answer C), are types of sensory input that have direct arousing effect on the nervous system. Blocking out all light (answer D) may produce arousal as a result of fear generated by total darkness. See reference: Case-Smith (ed): Cronin, AF: Psychosocial and emotional domains of behavior.

11. (B) a local wheelchair equipment vendor. Although any community resource may be helpful to a child and family with a severe physical disability, answer B is correct because of the possible breakdown of this already purchased piece of equipment. The OT practitioner needs to consider this possible problem and provide local support for a solution. Therefore, although answers A, C, and D may serve as resources for other needs of the child, only a specialist in wheelchair equipment would be able to solve mechanical problems that arise. See reference: Case-Smith (ed): Wright-Ott, C and Egilson, S: Mobility.

12. (B) In a written report. The OTR can read the written report at her leisure. Confidential information about an individual must be respected by OT practitioners and should not be discussed in public places (answer C). A phone call (answer A) and a discussion in the OT office (answer D) would both require time the OTR does not have available. See reference: Early: Data collection and evaluation.

13. (C) The infant is exhibiting ulnar palmar grasp. Ulnar palmar grasp precedes the other types of grasp. The infant first grasps on the ulnar side of the hand against the palm, then with all four fingers against the palm (palmar grasp), and finally the grasp moves to the radial side of the hand (radial grasp). The highest level of grasp is pincer grasp, in which the pad of the index finger meets the opposed thumb. See reference: Case-Smith (ed): Exner, CE: Development of hand skills.

14. (C) prosthetist. Prosthetists are professionals trained to make and fit artificial limbs. The physiatrist (answer A) is a physician with specialized training in physical medicine. The orthotist (answer B) specializes in fitting and fabricating permanent splints and braces. The physical therapist (answer D) is a rehabilitation professional trained to administer exercise and physical modalities to restore function and prevent disability. See reference: Case-Smith (ed): Rogers, L, Gordon, CY, Schanzenbacher, KE, and Case-

Smith, J: Common diagnoses in pediatric occupational therapy practice.

15. (C) Following directions about objects located in front, in back, and to the side. Answer C is correct because a deficit in "position in space" refers to difficulty in perceiving the relationship of an object to the self. Answer A, identifying letters on a distracting page, is not correct because it refers to a problem of recognizing size and shape (form) constancy. Answer D, making judgments about moving through space, is incorrect because it refers to a problem in perceiving spatial relationships. See reference: Case-Smith (ed): Schneck, CM: Visual perception.

16. (D) redirect the individual to a more neutral topic. In depth discussion of physical symptoms is not helpful for individuals with anxiety disorders, and they should be redirected, not encouraged (answer C), to speak further about somatic symptoms. It is best to "focus on what clients are concerned about, listen to their fears, and then gradually turn their attention to a neutral topic or something more constructive" (p. 241). Because individuals with anxiety often fixate on their physical symptoms, and because they occurred the previous day, it is probably not necessary to report them to the OTR or physician (answers A and B). See reference: Early: Responding to symptoms and behaviors.

17. (C) by tilting backwards up to 60 degrees while rocking. By lowering the child backwards from the sitting position, the child is required to activate increasing degrees of antigravity control in the neck musculature. As the child's strength increases, the degree of incline can be increased. Answers A, B, and D do not address antigravity control using neck flexor musculature. See reference: Case-Smith (ed): Nichols, DS: Development of postural control.

18. (B) stress bilateral play and school activities incorporating the prosthesis. Two-handed activities for play, school and self-care should be used to incorporate the prosthesis into the child's body image and to help develop bilateral skills. Activities that avoid the use of the prosthesis, as in answers A, C, and D, would not help the child to integrate the prosthesis into normal patterns of use. See reference: Case-Smith (ed): Rogers, SL, Gordon, CY, Schanzenbacher, KE, Case-Smith, J: Common diagnoses is pediatric occupational therapy practice.

19. (B) Obtain as much information as possible from the chart. By reviewing the individual's medical records before the interview, the COTA can determine what information has already been obtained. This will enable the COTA to make the best use of the available time, and to avoid asking the individual to answer the same questions twice. With such a limited attention span, it would probably be more efficient to schedule two 15-minute sessions

rather than one 30-minute session (answer A). Answers C and D are both essential to good interview technique, but would occur at the time of the actual interview, after collecting data from the chart. See reference: Early: Data collection and evaluation.

20. (D) shallow spoon. The use of a shallow spoon encourages the development of upper lip control because it makes it easier for the lip to remove all of the food on the spoon. It would be more difficult for the child to get food off a deep spoon (answer C). Straws (answer A) can be used to develop sucking. A "spork" (answer B) is a device that combines the qualities of a fork and a spoon and is useful if the child can only manage one utensil. See reference: Case-Smith (ed): Case-Smith, J and Humphry, R: Feeding intervention.

21. (C) Modify the environment to protect the infant from excessive and/or inappropriate sensory stimulation prior to direct intervention. Preterm infants with histories of maternal drug abuse have multiple sensory needs often resulting in poor self-regulation and behavioral organization. Answers C and D both incorporate sensory integration approaches. However, answer C best demonstrates an initial intervention to promote the neurobehavioral organization required to tolerate direct handling. Answers A and B are important in determining appropriate treatment plans for the infant and family. However, a social work referral should be made after initial assessments are completed, to make the most appropriate recommendations for social service involvement, if needed. Although identifying maternal medical status and treatment compliance issues are of great importance to best determine eventual educational and disposition recommendations, it is not the primary sensory intervention focus of the OT team. See reference: Case-Smith (ed): Hunter, JG: Neonatal intensive care unit.

22. (A) Subjective section. The subjective portion of a SOAP note (answer A) includes what the patient reports or comments about the treatment. The objective portion of the SOAP note (answer B) focuses on measurable and or observable data obtained by the OT practitioner through specific evaluations, observations or the use of the therapeutic activities. The assessment part of the SOAP note (answer C) addresses the effectiveness of treatment and any changes needed, the status of the goals, and justification of continuing occupational therapy treatment. The plan section of a SOAP note (answer D) includes statements related to continuing treatment, the frequency and duration of the treatment, suggestions for additional activities or treatment techniques, the need for further evaluation, and the recommendations for new goals as needed. See reference: Early: Medical records and documentation.

23. (D) Playing "Simon Says." Playing "Simon Says" is the most appropriate choice because it promotes a gross motor activity, a major component of the physical or "rough and tumble" form of play. "Children from 2 to 5 years of age are extremely active and almost always ready to engage in rough and tumble play...activities such as running, hopping, skipping and tumbling are performed without any typical goal" (p. 86). The game of "Simon Says" can be downgraded so children can play from a wheelchair, mat or standing position. Drawing and putting together puzzles, and constructing towers out of blocks (answers A and B), are activities typically introduced to encourage constructive play (activities used to encourage creativity with construction). Although answer C, role playing (telling stories within the group, playing dress up and imaginary play), is an activity utilized to support the concept of dramatic play, it is not necessarily physical in nature. See reference: Case-Smith (ed): Case-Smith, J: Development of childhood occupations.

24. (B) Crawling over and along a rope taped to the floor. The crawling activity requires both sides of the body to work together in either reciprocal or bilateral movements. Weight bearing provides proprioceptive input and having the rope between arms and legs develops awareness of body sidedness from a visual standpoint. The remaining choices do not provide reciprocal or bilateral movement, which would develop coordination of the body sides in rhythmic patterns. See reference: Case-Smith (ed): Parham, LD and Mailloux, Z: Sensory integration.

25. (D) Encourage group members to share similar experiences and reactions with each other. Answer D is a strategy designed to develop cohesiveness among members. Many people have reported that recognizing one's similarities with other people is a very valuable experience. Answers A and C are designed to impart information. Answer B is an example of catharsis, which may not be helpful to all members. Moreover, the OT practitioner must be aware of, and understand, the precautions necessary for the use of catharsis. See reference: Early: Group concepts and techniques.

26. (B) Verbal and gestural cues. The next least intrusive level of cues consists of the combination of verbal and gestural cues. Physical cues (answers C and D) are the most intrusive, and only verbal cues (answer A) are the least intrusive. See reference: Case-Smith (ed): Shepherd, J: Self-care and adaptations for independent living.

27. (C) Toothbrush with built-up handle. An individual with C7-C8 quadriplegia has the hand strength to hold a toothbrush with a built-up handle. An alternate method can be to position the toothbrush between the fingers. An individual with a C5 injury may require a MAS for brushing teeth (answer A). Other individuals with injuries at the C5-C6 level may be able to use a universal cuff (answer B), or a wrist support with a utensil holder (answer D), to hold the toothbrush. See reference: Christiansen (ed): Garber, SL, Gregorio, TL, Pumphrey, N, and Lathem, P. Self-care strategies for persons with spinal cord injuries.

28. (D) managing stigma. More stigma is attached to issues surrounding mental health than physical health, and individuals with mental illness frequently experience prejudice. It is important for individuals re-entering the community to be prepared for this with strategies that will enable them to cope with stigmatization. Self-esteem, assertiveness, and anger management (answers A, B, and C) are skills, which together, enable the individual with mental illness to effectively manage stigma. See reference: Cottrell (ed): Van Leit, B: Managed mental health care: reflections in a time of turmoil.

29. (B) identify the abilities, needs, and life goals of the client. Identifying the abilities, needs, and life goals of the client occurs before any other steps in the process in order to make a match between the client's abilities, environmental demands, and the appropriate technology to carry out desired daily occupations. Answers A, C, and D are steps which would come later in the process. See reference: Christiansen and Baum (eds): Trefler, E and Hobson, D: Assistive technology.

30. (A) Incorporate activities such as wiping the tables after lunch, which are concrete, consistent, and predictable. Many of these clients have never held a job. Those who have held jobs have most likely experienced failure when attempting to work. In addition to inadequate skills for job performance, bizarre behavior and appearance, resulting from poor social and self-care skills, have led to stigma and rejection in the past. Work activities for these individuals must be concrete, predictable, consistent and meaningful. These individuals are usually unable to generalize learning from one environment or situation to another, therefore answers B and C, which involve generalization of new learning, are impractical. In addition, sorting nuts and bolts is not a meaningful activity. Mail management activities (answer D) are a good choice for this population, but this answer is less than optimal because "when available" does not provide the necessary consistency. See reference: Cottrell (ed): Coviensky, M and Buckley, VC: Day activities programming: Serving the severely impaired chronic client.

31. (C) Modify the activity to make it less challenging. The COTA should recognize subtle signs of fatigue, such as frustration, slowing down, hurrying to finish, lessening range of motion, and use of substitution movements, which indicate the training level was too difficult and should be downgraded. Other signs include the individual's heart rate exceeding the target heart rate; increase of more than 20 bpm above resting pulse; failure to return to resting heart rate after a 5 minute rest; systolic pressure that does not increase at all, or that increases more than 20 mm Hg from baseline. Stopping the activity (answer A) is necessary if the individual experiences symptoms such as dyspnea, chest pain, lightheadedness, or diaphoresis. The activity should be upgraded (answer B) only when the individual is able to perform the activity without signs of fatigue or cardiac symptoms. Isometric exercises (answer D), which interfere with bloodflow through the muscles and create a heightened demand on the cardiovascular system, should not be used in individuals with cardiac conditions. See reference: Dutton: Introduction to biomechanical frame of reference.

32. (A) A craft activity using increasingly heavy hand tools. Progressive resistive exercise is the most effective method for increasing strength in a muscle with fair plus strength. Mildly resistive activities that are stopped as soon as the individual begins to experience fatigue (answer B), are appropriate for maintaining or improving strength in individuals with conditions in which fatigue should be avoided (e.g., MS, ALS, and Guillain-Barré syndrome). Electric stimulation (answer C) is appropriate for increasing strength in very weak muscles. When performing resistive active range of motion with this individual, the COTA would use maximal resistance. In addition, a craft activity that can be performed against increasing resistance for prolonged periods of time, would be more effective than resisted active range of motion (answer D), which is usually only performed once or twice a day. See reference: Dutton: Biomechanical postulates regarding intervention.

33. (C) Interview a reliable informant instead of the individual. Individuals who are unable to think clearly, or who are experiencing memory loss, are often disturbed or frightened by this change, and may confabulate stories or answers to cover themselves. When an individual is unable or unwilling to provide accurate information, it may be necessary to use a reliable informant (answer C). This is often someone who lives with the individual and is able and willing to provide the necessary information. Using closed-ended questions (answer A) with this individual would not necessarily yield more accurate information, but can be useful when specific information is being sought, or to more effectively structure or control an interview situation. This individual is unlikely to do any better with a written questionnaire than an oral interview. However, written questionnaires (answer D) may be used effectively with individuals with the requisite cognitive skills. There is no reason to think the individual would be any more reliable the next day (answer B). See reference: Early: Data collection and evaluation.

34. (A) Chaining. Chaining with the child who demonstrates a cognitive disability shows the entire process of a task with all sequences. Initially, the child performs only the beginning or end of a task. Thus, the child concentrates on only a small part of the

task, but gradually increases participation in all sequences in their correct order. Answers B, C, and D are other methods that can be used, but forward and backward chaining are particularly successful instructional methods for individuals who are mentally retarded. See reference: Early: Medical and psychological models of mental health and illness.

35. (D) set clear expectations for behavior and enforce consequences, such as a time-out, if the child loses control. The behavioral frame of reference can be useful in helping children with maladaptive behavior to learn to modify their behaviors and to learn new more adaptive behaviors through the principle of reinforcement. To use this effectively, the child must clearly understand the expectations for behavior (or rules), and that there will be consistent consequences for behaviors that break the rules. Answers A and B, allowing the child to express his anger and ignoring the behaviors, would not help the child to learn new behaviors and could cause an increased loss of control. A child who is out of control and responding to impulses is not able to respond to an insight-based approach such as reasoning. See reference: Sladyk, K and Ryan, SE (eds): Florey, L: A second-grader with conduct disorder.

36. (D) stenciling project on poster board. Stenciling on poster board is the safest craft choice because it is free of sharp, toxic, and cordlike materials. A ceramic object (answer C) could be broken into sharp pieces that an individual could use to harm themself. Craft projects that contain rope or cordlike materials that can be used for hanging (answers A and B) should also be avoided. See reference: Early: Safety techniques.

37. (A) Use pictures, music, and discussion to encourage discussion of memories. Remotivation approaches are used to encourage the expression of thoughts and feelings related to intact long-term memories. The topic should be linked to the group's past experiences and should be easy to understand. The reality orientation approach is designed to maintain or improve awareness of time, situation, and place, and often uses activities related to holidays and other temporal concepts (answer B). The environmental adaptation approach (answer C) promotes independence, but has no relevance to remotivation. Interpersonal skills (answer D) are most effectively addressed through role-playing and discussion groups. See reference: Early: Cognitive and sensorimotor activities.

38. (B) interest checklist. An interest checklist is frequently used to initiate discussion of how a patient usually spends his leisure time and to identify areas of specific interest. Although the evaluations of living skills and self-care (answers A and D) address the use of leisure time, they are used primarily to assess skills in personal care, safety and health, money management, transportation, use of the telephone, and work. An activity configuration (answer C) is used to assess the patient's use of time and his feelings about all of the activities he performs in a typical day or week. See reference: Early: Data gathering and evaluation.

39. (D) Reinforcement of competence. According to Erikson, an 8-year-old child is usually at the stage of industry versus inferiority, during which time he or she develops a sense of competency. For a client who is expected to lose motor function gradually, a treatment plan that will provide an ongoing sense of competence (possibly in other areas) is especially relevant. Answers A, B, and C describe other developmental issues identified by Erikson that are typically achieved at other ages: basic trust (answer A) in infancy; initiative (answer B) during the toddler years; and self-identity (answer C) during adolescence. See reference: Case-Smith (ed): Law, M, Missiuna, C, Pollock, N, and Stewart, D: Foundations of occupational therapy practice with children.

40. (B) source of the referral, the reason for the referral, and the date the referral was received. The initial note is used to record basic information, results of initial evaluations and, often, the treatment plan. In addition to documenting the items in answer B, the COTA may also contribute data collected from assessments she or he has performed. The OTR is responsible for analyzing an individual's assets and deficits, developing a treatment plan, and for projecting the outcome of treatment (answers A, C, and D). See reference: Early: Medical records and documentation.

41. (A) A problem with learning new motor skills. Answer A is correct because it describes the central problem of dyspraxia—difficulty in performing skills not previously mastered where motor planning is required. Answer B is not correct because, although developmental dyspraxia is considered a sensory integration problem, it does not explain what problems the child faces, which are praxic in nature. Answers C and D are incorrect because, although reflex integration and balance problems may be present with developmental dyspraxia, they are not problems of praxis or motor planning. Answers C and D are automatic motor activities, and dyspraxia is a problem of mastering motor activities that must be learned. See reference: Case-Smith (ed): Parham, LD and Mailloux, Z: Sensory integration.

42. (A) single pressure switch, firmly mounted within easy reach. A child with fluctuating muscle tone lacks stability and demonstrates extraneous movement, therefore, deliberate motor action is most effectively executed on a securely mounted device using simple movement patterns. Answers B, C, and D involve devices that would respond to slight touch, and would therefore not be effective for a person with extraneous movement and difficulty grading motor action. See reference: Case-Smith (ed):

Swinth, Y: Assistive technology: Computers and augmentative communication.

43. (B) floor sitter. "A floor sitter may enable the child with cerebral palsy to play on the floor near his or her typically developing peers" (p. 725). Occupational therapy practitioners can recommend and provide appropriate adapted equipment and positioning devices when working in an early intervention setting. A hammock (answer A) would not allow the child to feel as if he "fits in." The child verbalized the desire to sit on the floor like his peers, whereas the hammock may make the child feel even more different then when he sits in his wheelchair. Hammocks are typically utilized in therapy to provide sensorimotor/vestibular input, and would not be indicated in this situation unless no other viable options were available. Introducing an adapted wheelchair insert and a prone stander (answers C and D), would be ignoring the child's desire to sit on the floor with his peers. Wheelchair inserts are often used for positioning a child in a wheelchair to permit increased trunk support and stability, thus allowing for more independent use of the upper extremities. A prone stander would allow a child to assume a standing or weight bearing position, but would not assist with positioning the child while sitting on a mat. See reference: Case-Smith (ed): Stephens, LC and Tauber, SK: Early intervention.

44. (D) drink juices and caffeine-free colas when thirsty. Continual dry mouth and thirst are a common side effect of many drugs. Juices and caffeine-free drinks are preferable for preventing dehydration. Caffeinated drinks (answer B) can intensify the dehydrating effects of this medication. Photosensitivity, an increased sensitivity to the sun, is another side effect often associated with neuroleptic medications, and can be addressed by limiting sun exposure (answer A). Answer C is a strategy that can be used to avoid postural hypotension, a sudden drop in blood pressure resulting in feeling faint, or loss of consciousness when moving from lying or sitting to standing. All of the answers are strategies for managing possible side effects of neuroleptic medications, but answer D is most important because it addresses the only side effect the individual has experienced. See reference: Early: Psychotropic medications and somatic treatments.

45. (A) provide each patient with an individual project and have him or her choose a tile color. The activity should begin with the most basic level of decision-making. Each of the other choices provide increasingly more challenging decision-making abilities. Choosing from an assortment of projects (answer B) requires higher level decision-making ability than only selecting a color. Answer C requires not only decisions on design, color, and size, but also involves decision making among group members. Answer D involves decision making on two separate aspects, pattern and colors, resulting in a higher level of complexity than answer A. See reference: Early: Analyzing, adapting, and grading activities.

46. (D) Meeting the vocational instructor weekly to discuss adaptations to work tasks. Effective consultation involves ongoing communication that helps team members problem solve more effectively. Answers A and B are activities typically done by the vocational teacher. A vocational instructor should already be able to perform assessments (answer C). See reference: Case-Smith (ed): Spencer, K: Transition services: From school to adult life.

47. (B) discuss the meaning and value of the client's doing her own laundry with the mother and client. By discussing the intervention plan options with caregivers, the COTA can determine whether the goals and intervention are meaningful and relevant to the individuals involved. Unilaterally explaining the importance of independence to the mother (answer A), and asking the father to intercede (answer C), are actions that do not ascertain the value or significance of the goal, which, if not valued by the client and caregivers, is inappropriate. After speaking with the mother and client, the COTA may determine later that independence in laundry skills is not an appropriate goal (answer D). See reference: Early: Who is the consumer?

48. (C) Relationships with others. The primary problem area for most individuals with a personality disorder is their ability to interact with others. Specific personality disorder categories indicate that there is some variation among the types of relationships that are impacted. For example, authority relationships seem particularly dysfunctional in those with antisocial personality disorders, and difficulty in establishing relationships is linked to avoidant personality disorders. Answers A and B (ADLs) are often problems for individuals with mood and thought disorders. Answer D is often a problem in those with schizophrenia. See reference: Early: Understanding psychiatric diagnosis: The DSM-IV.

49. (C) Creating a written and specific supervisory plan based on competency levels for both practitioners. Medicare certified home health agencies have extensive requirements for OT supervision of the OTA. In addition to requiring adequate competency on the part of the supervising OT and the practicing OTA, Medicare may request to see specific supervisory plans that detail the type and frequency of supervision provided. Supervision options include documentation review, joint visits or telephone consultation. Countersignature alone for documentation (answer B) does not necessarily constitute adequate supervision. Individual states may have additional specific guidelines. A handout (answer D) may provide useful information to the client and caregivers about OT services, but is not a critical component is establishing a collaborative relationship. See reference: Glantz and Richman:

50. (C) time management and use of leisure time. One of the lifestyle characteristics of people with substance abuse problems is that most time and effort eventually becomes structured around obtaining and using of the abused substance. Time management and use of leisure time are very important areas for the OT practitioner to address with a newly sober client who has been counseled to avoid situations and people associated with drinking alcohol. Identifying leisure interests and establishing plans for structuring large amounts of time without drinking can help support attempts to remain substance free. Answer A, work performance, would also be an area to explore, but would probably not be an area of skill development introduced early in the OT intervention process. Answer B, self-care skills, may need to be addressed as part of daily living skills performance, but would not impact as directly on avoiding substance abuse. Medication is not typically a feature of treatment for substance abuse, so answer D is also incorrect. See reference: Early: Understanding psychiatric diagnosis: The DSM-IV.

51. (B) Does the client want to paint the project blue or white? The COTA should provide an individual who is just beginning to make decisions with limited, simple choices. The client is not yet ready to choose from four broad categories of activities (answer A); it would be better to ask him if he would like to make a leather key ring or a wooden coaster. Projecting about what the client will want to do with the finished project (answer C) is premature. The decision to work alone or in a group (answer D) should be made by the COTA, not the client, depending on how the environment would be best structured to benefit the individual. See reference: Early: Analyzing, adapting and grading activities.

52. (A) Give him a guitar to play during break under the supervision of the COTA. Participation in meaningful activity will promote self-esteem and self-concept. This will also facilitate development of rapport with the COTA, while providing a safe environment for the individual. Activities such as answers B and D isolate the individual from the group process, and would be contraindicated for an individual who recently attempted suicide. The responsibility of composing music (answer C) would probably be too challenging at this time. See reference: Early: Leisure skills.

53. (B) providing staff education, recommendations, and support for restraint alternatives. Providing education on the effects of restraints, and recommendations, and program support for alternatives to the use of restraints, such as activities, distraction techniques, and environmental adaptations would be the MOST appropriate functions for the OT practitioner to provide. Answers A, C, and D would be elements of a facility's restraint reduction efforts, but would not be likely to be performed by the OT practitioner. See reference: Hellen: Physical wellness: Mobility and exercise.

54. (C) Position the stander at 75 to 90 degrees from the floor. Answer C is correct because by adjusting the prone stander nearest to vertical (the least effect of gravity on the head or posture), the child will be able to tolerate working on head righting. Answer A is not correct because while working on the floor in prone, the head and neck are doing the most work against gravity. Answer D is not correct because the head and neck work the least against gravity in the standing or upright position. See reference: Kramer and Hinojosa (eds): Colangelo, CA: Biomechanical frame of reference.

55. (C) Constructional. Constructional play involves building and creating things. It is in this area of play that children develop a sense of mastery and problem-solving skills. Sensorimotor play (answer A) generally develops a child's body awareness and sensory experience. Imaginary play (answer B) involves manipulating people and objects in fantasy as a prelude to dealing with reality. Game play (answer D) requires the ability to learn and apply rules in play. See reference: Kramer and Hinojosa (eds): Luebben, AJ, Hinojosa, J, and Kramer, P: Legitimate tools of pediatric occupational therapy.

56. (B) conditional reasoning. Conditional reasoning is a form of clinical reasoning that takes into account various systems and dynamics involved with the patient and his or her illness or injury. This approach is more "holistic," in that it takes into account the "whole patient" as he or she functions and interacts within his or her environment. Reasoning based on corresponding an individual's deficits and physical symptoms with a procedure that may benefit the area of need is referred to as procedural reasoning (answer A). Interactive reasoning (answer C) is a process by which the practitioner and patient collaborate, so that the practitioner may better understand the patient's environment or situation. Narrative reasoning (answer D) is a form of "story telling" in which practitioners share similar experiences, allowing for problem solving to occur. See reference: Mattingly and Fleming: Fleming, MH: The therapist with the three-track mind.

57. (C) level of arousal. Timing of group activities is very important. Individuals, especially the elderly, often become sleepy after eating lunch. Activities that require the highest levels of arousal should be planned for earlier in the day. Nonparticipation may also be caused by lack of motivation or interest (answers A and B), and a poor attention span may limit an individual's ability to participate, but the age of the group members and the timing of the group provide clues to the correct answer. See reference: Neistadt and Crepeau (eds): Crepeau, EB: Activity analysis: A way of thinking about occupational performance.

58. (A) a can of soup. Grading activities according to complexity is an important part of the therapist's selection of appropriate activities for each individual. Complexity increases as the number of steps, number of different ingredients or tools used, and time to complete the task increases. Answers B, C, and D all require more steps, materials, and time than preparing a can of soup. See reference: Neistadt and Crepeau (eds): Neistadt, ME: Overview of treatment.

59. (A) from a home health OTR or COTA. Home health services, which may include nursing, OT, PT and speech therapy, are provided in the patient's home. Individuals who require continued care following discharge from the hospital may be appropriate for home health services if they are unable to travel to the hospital for outpatient services. If the decision to discharge the person has already been made, recommendations for a continued stay in the acute care hospital, or transfer to a rehabilitation center (answer B and C), are not appropriate. The patient's weakness and continuing requirement for IV drug therapy would make it extremely difficult for this patient to return to the hospital for outpatient therapy (answer D). See reference: Neistadt and Crepeau (eds): Griswold, LS: Community-based practice arenas.

60. (B) a cheese sandwich. The most basic level of meal preparation is accessing a prepared meal, which involves tasks such as opening a thermos and unwrapping a sandwich. When an individual becomes proficient at this level, he or she can, and should, progress to a higher level. More advanced meal preparation activities can be structured to increase in complexity in the following sequence: prepare a cold meal (answer B); prepare a hot one dish meal (answers A and C); and prepare a hot multi-dish meal (answer D). See reference: Neistadt and Crepeau (eds): Rogers, JC and Holm, MB: Evaluation of activities of daily living (ADL) and home management.

61. (B) remain matter of fact and consistent in approach. Individuals with borderline personality disorder demonstrate inconsistent behavior, have difficulty maintaining stable relationships, and have poor self image. Practitioners usually need to work hard to remain consistent and trustworthy to those individuals. It is important in this case that the OT practitioner recognizes this behavior as part of the pathology and not take it personally. Because the accusation is a result of pathology, the COTA has nothing to apologize for, and is unlikely to uncover any reasonable explanation for a misunderstanding (answer D). In addition, the practitioner should not complain of hurt feelings to a client (answer A). Delving into exploration of the individual's past (answer C) is not a recommended approach for occupational therapy. See reference: Neistadt and Crepeau (eds): Ward, JD: Psychosocial dysfunction in adults.

62. (B) Stress management. Many addicts use drugs and alcohol as a way to fill leisure time and to manage stress or boredom. When this individual experienced frustration with the birdhouse project, he was unable to manage this stress, became agitated, escaped the challenge, and sought out an addictive substance (the cigarette). Individuals with problems related to eye-hand coordination, visual perception, or fine motor performance (answers A, C, and D) may also have difficulty gluing pieces of a birdhouse together. However, the behaviors described above in combination with the diagnosis of substance abuse make B the most likely answer. See reference: Neistadt and Crepeau (eds): Ward, JD: Psychosocial dysfunction in adults.

63. (A) Practice regular skin inspection. Children with lower extremity paralysis resulting from myelomeningocele usually experience impaired lower extremity sensation, placing them at risk for developing decubitus ulcers or burns due to contact with hot water or objects. Generally, children with myelomeningocele do not have oral motor or eating problems (answer B) or apnea episodes (answer C), unless Arnold-Chiari deformity is present. Tactile defensive behaviors and other sensory integrative disorders (answer D) can be present in children with spina bifida and myelomeningocele, but the issue of skin breakdown is more important at this time. See reference: Neistadt and Crepeau (eds): Erhardt, RP and Merrill, SC: Neurological dysfunction in children.

64. (D) Encourage the patient to speak with the rehabilitation psychologist to discuss his concerns. OT practitioners often need to address functional issues related to sexuality when working with individuals who have been seriously injured or disabled, and should be well versed and comfortable with the topic. Rather than moving into an area requiring skills beyond the scope of the COTA (answer A), the COTA should refer the individual to the psychologist, whose role it is to provide more extensive sexual or marital counseling, which appears to be what is required in this situation. The physiatrist (answer C), a physician specializing in rehabilitation, is responsible for attending to the medical needs of the individual and coordinating the rehabilitation process. Discussing the increased chances of divorce (answer B), while true, would not be helpful to this individual at this vulnerable time. See reference: Neistadt and Crepeau (eds): Cohn, ES: Interdisciplinary communication and supervision of personnel.

65. (C) give simple directions and patiently wait for responses. Severe depression can result in slowing of cognitive and motor functions, known as psychomotor retardation. The OT practitioner must not rush the individual (answer A), but should give her or him time to process information and respond. Too much stimulation (answers B and D) may cause the individual to withdraw even further. See reference: Neistadt and Crepeau (eds): Ward, JD: Psychosocial dysfunction in adults.

66. (B) Learning proper body mechanics. Learning proper body mechanics (along with achieving a good fitness level) is one of the first steps to reducing the risk of reinjury in a work program. Answer C, work hardening, is appropriate to implement after the physical demands of the job's specific tasks are achieved. Answer D, engaging in vocational counseling, is appropriate after it is determined that a client cannot return to the same job or employer. Answer A, a prework screening, is typically completed by the practitioner before the employer offers the new employee a job. See reference: Neistadt and Crepeau (eds): Fenton, S and Gagnon, P: Treatment of work and productive activities: Functional restoration, an industrial approach.

67. (B) environmental adaptations and assistance for ADL. A patient who exhibits no capacity for new learning will be unable to benefit from therapy interventions that require the ability to transfer learning (answers A, C, and D). A compensatory approach of adapting the environment and recommending assistance for safe performance of daily activities is the most appropriate intervention. See reference: Neistadt and Crepeau (eds): Neistadt, ME: Theories derived from learning perspectives.

68. (C) Making a checklist of steps in the process, then consulting the list while doing laundry in the actual setting. Making a checklist and having the person use the checklist during the activity, would provide an external memory aid during practice of the functional activity. This would provide compensation for cognitive deficits during task training in the specific context where it will be performed. Answers A, B, and D are methods that require a person to be able to transfer learning of skills from one context to another. See reference: Pedretti and Early (eds): Wheatley, CJ: Evaluation and treatment of cognitive dysfunction.

69. (C) steps, width of doorways, and threshold heights. The first area of evaluation would be the steps, width of doorways, and presence and height of door thresholds to determine whether the wheelchair user will be able to enter or exit interior spaces in the wheelchair or whether structural modifications are required. Answers A, B, and D reflect areas that will also need to be evaluated, however, they are not as critical to initial interior access. See reference: Pedretti and Early (eds): Foti, D: Activities of daily living.

70. (A) putting blankets in the overhead compartments. When distributing magazines, the flight attendant uses negligible reaching and bending. Upgrading the activity increases the degree of reaching and bending and adds more resistance than that provided by magazines. Putting blankets in the overhead copmartments (answer A) would be an appropriate gradual upgrade. Handling full meal trays (answer B), which are significantly heavier than magazines, extending them to passengers especially in window seats, is more than a gradual increase or upgrade. Putting luggage into the overhead compartments (answer D) would be the final step in the work hardening process, because it involves the most weight and the riskiest back position. Distributing magazines to half of the passengers (answer C) would be downgrading the activity. See reference: Pedretti and Early (eds): Smithline, J and Dunlop, LE: Low back pain.

71. (C) Ulnar styloid, distal head of radius, and thumb CMC joint. The ulnar styloid, distal head of the radius, and thumb CMC joints are the most common sites for pressure because of their overt bony prominences. Answers A, B, and D are also areas that could potentially be susceptible to skin breakdown, but are not primary sites of pressure when fabricating a resting pan splint. See reference: Pedretti and Early (eds): Belkin, J and Yasada, L: Orthotics.

72. (C) environmental modification. Environmental modification is the area of intervention that can best assist in maintaining safety and supporting function at home by providing the physical and sensory environments to compensate for deficits. Strength and endurance activities (answer A) will have no direct effect on safety in the home. Cognitive rehabilitation techniques (answer B) are not indicated for conditions with progressive cognitive deterioration. Use of assertiveness skills (answer D) would be inappropriate for dealing with the kinds of communication problems encountered with persons who have Alzheimer's disease. See reference: Pedretti and Early (eds): Glogoski, C: Alzheimer's disease.

73. (A) Prevent loss of joint and skin mobility. During the acute stage, when burn wounds are partial or full thickness in nature, maintenance of joint range of motion and skin mobility is the primary goal of intervention. Providing adaptive equipment (answer B) is typically performed during the surgical or postoperative stage, and compression and vascular garments (answer C), and the prevention of scarring (answer D) are goals most commonly implemented during the rehabilitation phase. See reference: Pedretti and Early (eds): Reeves, SU: Burns and burn rehabilitation.

74. (C) Provide a transfer tub bench and install grab bars. The best adaptation to achieve access to the tub would be providing the client with a transfer tub bench, which is recommended for individuals who cannot step over the edge of the tub. Bathroom grab bars should also be installed to provide stability during the move into the tub. Answer A, repositioning the light switch would help to enhance visual cues and safety. Providing long handled adaptive devices

(answer B) would enhance bathing performance if the individual had difficulty with reaching their legs and feet. Answer D, nonskid decals and mats, are primarily safety measures to prevent slipping and falling. See reference: Pedretti and Early (eds): Smith, P: Americans with Disabilities Act: Accommodating persons with disabilities.

75. (A) Remove all throw or scatter rugs. Regardless of whether an individual with instability walks with the help of a walker, cane, or no equipment, the floor should be cleared of any obstacles that could cause them to slip or trip. A person's foot or on the tip of an assistive device may catch on scatter or throw rugs. Also, rugs may not be firmly taped down or secured with nonskid backing, causing a further safety hazard. Installing lever handles, a ramp, or a handheld shower (answers B, C, and D) would make certain tasks easier for a patient, but they would not be necessary for safety. See reference: Pedretti and Early (eds): Foti, D: Activities of daily living.

76. (C) A phone with extra large buttons. "Phone companies offer adapted phone systems for children and adults who have various limitations…some phones have extra large buttons for those with incoordination or visual impairments" (p. 267). A phone with extra large buttons would most likely be the best solution for the child with mild visual impairments who desires to use the phone without assistance. Answers A, B, and C would assist individuals who are unable to hold the phone independently due to incoordination, weakness or loss of function in the hand or upper extremity. See reference: Solomon (ed): Jones, LMW and Machover, PZ: Occupational performance areas: Daily living and work and productive activities

77. (C) Trim lines of the splint should extend proximal to the MCP crease. Trim lines of a splint that extend proximal to the MCP crease allow for adequate MCP digit extension and flexion. Answers A, B, and D fall distal to the MCP crease, thus restricting full extension and flexion of the digits at the metacarpal heads. See reference: Pedretti and Early (eds): Bekin, J and Yasuda, L: Orthotics.

78. (B) Obtain a raised toilet seat. The individual will most likely continue to require a raised toilet seat for several months in order to avoid flexing the hip past the designated range. A handheld shower (answer D) is not always necessary, however, a shower chair with adjustable legs and grab bars could be helpful. High contrast tape (answer C) may help to make ascending and descending stairs safer for individuals with limitations in vision. Moving items from low cabinets to higher locations may help this individual comply more readily with the necessary hip precautions, but moving objects from high to lower cabinets (answer A) would not. See reference: Pedretti and Early (eds): Coleman, S: Hip fractures and lower extremity joint replacement.

79. (A) are more easily performed if coordinated with consistent timing of medications. A patient with Parkinson's disease needs to learn to use the period of reduced symptoms and improved mobility resulting from medication use, to best advantage for performing ADL. Medications taken regularly and consistently aid the establishment of routines for self-care. Performance of self-care activities before medications (answer B), and stretched out throughout the day (answer D), would not make best use of the medication's positive effects. Answer C is incorrect because it discourages attempts for independent functioning. See reference: Pedretti and Early (eds): Schultz-Krohn, W, Foti, D and Glogoski, C: Degenerative diseases of the central nervous system.

80. (A) Use socks with a wide opening. "A wide sock opening can prevent frustration during the most difficult part of putting on socks, which is inserting the toes" (p. 235). Answer B, a sock aid, may be a viable option, but at times, "these aids can be difficult to use...however, they may benefit children with limited reaching, coordination, and lower extremity functioning" (p. 235). Answer C, nylon tights, are typically more difficult to put on independently because of the elastic quality of the material and the high level of balance required. Answer D, utilizing a sock with a narrow opening, will also make it more difficult to put on because the child will not have as much room to insert her toes. See reference: Solomon (ed): Jones, LMW and Machover, PZ: Occupational performance areas: Daily living and work and productive activities.

81. (B) 33 to 36 inches. This is the proper height for grab bars to allow for the upper extremities to lift the body with enough clearance to transfer onto the toilet seat. A height of 28 to 32 inches (answer A) would be too low to allow the body to clear the toilet seat when the arms are straightened. A height of 38 to 41 inches or 43 to 46 inches (answers C and D) would be too high to effectively push down with the arms to lift the body onto the toilet seat. See reference: Rothstein, Roy, and Wolf: American's with disabilities act and accessibility issues.

82. (D) arm trough. An arm trough would provide a stable surface that would keep the individual's arm in a safe and appropriate position. In addition, an arm trough approximates the humeral head into the glenoid fossa at a natural angle. If the individual has edema in his hand, a foam wedge may be placed in the trough to elevate the hand. A lap tray (answer A) would provide support, but is more restrictive than an arm trough, which should be attempted first. The fact that the individual's arm was seen dangling by the side of the wheelchair indicates that the wheelchair armrest alone (answer B) is inadequate. Answer C, an arm sling, would provide support for his

arm, but would immobilize it in adduction and internal rotation. Current literature supports the use of slings only when necessary, such as during ambulation when a flaccid upper extremity may sublux or cause loss of balance. See reference: Pedretti and Early (eds): Gillen, G: Cerebrovascular accident.

83. (B) Use heavy utensils, pots, and pans. Using heavy kitchen items (answer B) increases stability for individuals with incoordination. Other suggestions include using prepared foods, nonskid mats, easy open containers, serrated knives, and tongs. Built-up-handles (answer A) are useful for individuals with limited grasp. A high stool (answer C) benefits those who fatigue easily. Placing the most commonly used items on shelves just above and below the counter (answer D) is a useful way to adapt the environment for individuals with limited reach. See reference: Pedretti and Early (eds): Foti, D: Activities of daily living.

84. (D) Role playing a tea party with "Barbie" dolls. Answer D, role playing with dolls, is the most appropriate choice because the COTA is encouraging the child to partake in pretend play. "Playfulness, like play, encompasses intrinsic motivation, internal control, and freedom to suspend reality" (p. 296). Role playing is focused primarily on the activity at hand, rather than the end product, such as in answer A (playing a game of "Go Fish") and answer B (playing a game of checkers). Answer C, jumping rope, might frustrate the child secondary to her difficulty with motor tasks. The end goal of an occupational therapy treatment would be to increase the child's play skills in the hopes that the child will begin to interact more comfortably within the home, school and peer environment. See reference: Solomon (ed): Clifford-O'Brien, J: Play.

85. (D) use brochures, posters, videotapes, and films available from the AOTA to enhance the presentation. The emphasis of this question is that it is every OT practitioner's responsibility to promote the profession. Simple, daily public relations activities occur each time an OT practitioner (whether it is a COTA or an OTR) describes the services to be provided to patients and families. More complex public relations may include developing a plan to promote community awareness regarding the profession. A public relations program is designed to increase public awareness about the role and importance of OT services. See reference: Sladyk, K (ed): Bowler, DF: OT and political action.

86. (B) Confront the individual's behavior and ask, "Are you aware that your frequent interruptions prevent others from having a chance to contribute?" In general, the group leader should try answers A, C, or D before confronting the individual who is monopolizing the conversation. However, considering that these more conservative attempts have failed the practitioner, Answer B, confronting the behavior, would be the best approach for the

COTA to take to modify the behavior. See reference: Posthuma: What to do if....

87. (B) labels with white print on a black background. White print on a black background is easier to see for individuals with poor vision. Using Braille labels (answer A) is not appropriate for individuals with peripheral neuropathy, because they have decreased tactile sensation in their fingertips. A pill organizer box (answer C) is useful for taking pills on schedule and is particularly helpful for individuals who have memory deficits or complex medication regimens. If the pills were presorted in the box, the client could safely take them without actually identifying them. Using the pill organizer, however, does not address the issue of medication identification. Brightly colored pills (answer D) would make it easier for identifying different medications, however, the therapist has no control over how pills are manufactured and what colors are used. See reference: Sladyk, K and Ryan, SE (eds): Jamison, PW: A retired librarian with sensory deficits.

88. (A) Position the child's trunk, head, neck, and shoulders in proper alignment. Proper positioning is the first thing the COTA must address prior to feeding the child. "Proper positioning is vital for tongue control. The trunk, head, neck, and shoulders need to be stable and aligned" (p. 224). Answer B, hyperextend the child's head, would be contraindicated because "abnormal tongue movements tend to occur more frequently when the head is hyperextended" (p. 224). Answers C and D are techniques commonly utilized to facilitate proper feeding techniques, but they should not be initiated until after the child is appropriately positioned. See reference: Solomon (ed): Jones, LMW and Machover, PZ: Occupational performance areas: Daily living and work and productive activities

89. (B) Sterilize it before using it again. OSHA has set out strategies to protect individuals from potential exposure to HIV and hepatitis B virus. This situation would be an example of an engineering control. These controls are to modify the work environment to reduce risk of exposure. Other examples are using sharps containers, eyewash stations, and biohazard waste containers. Answers A, C, and D would not meet guidelines set forth by OSHA regarding equipment that has come into contact with open wounds. See reference: Pedretti and Early (eds): Buckner, WS: Infection control and safety issues in the clinic.

90. (B) Gently touch the infant's lips to encourage her to open her mouth and begin sucking motions. Answer B, gently touching the infant's lips would most likely facilitate the suck-swallow reflex. "When the infant's lips are touched, the infant's mouth opens and sucking movements begin" (p. 91). Answer A, touching the infants cheek before feeding, would most likely facilitate the rooting reflex.

Answer C would most likely facilitate the phasic-bite reflex, and answer D, rubbing the infant's lips and cheeks simultaneously, would most likely frustrate the infant, because several different reflexes are being encourage at the same time (e.g., the rooting reflex and phasic-bite reflex). See reference: Solomon (ed): O'Brien, JC, Koontz Lowman, D, and Solomon, JW: Development of occupational performance areas.

91. (A) A small spoon. According to Solomon "by 24 months, children can hold a spoon and bring it to the mouth with the wrist supinated into the palm-up position...at 30-36 months children experiment with forks to stab at food" (p. 92), thus making answer D, a small fork incorrect. The COTA may allow the child to eat with his fingers (answer B), however the child would most likely be developmentally ready to attempt to use a spoon. Answer C, a swivel spoon, would be indicated when a child is unable to deviate the wrist radially and/or supinate the forearm. See reference: Solomon (ed): O'Brien, JC, Koontz Lowman, D and Solomon, JW: Development of occupational performance areas.

92. (B) left unilateral neglect. This is the inability to respond or orient to perceptions from the left side of the body. Evidenced as left unilateral neglect (answer B), this deficit is also apparent in the draw-a-man test, flower-copying test, house test, and completing a human figure or face puzzle. Unilateral neglect is contralateral to the side of a brain lesion, therefore, left unilateral neglect would result from right-sided brain damage. Left neglect occurs most commonly in right hemisphere lesions. A cataract (answer C) would cause a visual impairment with detail on both sides of a page. Bitemporal hemianopia (hemianopia is also referred to as hemianopsia), also known as "tunnel vision," occurs when the individual's peripheral vision lost (answer A). The individual would still be able to cross midline with cataracts or bitemporal hemianopsia (answer D). A right neglect would not see the right side, and this type of patient would draw all the figures on the left side of the page. Visuospatial deficits are an important factor influencing functional independence outcomes. Visuospatial ability should be taken into account when establishing treatment goals as well as during discharge planning. See reference: Trombly (ed): Quintana, L: Evaluation of perception and cognition.

93. (B) A call system for emergency and nonemergency use. A call system (answer B) is necessary for a person with a high level spinal cord injury to allow the caretaker to leave the room, but remains available to answer calls for assistance with daily needs or an emergency. This is frequently the first opportunity that a person with a spinal cord injury would have to control some part of his or her life, giving some feeling of independence or choice. An ECU (answer A) does allow independence in operating appliances, lights, and so on through the use of switches or voice control, but would not be a necessity for safety. A remote control power door opener that would allow a caretaker to enter would be useless if the individual is unable to call for assistance. An electric page turner (answer D) is useless without the ability to call for someone to position or replace reading material. See reference: Trombly (ed): Dow, PW and Rees, NP: High-technology adaptations to overcome disability.

94. (B) teach the client to use a diary or log. Compensation techniques are used to work around a deficit area by using alternative methods to accomplish the same task. Teaching the use of a diary or log (answer B) is an example of an external memory aid which provides cues to compensate for memory deficits. Answers A and C are incorrect, because they are examples of internal memory strategies (retracing and rehearsal) which rely on mental effort. Answer D, use of a memory training computer program, is a technique for remediation of memory skills and, therefore, not an example of a compensation method. See reference: Trombly (ed): Quintana, LE: Remediating cognitive impairments.

95. (C) anterograde amnesia. Anterograde amnesia is the inability to recall events after a trauma. Retrograde amnesia (answer D) is the inability to recall events prior to trauma. Long-term memory (answer B) is the storage of information for recall at a later time. Orientation (answer A) is the awareness of person, place, and time. See reference: Trombly (ed): Quintana, LA: Evaluation of perception and cognition.

96. (D) built-up handles. Built-up handles, without adding extra weight, allow a comfortable grasp that regular utensils do not provide. A weighted handle would cause more rapid fatigue and strain to the joints. An arthritic person most likely has adequate grasp and release with a built-up handle, making it easier to use than a universal cuff. See reference: Trombly (ed): Feinberg, JR and Trombly, CA: Arthritis.

97. (D) decreased attention. An attention deficit (answer D) is indicated if the individual recognizes a letter and marks it accurately on both the right and left sides of the page but misses letters in a random pattern. A visual field cut (answers A and B) is evidenced by missed letters appearing close together in one area, on either the left or right side of the page. Illiteracy (answer C) is unlikely because the individual is a high school teacher. See reference: Trombly (ed): Quintana, LA: Remediating perceptual impairments.

98. (D) A pediatric weighted utensil holder. "Children who lack sensory discrimination skills in the hands use the weighted holder. The weight increases proprioceptive (deep-pressure) feedback to the joints and muscles in the hand and wrist, adding

to children's awareness of the position and movement of the hand, fingers, and wrist in relation to the pencil and paper" (p. 264). Answers A and C, a wide pen and soft triangle grip, would assist a child with decreased grip, while answer B, rubber bands, would assist a child who has difficulty opposing their thumb into the web space. See reference: Solomon (ed): Jones, LMW and Machover, PZ:Occupational performance areas: Daily living and work and productive activities

99. (C) Biomechanical. The biomechanical approach uses voluntary muscle control during performance of activities for individuals with deficits in strength, endurance, or range of motion. The biomechanical approach focuses on decreasing deficits in order to improve performance of daily activities. The neurophysiological approach (answer A) is applied to individuals with brain damage. Emphasis is on the nervous system and methods for eliciting desired responses. The neurodevelopmental approach (answer B) also focuses on the nervous system, but emphasizes eliciting responses in a developmental sequence. The rehabilitative approach (answer D) teaches an individual how to compensate for a deficit on either a temporary or permanent basis. See reference: Trombly (ed): Zemke, R: Remediating biomechanical and physiological impairments of motor performance.

100. (B) figure-ground perception. Figure-ground perception is the ability to visually separate an object from the surrounding background. An example of this would be the ability to find a button on a plaid shirt. A problem with spatial relations (answer A) is seen in dressing when a person overestimates or underestimates reach because of an inability to judge the relationship between the object and the body. Body image (answer C) is a mental picture of the person's body that includes how the person feels about their body. Visual closure (answer D) is the ability to recognize an object even though only part of it is seen, e.g., recognizing a partially covered button. See reference: Zoltan: Visual discrimination skills.

101. (D) Chaining. Teaching a task one step at a time, gradually adding more steps as each are mastered, is called chaining. Chaining is frequently used when teaching a multistep task, because it is easier to learn one step at a time than it is to learn a complete activity. Repetition and rehearsal (answers A and C) involve repeating the whole activity repetitively until the activity is learned. Cueing (answer B) uses an external source to remind a person of the next step or part of that step. See reference: Zoltan: Executive functions.

102. (C) Play activities which incorporate tapping, application of textures, and weight bearing to the residual limb. Massage, tapping, use of textures, and weight bearing on the distal end of a residual limb are techniques used to develop tolerance to touch and pressure in the hypersensitive limb. Answers A and B will not affect hypersensitivity, and answer D is incorrect because the child is in the preprosthetic phase and does not yet have access to the prosthesis. See reference: Trombly (ed): Celikol, F: Amputation and prosthetics.

103. (A) work locks and latches on doors and windows. The ability to manipulate the locks and latches is a safety concern because the individual may be unable to open them to let family members into the home or close them to keep intruders from entering. Built-up handles (answer B), energy conservation techniques (answer C), and adaptations to clothing fasteners (answer D) are not safety issues. See reference: Trombly (ed): Feinberg, JR and Trombly, CA: Arthritis.

104. (A) within normal limits. Normal range of motion for internal rotation is 70 degrees (answer A). Rotation can be assessed with the humerus adducted against the trunk or with the shoulder abducted to 90 degrees. If the humeral movements for internal or external rotation are observed during the performance of activities and found to be adequate for performance of functional activities, range of motion may be noted as WFL (answer B). The OT practitioner may choose not to perform a formal joint measurement if the joint is WFL, even though the end of the range may be lacking a few degrees, because the loss of movement may not be significant to the individual. Hypermobility (answer C) at a joint is motion past the average range of motion, which at the shoulder would be past 70 degrees of internal rotation. If hypermobility is caused by an unstable joint as might occur after a surgical repair or a disease process, then splinting or another form of stabilization or immobilization can be used to correct the problem. If the practitioner observes hypermobility during range of motion, they should compare the range of motion to that on the individual's opposite side in order to assess normal range. A limitation of internal rotation (answer D) at the shoulder would be less than 70 degrees of motion. If a limitation is apparent, the rehabilitation team may choose not to treat it unless it interferes with the function of the upper extremity. See reference: Trombly (ed): Trombly, CA: Evaluation of biomechanical and physiological aspects of motor performance.

105. (A) skin inspection. Visual inspection of an insensate area is essential for preventing pressure sores, which may develop when there are no sensory cues to alert a person to skin breakdown. Nail trimming (answer B) is an important issue to address with individuals with diabetes, but is secondary to skin inspection in importance. Many individuals with diabetes have abnormalities in nail growth, and instead of trimming their own nails they have them trimmed by a podiatrist. Moreover, the nursing staff may address this issue with the patient. Retirement

planning (answer C), and returning to work (answer D), are issues that may be addressed when discussing discharge plans. See reference: Trombly (ed): Bentzel, K: Remediating sensory impairment.

106. (D) protective extension response. "Protective extension responses are postural reactions that are used to stop a fall or to prevent injury when equilibrium reactions fail to do so" (p. 74). Equilibrium reactions (answer C) involve "automatic, compensatory movements...used to maintain the center of gravity over the base of support" (p. 74). Righting reactions (answer B) "bring the head and trunk back into an upright position" (p. 74). Primitive reflexes (answer A) are automatic movements that occur involuntarily and disappear as the infant matures. See reference: Solomon (ed): Lowman, DK: Development of occupational performance components.

107. (D) The individual traces letters through a pan of rice with her fingers. This method involves greater input of sensory information to the brain by performing a gross movement in a more stimulating environment. A verbal description of how to make a letter (Answer A), watching her grip (answer B), or performing strengthening exercises (Answer C), would not give the individual proprioceptive feedback on her letter formation through tactile input. See reference: Trombly (ed): Bentzel, K: Remediating sensory impairment.

108. (A) wrist cock-up splint. Carpal tunnel syndrome is a condition that results from compression of the median nerve at the wrist. A wrist cock-up splint positions the wrist in 10 to 20 degrees of extension to alleviate symptoms and prevent further damage. Answer B refers to splints made out of thermoplastic materials, and does not indicate a splint type specific to carpal tunnel syndrome. Resting hand splints (answer C) are typically used to prevent deformity development in individuals with arthritis or quadriplegia. Dynamic MP flexion splints (answer D) are used to assist flexion at the MP joints when this motion is weak or absent. See reference: Trombly (ed): Trombly, CA and Linden, CA: Orthoses: Kinds and purposes

109. (B) Teach the child to sit in a chair and lift and place the affected foot up on a small stool. "For a child with hemiplegia or limited balance, sitting with back support may be the best starting position for putting on and removing socks. The child lifts the affected leg onto a box or step to bring the foot closer to the unaffected hand" (p. 235). Answer A, encourage the child to wear tight fitting socks, would make it more difficult for the child to put on and take off his or her socks. The child would benefit more from socks that have a wide opening. Answer C, encourage the child to lay on his back in bed when putting on socks, and answer D, placing the unaffected foot on a small stool, would not assist in dressing skills independence for this child. See reference: Solomon (ed): Jones, LMW and Machover, PZ: Occupational performance areas: Daily living and work and productive activities

110. (A) Continue to perform PROM and then position and elevate the affected extremity. Positioning, the use of a compression glove, edema massage, and PROM exercises are all effective methods for reducing edema and preventing further edema. The goal is to promote the movement of fluid back into normal circulation, rather than allowing it to collect in one area or body part. Gentle PROM is necessary to help maintain joint structure and provide nutrients to the joint. The actual movement of the extremity may serve as a "pump" to assist in moving excess fluid back into the body. These techniques are contraindicated for individuals who have deep vein thrombosis. Edema is caused in part by the loss of movement in an extremity because there is no contraction of muscles, which helps to pump the fluid to the heart. Splinting (answer B) is effective in preventing deformity, but compression gloves are more effective in reducing edema. Taking no action (answer C) could result in permanent damage to the tissue of the involved extremity. Having the individual attempt to squeeze a ball (answer D) would be inappropriate because the left arm is flaccid. See reference: Trombly (ed): Woodson, AM: Stroke.

111. (B) perform the evaluation over several sessions. Upper extremity evaluation is lengthy and can be fatiguing, and fatigue should be avoided with individuals with Guillain-Barré syndrome. In addition, results may be invalid if the individual is fatigued and not performing at the highest level possible. Strength, range of motion, and sensory testing (answers A, C, and D) are all important when evaluating an individual with Guillain-Barré syndrome, but must be administered using a method that will yield valid results. See reference: Pedretti and Early (eds): Lehman, RM and McCormack, G: Neurogenic and myopathic dysfunction.

112. (A) A game of rhythmic exercises performed to music. Rhythmic activities facilitate motor performance in individuals with Parkinson's disease, especially when performed to music. Time capsules (answer B) are a meaningful activity for those who are approaching the end of life, but the description of the activity provides no rationale for why it would benefit the motor skills of those individuals with Parkinson's disease. Races (answer C) are generally not a good idea for this population because of the difficulty they often have stopping during ambulation. Reading out loud (answer D) is an effective intervention for addressing the communication, not motor deficits, frequently experienced by these individuals. Group activities are particularly beneficial because of the added advantage of social interaction. See reference: Sladyk, K and Ryan, SE (eds): Eberhardt, KM: A homemaker and volunteer with Parkinson's disease.

113. (C) train the client in the operation of the AT system and in strategies for its use. Training activities in the use of the assistive devices are the next critical step after setup of the system, and are essential because the complex nature of assistive technologies can require many hours of practice to master. Evaluating how well the whole system works (answer A) usually occurs after training is completed during the follow-up phase. Evaluating the match between the client and the technology (answer B) is done earlier in the process to ensure maximum success and because expensive technological devices may only be ordered once. Funding sources (answer C) are also determined before ordering equipment. See reference: Pedretti and Early (eds): Anson, D: Assistive technology.

114. (B) side-lying on a mat. "Side-lying is a good positioning choice for children whose muscle tone becomes too high or low in prone or supine positions. Side-lying positions also give children a stable, midline head position and keep their hands in their line of vision...hands remain free to reach for and manipulate objects without having to resist the pull of gravity" (p. 354). Answer A, long-sitting, answer C, supine positioning, and answer D, prone positioning, all require the child to work against gravity, and would most likely be too difficult for the child to maintain while engaging in play activities secondary to low tone. See reference: Solomon (ed): Wandel, JA: Positioning and handling.

115. (A) elevate the arm on pillows so it rests higher than the heart. Elevation, contrast baths, retrograde massage, pressure wraps, and active range-of-motion are effective methods for managing edema. When massaging an edematous extremity, stroking should be performed from the distal area to the proximal, not the reverse (answer B). Because active and PROM can both be beneficial to managing edema, instructing the patient to avoid range-of-motion activities (answers C and D) would be incorrect. See reference: Pedretti and Early (eds): Kasch, MC and Nickerson, E: Hand and upper extremity injuries.

116. (B) Objective. The objective portion of the SOAP note (answer B) focuses on measurable or observable data obtained by the OT practitioner through specific evaluations, observations, or use of therapeutic activities. The subjective portion of a SOAP note (answer A) should feature relevant patient reports or comments. The assessment part of a SOAP note (answer C) addresses the effectiveness of treatment and changes needed, the status of the goals, and the justification for continuing OT treatment. The plan section of a SOAP note (answer D) includes statements related to continuing treatment; the frequency and duration of the treatment; suggestions for additional activities or treatment techniques; the need for further evaluations; and, when needed, recommendations for new goals. See reference: Sabonis-Chafee and Hussey: Treatment planning and implementation.

117. (B) Introduce active range of motion exercises through gentle swaying/dancing with the child's favorite music. By introducing gentle, nonthreatening activities (such as dancing to his favorite music), the child will have time to develop trust with the COTA in addition to having some sense of power over the situation by choosing his own type of music. Informing the child that he will most likely scar if he does not participate in therapy is not the first thing the COTA should do (answer A). This may make the child feel scared, and given his age, even more frightened to participate in therapy. Patient education, especially when done with children, is something that should be done slowly and in a non-threatening manner. Answer C, introducing passive range of motion, does not assist the child to move actively, a crucial component to resuming activities of daily living post burn injury. While positioning the child over a bolster (answer D) is a viable option, it would not be the first activity to select in this particular case, because the child is unlikely to allow the COTA to touch his body in order to appropriately position him until further trust is established. See reference: Richard and Staley (eds): Reeves, SU, Warden, G and Staley, MJ: Management of the pediatric burn patient.

118. (C) folding laundry. Sorting and folding laundry (answer C) challenge balance and upper extremity function in ways that are more functional than stacking cones or throwing a ball. Rather than seeking contrived activities (answers A, B, and C) that challenge single component deficits, the focus of home care is to find ways for the patient to actually perform the daily activities that are presenting the challenges. Because this patient is a mother of four teenagers, it is presumed that her occupational role includes homemaking activities. See reference: Piersol and Ehrlich (eds): Seibert, C: The clinic called home.

119. (A) Read the facility's infection control plan. An infection control plan most likely incluldes appropriate techniques and procedures for storing and handling foods within the OT department. Such plans specify the shelf lives of certain foods, standards for storage of food, use of hair nets, and cooking temperatures and times. A risk management plan (answer C) addresses the issue of liability in reference to negligence and malpractice issues. The dietary department (answer B) would not be likely to have information regarding the handling and storage of food. Cooking with only canned foods (answer D) would still require the COTA to apply the principles of infection control. See reference: Sladyk, K and Ryan, SE (eds): Leary, CJ: Management issues and models.

120. (C) Eat six small meals a day. An individual with ALS who becomes fatigued eating three full meals a day should attempt eating six smaller meals a day before resorting to tube feedings or pureed diets (answers A and D). Eating regular food is usually more enjoyable and is therefore likely to enhance the quality of life. An upright position is optimal when feeding individuals with dysphagia. A semi-reclined position (answer B) can make swallowing more difficult or dangerous. See reference: Pedretti and Early (eds): Schultz-Krohn, W, Foti, D and Glogoski, C: Degenerative diseases of the central nervous system.

121. (D) set personal boundaries appropriate to the therapist–patient relationship. It is important to acknowledge the individual's need for sexual expression, while supporting the sense of self, and identifying acceptable relationships and behaviors. Setting boundaries while accepting the individual is the most appropriate therapeutic response. Outright rejection (answer A) may cause an individual to believe he or she is sexually undesirable or unlovable. Flirting back (answer B) may imply that a sexual relationship between COTA and the patient is acceptable. Although the individual may need to know how SCI affects sexual functioning (answer C), the behavior that requires a response is not about a lack of knowledge, but rather about how to appropriately express sexual interest and the need for reinforcement of a sexual identity. See reference: Pedretti and Early (eds): Burton, GU: Sexuality and physical dysfunction.

122. (B) adult day care. This environment in answer B provides programming for an elderly patient that is psychosocial in nature and focuses on vocational skills and social activities. Partial hospitalization (answer A) is a type of outpatient program that serves as a transition to community living. It offers most of the structure and services available on an inpatient unit, while allowing individuals to live in the community. Home health care (answer C) provides treatment services to individuals who have chronic or debilitating illnesses in their own homes in order to increase their functional independence. Although most individuals who receive home health services have disabilities that are primarily physical, secondary psychiatric disorders are quite common. Psychosocial rehabilitation centers (answer D) focus on the social rather than the medical aspects of mental illness. Psychosocial clubs and rehabilitation centers provide socialization programs, daily living skills counseling, prevocational rehabilitation, and transitional employment. See reference: Early: Treatment settings.

123. (D) a weighted pen and weighted wrists. Weighting body parts and utensils (e.g., writing tools) are effective for individuals with ataxia to improve control during performance of a task. Hitting the keys on a keyboard (answer A) would be difficult for such a client, although weighting the wrists could make performance of the activity possible. A keyboard is a good alternative for individuals with difficulty writing due to weakness, limited range of motion, or incoordination. A universal cuff with a pencil holder attachment (answer B) would be appropriate for an individual with hand weakness who uses a universal cuff for other tasks. A balanced forearm orthosis (answer C) is appropriate for individuals with severe muscle weakness. In addition, individuals with muscle weakness find felt tip pens easier to write with than ballpoint pens. See reference: Pedretti and Early (eds): Gutman, SA: Traumatic brain injury.

124. (D) Just before discharge. Because the prognosis for patients with Guillain-Barré syndrome is usually good, equipment should be ordered just before discharge to accurately determine the individual's needs. Equipment ordered during the first week of therapy, or as soon as approved (answers B and C), may not be necessary at the time the individual is discharged. Although collaborating with the patient and family on decisions about ordering equipment is essential, acceptance of the disability (answer A) may not necessarily correspond with the appropriate time for ordering equipment. See reference: Pedretti and Early (eds): Lehman, RM and McCormack, GL: Neurogenic and myopathic dysfunction.

125. (B) wear gloves. Wearing gloves places a barrier between the practitioner and any possible infective agent on the patient's hand. A mask (answer A) is more effective as a barrier for airborne pathogens, or for protection from splashes of bodily fluids. Refusing to work with the patient (answer C) is not an option, as indicated in the *OT Code of Ethics*. Individuals fearful of infection should educate themselves about appropriate precautions and procedures, and should seek employment in environments in which they can provide intervention to all patients served by the facility. Although handwashing before and after treatment (answer A) should be the rule with all patients, and is effective in protecting the patient and practitioner from contamination, that precaution would not be effective in protecting the practitioner during patient treatment. See reference: Pedretti and Early (eds): Buckner, WS: Infection control and safety issues in the clinic.

126. (D) sensory compensation. When protective sensation is severely decreased or absent, the primary focus of intervention becomes protection of the insensate part through educational methods, to increase awareness of potential injury dangers, teach safety procedures, and train in the use of vision, to compensate for sensory loss. Sensory re-education (answer A) is a remedial retraining technique which focuses on helping the patient correctly interpret sensory impulses through a program of graded sensory stimuli. Sensory desensitization (answer B) involves a program of graded sensory stimuli to gradually decrease hypersensitivity to sensory stimuli. Sensory bombardment (answer C) is a sensory retraining method of stimulating many senses. See reference: Pedretti and Early (eds): Iyer, MB

and Pedretti, LW: Evaluation of sensation and treatment of sensory dysfunction.

127. (A) remedial treatment, such as rubbing or stroking the involved extremity. When sensation begins to return, it is appropriate to initiate remedial activities for sensory retraining. Stimulating the involved extremity by rubbing or stroking (to provide tactile input), or through weight-bearing activities (to provide proprioceptive input), are examples of remedial activities. Compensatory activities, which are essential for individuals with decreased or absent sensation, would have been part of the original treatment plan. Answers B, C, and D are all examples of compensatory strategies. See reference: Pedretti and Early (eds): Iyer, MB and Pedretti, LW: Evaluation of sensation and treatment of sensory dysfunction.

128. (B) decrease the effects of prolonged inactivity. Some of the main objectives of inpatient cardiac rehabilitation include decreasing the effects of prolonged inactivity, such as thromboembolism, orthostatic hypotension, and muscle atrophy; safely providing a program of monitored activity performance to maximize function; reinforcing cardiac precautions; and providing instruction in energy conservation techniques. It is acceptable and expected to encounter fatigue in this population after activity (answer A); however, activities that produce cardiac symptoms should be avoided. Activities that promote endurance and strength are beneficial, but ROM (answer C) is not usually an area of concern. Most individuals do not need to relearn activities, other than applying energy conservation techniques, therefore, independent performance (answer D) is not a primary concern. See reference: Pedretti and Early (eds): Matthews, MM: Cardiac and pulmonary diseases.

129. (C) "I see you've finished the project, is there anything else you'd like to do with it?" This comment is best because it acknowledges the patient's effort to engage in the activity, rather than the quality of the finished product. Craft projects completed by depressed patients may show inattention to detail, and minimal effort as a result of their low energy level. Answer A provides false praise which the client would probably recognize as unrealistic and untrustworthy. Answer B would put pressure on the client to improve performance, which could reinforce feelings of low self-esteem. Answer D minimizes the effort which the client put forth in attempting and completing the activity. See reference: Early: Responding to symptoms and behaviors.

130. (B) Positioning, adaptive equipment, and patient education. Positioning and adaptive equipment are necessary to maintain the integrity of the musculoskeletal system and to prevent deformity. Patient education about the disease and ways of dealing with its effects can also be started at this stage. Resistive exercises (answer A) are not appropriate if there is joint swelling and inflammation, and are always used cautiously with individuals with RA because of the potential for tissue damage. Discharge planning would be more relevant at a later time (answer C). Surgical intervention (answer D) would not be needed in the early stages of rheumatoid arthritis. It may be offered later as a corrective measure for long-standing deformities. See reference: Pedretti and Early (eds): Buckner, WS: Arthritis.

131. (C) Wrist splints to promote development of tenodesis. Hand splinting to promote tenodesis is implemented in the acute phase of rehabilitation. A tenodesis grasp is developed by allowing the finger flexors to shorten. The patient is then able to achieve a functional grasp by extending the wrist. This improves the ability of an individual with a C6 or C7 spinal cord injury to grasp and hold objects. A volar pan splint (answer A) would not allow finger flexors to shorten, and would interfere with the development of tenodesis. Interventions related to promoting independent performance (answer B) should begin as soon as possible, but issues related to positioning must be addressed first. An individual would not be instructed in bed mobility (answer D) until after the acute phase. See reference: Pedretti and Early (eds): Adler, C: Spinal cord injury.

132. (A) safety and stability. Incoordination, tremors, ataxia and athetoid movements may result from conditions that affect the central nervous system, such as Parkinson's disease, CP, multiple sclerosis, and head injuries. "The major problems encountered in ADL performance [for people with incoordination] are safety and adequate stability of gait, body parts and objects to complete the tasks" (p. 148). Strength (answer C) was not identified as an area of concern for this individual. The ability to reach and bend (answer B) is of primary concern for those with limitations in range of motion. Endurance level (answer D) is a primary concern for individuals with MS, Guillain-Barré syndrome, ALS, and other neurological conditions that cause them to fatigue quickly. See reference: Pedretti and Early (eds): Foti, D: Activities of daily living.

133. (D) Add a thickening agent to liquids. Individuals with swallowing problems usually have more difficulty with thin liquids than with thicker ones. A straw (answer A) is useful for individuals who are unable to lift a cup or glass to their mouth. "Sippy cups" (answer B) benefit individuals who tend to spill when they are drinking. It may be important to monitor fluid intake (answer C) for individuals who drink too much or don't drink enough. See reference: Neistadt and Crepeau (eds): Holm, MB, Rogers, JC, and James, AB: Treatment activities of daily living.

134. (C) marking the end of each step with high contrast tape. Difficulty in seeing contrast and col-

or are two forms of decreased visual acuity that cannot be addressed by corrective lenses. Two effective environmental adaptations to these deficits are increasing background contrast and illumination. Using tape or paint to make the edge of each step contrast sharply with the rest of the step is an inexpensive way to adapt the environment. Installing a stair glide or handrails (answers A and B) are more costly adaptations that do not address the problems of decreased visual acuity. Instructing the patient to take only one step at a time may cause the individual to be unnecessarily slow, and does not address the problems of decreased visual acuity. See reference: Pedretti and Early (eds): Warren, M: Evaluation and treatment of visual deficits.

135. (B) Moro reflex. The Moro reflex is characterized by abduction, extension, and external rotation of the arms. The rooting reflex (answer A) is the turning of the head toward tactile stimulation near the mouth. The flexor withdrawal reflex (answer C) is characterized by flexion of an extremity in response to a painful stimulus. The neck righting reaction (answer D) involves body alignment in rotation after turning of the head. Only the Moro reflex causes an extension movement. See reference: Neistadt and Crepeau (eds): Kohlmeyer, K: Evaluation of performance components.

136. (D) Provide the client with several outfits similar to the preferred one. This option meets the client's need to wear the outfit of her choice, while having enough clean outfits. Answers A and C limit the client's freedom of choice, and will result in an unhappy individual. Washing the outfit each night (answer B) is burdensome for the caregiver and will quickly wear out the outfit. See reference: Neistadt and Crepeau (eds): Holm, MB, Rogers, JC, and James, AB: Treatment activities of daily living.

137. (C) Design an individualized program directed at the underlying neurologic deficit. Sensory integration is a complex treatment modality that is a highly individualized form of treatment carried out by a therapist with advanced training and understanding in the area of neuroscience. Answer A is incorrect because the child's program is not being "individualized," but is included in a group program. Answer B is not correct because sensory integration treatment is active and requires an adaptive response from the child. Answer D is not correct because sensory integration is directed at improving underlying neurologic, functioning rather than skill development. See reference: Neistadt and Crepeau (eds): Baloueff, O: Sensory integration.

138. (A) increasing self-awareness through expressive activities. Increasing self-awareness would be an initial goal area because people with eating disorders are often out-of-touch with their bodies as well as their psychological and social needs. Expressive activities address psychosocial needs to increase self-awareness by providing opportunities for emotional self-expression and self-assertion (answer A). Answer B is incorrect because preoccupation with "good" versus "bad" nutrition may be part of the eating disorder. Answer C is incorrect because school performance tends to be unaffected when individuals have eating disorders unless they are physically ill. Family therapy referrals are typically performed by other disciplines on the team at the time of discharge, so answer D is also incorrect. See reference: Neistadt and Crepeau (eds): Ward, JD: Psychosocial dysfunction in adults.

139. (C) flange the area around the ulnar styloid. Reddened areas indicate the splint is too tight in a particular spot. To reduce pressure, it is often helpful to flange splint edges. Lining the splint with any material, whether moleskin or foam (answers A and B), will only make a tight area tighter. Remaking the splint (answer D) is unnecessary and a waste of the COTA's time. See reference: Neistadt and Crepeau (eds): Fess, EE and Kiel, JH: Neuromuscular treatment: Upper extremity splinting.

140. (A) baking brownies. A correctly sequenced progression of difficulty in meal preparation is access a prepared meal; prepare a cold meal; prepare a hot beverage, soup, or prepared dish; prepare a hot one dish meal; and prepare a hot multidish meal. Making a fresh fruit salad (answer D) is a less challenging activity, because no cooking is involved. Although both involve heating an item, preparing toast (answer C) is simpler than heating soup because opening a plastic bag is a less complex task than opening a can. Baking brownies (answer A) is slightly more complex, because of the progression from stove top to oven, and the addition of several ingredients that need to be mixed. Therefore, this would be the appropriate upgrade. Making an apple pie (answer B) requires a higher level of task performance and complexity than brownies, and would be an appropriate task after the individual demonstrates competence in the less complex task of baking brownies. See reference: Neistadt and Crepeau (eds): Rogers, JC and Holm, MB: Evaluation of activities of daily living (ADL) and home management.

141. (D) Program evaluation. Program evaluation is a systematic collection and reporting of outcome data to document program effectiveness and cost-efficiency. Quality assurance (answer A) identifies problems and implements corrective actions. Peer review (answer B) is the system of other service providers assessing the provision of care to ensure appropriate interventions and documentation practices. Answer C, utilization review, is the process of analyzing the provision of services to promote the most economical delivery of service. See reference: Neistadt and Crepeau (eds): Perinchief, JM: Management of occupational therapy services.

142. (A) Biofeedback, distraction, and relaxation techniques. Biofeedback, distraction, and relaxation techniques are all examples of psychosocial measures that can be introduced to manage pain. Answers B and C, specific skill training and endurance building, are not directly related to pain management techniques and are often associated with cognitive or motor limitations. Answer D, cognitive retraining techniques, are also not directly related to pain management techniques. See reference: Neistadt and Crepeau (eds): Engel, JM: Treatment for psychosocial components: Pain management.

143. (A) restore and maintain performance of self-chosen occupations that support performance of valued occupational roles. The individual's depression is likely to be in reaction to the AIDS disease and major loss of functioning at stage 4. Stage 4 of AIDS generally means severe physical and neurologic changes. Because the change of function can be broad, answer A is the most comprehensive approach. Answers B and C are too restrictive to be a "major focus." Answer D, restoration of work, is typically unrealistic at stage 4 of AIDS. See reference: Neistadt and Crepeau (eds): Pizzi, M and Burkhardt, A: Occupational therapy for adults with immunological diseases.

144. (A) selected tasks in which aides have been trained, with intense close supervision. To maximize efficiency and cost-effectiveness of therapy services, there has been an increased use OT aides. Such aides must be very closely supervised, and are expected to receive site specific training in selected activities determined by the supervising OT practitioner, and must be utilized in accordance with state regulations. Activities and levels of supervision in answers B, C, and D are all beyond the scope of the OT aide. See reference: Neistadt and Crepeau (eds): Cohn, ES: Interdisciplinary communication and supervision of personnel.

145. (B) All group members construct one tower that incorporates all the pieces provided in a set of constructional materials (e.g., Lego blocks, Tinkertoys, or Erector set). Activities used in evaluation groups should require group collaboration that can be done in approximately 45 minutes and emphasize process rather than end product. The collage and crafts (answers A and D) are individual activities and do not demand group interaction. Making pizza for lunch (answer C) is an end product that serves the group as a whole and usually takes longer than 45 minutes. The pizza activity and format is typically not an evaluation group, but is better suited as a task oriented group activity in which self-awareness and self-understanding are primary goals. See reference: Mosey: Evaluation.

146. (D) home delivered meal services. Answer A, continued OT services to teach the patient to use the kitchen appliances safely, is incorrect because individuals diagnosed with dementia tend to decline over time, and interventions aimed at improvement are unrealistic. Volunteer companions (answer B), provide companionship to elders at home, but not skilled supervision of activities. Transporting to a community site for meals (answer C) on a daily basis could be inconvenient, overly challenging and taxing for an elder with beginning dementia. Answer D, in home meal delivery services, such as Meals-on-Wheels, would be the best and safest option for providing consistent access to food in the home. See reference: Larson, Stevens-Ratchford, Pedretti, and Crabtree (eds): Aitken, MJ and Lohman, H: Health care systems: Changing perspectives.

147. (C) Biomechanical. According to Colangelo, "The biomechanical frame of reference is applied when a person cannot maintain posture through appropriate automatic muscle activity because of neuromuscular or musculoskeletal dysfunction" (p. 257). This child's physical status has changed with decreasing postural control. Adaptive support devices need to be considered, and a biomechanical frame of reference provides this approach. Answer A is not correct because the neurodevelopmental treatment frame of reference is concerned with improving posture and movement, and supportive equipment is prescribed for that purpose. Answer B is not correct because the sensory integration frame of reference is concerned with sensory input in relation to posture and movement in children with sensory integration disorders, whereas Duchenne's disease is a neuromuscular disorder. Answer D is not correct because the visual perceptual frame of reference is concerned with guiding and compensating for visual perceptual problems, not postural delays. See reference: Kramer and Hinojosa (eds): Colangelo, CA: Biomechanical frame of reference.

148. (A) the therapist has the child play "sandwich" between heavy mats. The sandwich activity provides heavy touch pressure over the child's body, which can be inhibitory to a child experiencing sensory defensiveness. Answer B is incorrect because light use of a feather brush stimulates the light touch system, which is already impaired, and would be extremely uncomfortable for a child with tactile defensiveness. Answer C is not correct because the use of a blindfold, when a child is already reacting to unexpected touch, would most likely create a fearful response in a child with tactile defensiveness. Answer D, although not using a blindfold, has an unexpected touch from the back and this would also aggravate the child's existing problem. Answer A, the use of proprioceptive input to break through the protective response to light touch, will initially treat the child's defensiveness problem instead of stimulating further reaction. See reference: Kramer and Hinojosa (eds): Kimball, JG: Sensory integration frame of reference: Theoretical base, function/dysfunction continua and guide to evaluation.

149. (A) reminiscence group. In a reminiscence group, the focus is on providing social opportunities for sharing life stories and feelings, expressing pride in past life experiences, and gaining support for past life difficulties, all of which would enhance self-esteem and help the residents achieve acceptance of past and present life. Answers B, C, and D would address some of the goals stated, but not as comprehensively as a reminiscence group. See reference: Hellen: Appendix 9-10: Activity therapy care conference report form information: Therapeutic value.

150. (C) Feeding the camp pets. Camp can provide a normalizing environment for children with special needs who don't always have the opportunity to engage in normal children's activities. Taking care of pets, in particular, can provide these children with an opportunity to be responsible for the well-being of another, as well as the chance to be the caregiver rather than the care recipient. Amusement parks (answer A), which are highly stimulating environments, can challenge any child's sense of responsibility, and would not be appropriate for beginning level responsibility. Roasting marshmallow (answer B) involves responsibility for one's self near a fire. Lifeguarding (answer D) is an inappropriate activity for someone who is not qualified. See reference: Fazio: Intervention and support programming in day camps, sleep-away camps, and adventures.

151. (B) A pinch meter. A pinch meter is used to measure the strength of a three-jaw chuck grasp (also known as palmar pinch), in addition to key (lateral) pinch and tip pinch. These tests are performed with three trials that are averaged together and then compared with a standardized norm. Answer A, the aesthesiometer, measures two-point discrimination. Answer C, the dynamometer, measures grip strength. Answer D, the volumeter, measures edema in the hand. See reference: Pedretti and Early (eds): Kasch, M and Nickerson, E: Hand injuries.

152. (C) Passive ROM, positioning, and splinting. The initial phase of treatment for the individual with Guillain-Barré syndrome includes PROM, splinting, and positioning to protect weak muscles and prevent contractures. This should be followed by gentle, nonresistive activities and light ADLs (answer A) as tolerated. Resistive exercises, and balance and stabilization activities (answers B and D) should be implemented later after strength begins to improve. See reference: Pedretti and Early (eds): Lehman, RM and McCormack, GL: Neurogenic and myopathic dysfunction.

153. (C) Use a board game to introduce the concept of receiving and spending money. This activity provides an opportunity for the individuals to experience the value and purpose of money. Although it is important to introduce the actual value of coins and paper money, it is essential to combine this with concrete applications that a board game can supply. Answers A, B, and D are examples of graded activities to be used after the initial introduction of money concepts. See reference: Early: Activities of daily living.

154. (B) put the dried dishes away and begin to hand her wet dishes. Compensating for mistakes helps to increase the sense of self-worth and integrity of individuals with dementia. This approach is preferable to drawing attention to errors, especially in situations in which safety is not an issue. Answers A, C, and D all draw attention to the individual's errors. See reference: Early: Responding to symptoms and behaviors.

155. (C) Simple meal preparation group. Obtaining food is a basic survival need and is often the focus of a homeless individual's day. Therefore, although all the above groups may meet a need, activities related to food are likely to be more highly valued by this individual. Craft groups (answer A) may be useful in developing healthy leisure interests. Volunteer activities (answer B) can help develop necessary work habits. Social skills groups (answer D) address interpersonal skills necessary for living in society. See reference: Early: Who is the consumer?

156. (A) Scribble on a piece of paper. The Bayley scales on infant development suggest that a child will be able to scribble on a piece of paper (answer A) between the ages of 10 to 12 months. Copying a triangle (answer B) is a task that is not anticipated until the age of 5 to 6 years. Copying a horizontal line (answer C) is typically not seen until the age of 2, while copying numerals (answer D) is typically not observed until the age of 5 to 6 years old. It is important to appreciate that despite these age/developmental generalizations, each child's skill level can vary. See reference: Case-Smith (ed): Amundson, SJ: Prewriting and handwriting skills.

157. (B) aerobic exercise. Gross motor activities, involving either aerobic exercise or stretching and relaxation, can help to reduce the physical symptoms associated with anxiety. Although line dancing (answer C) involves all of the elements of gross motor activities, it requires the individual to follow specific steps and movements, which could cause the patient to become more anxious. Sewing and handcrafts (answer A) and woodworking (answer D) would not be the best recommendation for reducing physical symptoms of muscle tension, as they are primarily fine motor activities which require sustained attention. See reference: Early: Responding to symptoms and behaviors.

158. (C) attention span and social interaction skills. Conduct disorders often involve aggression toward people or animals and destruction of property. When working with this population, OT typically addresses the areas of attention span, impulse control, age appropriate social role performance, and

social skills. Children with developmental delays typically require intervention for perceptual-motor skills (answer A). Multiple role performance (answer D) is more developmentally relevant to adulthood than to adolescence. Although leisure and vocational interests (answer B) may be relevant to the adolescent population, the issues of attention span and social interaction would be more significant for an individual with conduct disorder. See reference: Early: Understanding psychiatric diagnosis: The DSM-IV.

159. (D) Assist clients in the selection of simple, short-term tasks. The skills required at the parallel level are the "ability to work and play in the presence of others comfortably and with an awareness of their presence" (p. 295). At this level, the COTA must be available to provide support, encouragement and assistance when indicated. Parallel group members (answer D) typically work together on individual tasks. Therefore, it would not be expected that the COTA encourage experimentation (answer A), because this level would require the client to be working at the project group level. This level focuses on the client working with another group member while encouraging trust. Answer C, the COTA participating as an active member, is also inappropriate. This level of assistance typically occurs during the mature group level, where individuals take on the roles necessary to achieve a balance between meeting the group task, and the emotional needs of the group. Answer B would also be an incorrect selection because the COTA must act as an authority figure in the parallel group in order to set limits, encourage interaction and assist the patient in feeling safe. See reference: Early: Group concepts and techniques.

160. (A) pull-to-sit, leaning back against a therapy ball. While all answers involve antigravity control, answer A addresses beginning control in neck and shoulders. Because control develops cephalocaudally, neck and shoulder control should be addressed first. By using an incline, the pull of gravity can be reduced, thus facilitating maximum control. See reference: Case-Smith (ed): Nichols, DS: The development of postural control.

161. (C) Report the incident to the client's physician. When an individual with depression and suicidal ideation gives away personal possessions, it may indicate she is considering suicide. The most important response is to notify the physician, although answers A, B, and D may all be appropriate. See reference: Early: Responding to symptoms and behaviors.

162. (D) Finishing a prefabricated wood birdhouse from a kit. A person experiencing a manic episode is likely to exhibit high energy levels, short attention span, poor frustration tolerance, difficulty delaying gratification and making decisions. Finishing a prefabricated wood birdhouse would be the most appropriate activity because it is a short-term, predictable activity with few steps. It also can be carried with the person if he or she needs to get up and move around during the activity. Answer A, a needle-point project, would require too high a degree of attention to detail for guaranteed success. Answer B, making a clay object, uses an unpredictable material and requires creative decisions, both of which are qualities that should be avoided. Answer C, watercolor painting, would not be a good choice because it is an unfocused activity involving artistic skill performance that could lead to frustration. See reference: Early: Responding to symptoms and behaviors.

163. (D) Discuss the observations with an OTR who is present. Although the COTA's own supervisor is absent, an OTR present would become the acting supervisor for the day. The COTA should always discuss concerns with the supervisor first. Going to the administrator (answer C) would not only disregard the chain of command, but could escalate a problem that should be handled internally. Training in ADLs is a skilled service beyond the scope of service of an aide. The COTA should not allow the aide to finish the treatment session (answer A). It may not be feasible for the COTA to complete the session (answer B), but it would also be inappropriate to terminate the aide when simple review of procedures and role delineations would be indicated in this case. See reference: Early: Supervision.

164. (D) During conversations with female group members, the client will make eye contact for 8 to 10 seconds, two times in each half-hour group. The short-term goal that describes appropriate verbal and nonverbal interactions with female peers (answer D) is the best answer. A goal set for 6 months (answer A) is a long-term goal. Awareness of thought processes (answer B) is more appropriate to a goal related to self-awareness. Attempting to develop skills with staff (answer C) can pose some confusing boundary and ethical questions in a long-term goal related to developing future personal relationships. See reference: Early: Understanding psychiatric diagnosis: The DSM-IV.

165. (A) Functional assessment of work-related skills, such as carrying and opening cartons and shelving items. Observation of the individual performing actual job responsibilities will provide more objective and measurable information about the individual's strengths and weaknesses in the area of job performance than a verbal interview (answer C) or task evaluation (answer D). Although a "dirty" medium may be contraindicated when initially working with an individual with OCD of the washing type, it would not be an issue for this individual because his OCD is of the checking type. There is nothing to indicate the individual has cognitive deficits, therefore a cognitive evaluation (answer B) would not be indicated. See reference: Early: Data collection and evaluation.

166. (B) The child demonstrated tongue thrust. "Tongue thrust" is an objective, well-defined term. The other answers are less objective. Answer A infers the child's emotional reaction. Answer C implies voluntary control and judges behavior. Answer D interprets data based on insufficient evidence. See reference: Early: Medical records and documentation.

167. (D) in private, explain the nature of the client-therapist relationship. It is inappropriate for the COTA to have more than a professional relationship with a client. Although self-disclosing some information to clients can be a therapeutic tool, there is some information that would be misinterpreted or inappropriate (e.g., giving out personal information [Answer A]). Ignoring the client's request (answer B) constitutes avoidance on the COTA's part and is unprofessional. Though a difficult situation, the COTA looses an opportunity to provide valuable feedback to her client. Whether the COTA has a boyfriend or not (answer C), she should not use this as an excuse for not giving out her number. It is be an easy way out, but unprofessional. See reference: Early: Therapeutic use of self.

168. (C) increase swimming time to 25 minutes or to tolerance. This individual's goal is to maximize strength and endurance. Although ALS is a progressive degenerative disease, improvements in strength and endurance are possible if the individual was not previously functioning at maximum capacity. This individual's performance indicates potential for further improvement. The program should therefore be upgraded, not downgraded (answer B). Methods for improving endurance include increasing the frequency, intensity, or duration of the activity. The correct answer (answer C) increases the duration of the activity while recognizing the importance of avoiding fatigue. Answer A continues the program at a maintenance level. Using adaptive equipment (answer D), such as a flotation belt, is an energy saving strategy that would be appropriate if the individual were experiencing fatigue during swimming. See reference: Dutton: Biomechanical postulates regarding intervention.

169. (D) Give the individual a rest break. Fatigue may cause additional structural damage in the acute stage of MS so should be avoided. Rest breaks need to be scheduled to avoid fatigue. Strengthening activities (answer C) do not need to be discontinued, but should be designed to benefit the patient without causing undue fatigue. See reference: Dutton: Biomechanical postulates regarding intervention.

170. (B) Improved verbal and nonverbal communication skills. Improved verbal and nonverbal communication skills would be the most relevant behavioral outcome indicating program effectiveness in the area of social skills development. Answers A, C, and D may all indirectly benefit as a result of improved social and communication skills, but these would not directly reflect positive outcomes for measuring effectiveness of social skill training programs. See reference: Cottrell (ed): Salo-Chydenius, S: Changing helplessness to coping: An exploratory study of social skills training with individuals with long-term mental illness.

171. (C) An electric toothbrush. According to Case-Smith, "for the child who independently brushes, an electric toothbrush enables more thorough cleaning. This is a good solution for children with limited dexterity, although for children with weakness, an electric toothbrush may be too heavy to manage" (p. 516). Answer A, using a soft bristle brush, would most likely assist a child with tongue thrust, while answer B, attaching a velcro strap to the toothbrush, would assist a child who has decreased grip strength in the hand. Answer D, encouraging the child to use a soft sponge-tipped toothette, is typically indicated in the child with oral hypersensitivity or defensiveness. See reference: Case-Smith (ed): Shepherd, J: Self-care and adaptations for independent living.

172. (D) Show a video about nutrition and keep a meal diary for a week. The psychoeducational model utilizes a teacher-student format as opposed to a learning by doing approach. It often includes a homework component. Answers A, B, and C can all be used to promote healthier eating, however, they all involve learning by doing. See reference: Cottrell (ed): Crist, PH: Community living skills: A psychoeducational community-based program.

173. (B) have the individual work at the keyboard for 30 minutes. Increasing the duration the individual is able to tolerate working on the computer is the most appropriate way to progress this individual. A heavier mouth stick (answer A) would make the task more difficult and yield no benefit. An individual with C4 quadriplegia would not have the potential to use a typing device that inserts into a wrist support (answer C). Teaching the individual how to correctly instruct a caregiver in use of the keyboard (answer D) would be downgrading the activity. See reference: Christiansen (ed): Garber, SL, Gregorio, TL Pumphrey, N, and Lathem, P: Self-care strategies for persons with spinal cord injuries.

174. (D) Conduct a group discussion about responsibilities people have when living in a group home. Discussion that heightens awareness in an attempt to modify behavior is one example of a cognitive intervention. Rewards and praise (answers A and B) are used when a behavioral approach is desired. Posting a schedule (answer C) is an example of an environmental adaptation that may facilitate compliance with chores, but does not represent a cognitive approach. See reference: Christiansen (ed): Self-care strategies in intervention for psychosocial conditions.

175. (A) Interview. Interviews provide "an opportunity for the parents to identify their values and priorities about the skills being evaluated by the therapist" (p. 207). Open-ended questions are best for eliciting information regarding the family's feelings about the intervention. Answers B, C, and D are structured observation methods, through which information on specific skills or functional levels is collected. See reference: Case-Smith (ed): Stewart, KB: Purposes, processes, and methods of evaluation.

176. (C) attainment of kindergarten readiness skills. The primary focus of intervention for a 5-year-old preschooler is to prepare the child for transition to kindergarten. The child's ability to perform the occupations related to that environment comprise readiness for kindergarten and include academic skills, as well as ADL (answers A and D) and social skills (answer B). A child who has achieved age-level skills in all these areas may benefit fully from the educational program and OT services can then be discontinued. See reference: Case-Smith (ed): Gartland, S and DuBoise, SA: Occupational therapy in preschool and childcare setting.

177. (A) Describe the treatment received. According to the 1991 *Role Delineations for OTRs and COTAs*, COTAs can record factual information at the time of discharge. Making referrals to outside agencies, comparing initial and final status, and independently making follow-up plans (answers B, C, and D) are not within the entry-level COTA's responsibilities. See reference: Early: Medical records and documentation.

178. (C) use headphones during work to reduce competing sensory input. Reducing competing sensory input is helpful in increasing visual attention. Increasing competing input (answers A and B), or reducing the amount of visual input (answer D), may reduce the ability to attend to visual stimuli. See reference: Case-Smith (ed): Schneck, CM: Visual perception.

179. (D) A scoop dish. A scoop dish is a plate with a high rim that provides a surface against which to push the food. The child would have less difficulty with controlling movement of food because the sides of the scoop dish would provide a shape that aids scooping of food onto the spoon. A swivel spoon (answer A) helps primarily when supination is limited. A nonslip mat (answer B) helps stabilize the plate itself, and a mobile arm support (answer C) positions the arm to help weak shoulder and elbow muscles to position the hand. See reference: Case-Smith (ed): Case-Smith, J and Humphrey, R: Feeding intervention.

180. (A) age appropriate. The child being observed is performing dressing activity which is age appropriate for a 5-year-old child. A typical child at this age can dress unsupervised and is able to tie and untie knots, but generally does not know how to tie a bow independently. See reference: Case-Smith (ed): Shepherd, J: Self-care and adaptations for independent living.

181. (C) encourage here-and-now explorations of member behaviors and issues, while promoting learning through doing. The purpose of task groups, as developed by Fidler, is to focus on the here-and-now; involve learning through doing, activity, and processing; and involve the development of daily living skills and work skills. Answer A describes an evaluative group, and answer B describes a topical discussion group, rather than a task group. Answer D describes the purpose of developmental group levels proposed by Mosey. See reference: Cole: A psychoanalytic approach.

182. (D) Hold him firmly when picking him up and dressing him. Holding the child firmly inhibits responses to light touch, which are usually uncomfortable for children with tactile defensiveness. Tickling (answer A), and light stroking (answer C), are also uncomfortable or intolerable for a child with tactile defensiveness. A strong stimulus such as loud music causes further discomfort during a time when the child is extremely vulnerable to the sensation of light touch (i.e., when clothing is being removed). See reference: Case-Smith (ed): Parham, LD and Mailloux, Z: Sensory integration.

183. (C) follow administration instructions and note changes in behavior. Although the tester may not deviate from the protocol, changes in behavior represent important test data and should be recorded. The responses described in answers A, B, and D may make the test results invalid by altering the sequence of test items, the grouping of items, or the actual test item itself. These may not be changed unless it is specified in the test manual. See reference: Case-Smith (ed): Richardson, PK: Use of standardized tests in pediatric practice.

184. (D) Recommend that the child wear an emergency alert system pendant around her neck. An emergency alert system would be the most likely solution for the COTA to recommend to the family. "Emergency alert systems, worn as pendants or stabilized on wheelchairs, are available for purchase with a service that places emergency calls when the system is activated" (p. 518). This intervention would be most effective because it can be placed on the client's body and does not require a great deal of dexterity to manipulate. This would also be especially appropriate if the teenager's parents were not home when the fire occurred. Answer A, positioning a wireless cell phone near the child, may be an effective solution, but would not be of much assistance if the child's dexterity is limited, in that she may not be able to push the buttons effectively. Answer B, establishing a quick exit routine in the event of a fire is something that the COTA and the client's

family should address, but in the event that no family members are home with the client when a fire occurs is potentially hazardous. Answer C, educating the client regarding fire prevention within the home, is something that should be reviewed by the COTA, but it does not address the immediate needs of responding to an actual fire via an emergency call system. See reference: Case-Smith (ed): Shepherd, J: Self-care and adaptations for independent living.

185. (B) Observe performance at the job site and make recommendations to increase productivity. One of the roles of the OT in transition services includes consulting with employers on adaptation to job activities to accommodate individuals with disabilities. The other members of the educational team can provide classroom-based instruction as in answers A, C, and D. See reference: Case-Smith (ed): Spencer, K: Transition services: From school to adult life.

186. (B) play and self-care activities. "When providing OT care for children with terminal illness, the underlying principle is to add quality to their remaining days. There are two performance areas that occupational therapists should address in children with terminal illness: (1) play activities; and (2) activities of daily living" (p. 838). Educational activities (answer A) would not address the emphasis of adding quality of life. Play activities help the child to focus interest and express feelings, and may incorporate socialization and motor activities (answers C and D), but neither of these types of activities alone would be the primary goal. Self-care activities allow the child to maintain independence and purposefulness. See reference: Case-Smith (ed): Barnstorff, MJ: The dying child.

187. (D) Provide a therapy ball to sit on while the child is playing a game of checkers. Answer D is the most appropriate recommendation because it contributes to the development of postural background movements. This is done by requiring the client to continually adjust to the subtle movements of a usable surface. Answers A, B, and C provide additional external support (i.e., they provide adaptations using a compensatory approach, rather than facilitating the development of new skills). See reference: Case-Smith (ed): Nichols, DS: The development of postural control.

188. (B) Dressing habits. Certain dressing habits may indicate tactile defensiveness, e.g., the child may show poor tolerance of certain textures or avoid wearing turtlenecks, socks, or shoes. Conversely, some children may never take off their shoes in order to avoid tactile overstimulation. Reading skills (answer A), friendships (answer C), and the choice of hobbies (answer D) could be affected secondarily, as a result of intolerance of certain textures or human touch or the inability to concentrate. However, because of the close connection between dressing and tactile tolerance, knowledge of the child's dressing habits (answer B) will give the OT practitioner the most reliable information. See reference: Case-Smith (ed): Parham, LD and Mailloux, Z: Sensory integration.

189. (A) begin with activities that have obvious solutions and high probabilities of success, and then gradually increase the complexity. This strategy is effective in developing problem solving skills. Gross and fine motor activities (answer B) can heighten awareness of self and develop coordination. Increasing the time spent on the activity (answer D) helps development of attention span. Structuring the number and kinds of choices (answer C) is a method for developing decision making skills. See reference: Early: Analyzing, adapting, and grading activities.

190. (C) cruising. The described pattern is cruising. Cruising occurs at approximately 12 months of age and directly precedes walking. Creeping (answer A) refers to four-point mobility in a prone position with only hands and knees on the floor, a pattern that occurs between the ages of 7 and 12 months. Crawling (answer B) is the term for the ability to move forward while in a prone position; this pattern occurs at about 7 months of age. Clawing (answer D), also called "fanning," is the ability to spread the toes to maintain balance in standing. See reference: Case-Smith (ed): Wright-Ott, C and Egilson, S: Mobility.

191. (B) Let the child sit at the front of the bus and use a tape player with earphones. A child who is seated in the front of the bus will experience less jostling by peers, resulting in less tactile and visual stimulation. Also, the earphones will reduce auditory overload. The method described in answer B addresses the underlying problem of the child's low tolerance for sensory stimulation. Answers A, C, and D are behavioral management techniques that do not take the child's hypersensitivity into account. See reference: Case-Smith (ed): Cronin, AF: Psychosocial and emotional domains.

192. (D) The effect of personal traits and the environment on role performance. Evaluation according to the Model of Human Occupation would focus on the effect of personal traits and the environment on role performance. Evaluation according to the Behavioral frame of reference identifies problem behaviors that need to be extinguished (answer A). The Object Relations frame of reference attempts to clarify thoughts, feelings, and experiences that influence behavior (answer B). An OT using the Cognitive Disability frame of reference should evaluate cognitive function, including assets and limitations (answer C). See reference: Bruce and Borg: Model of human occupation.

193. (A) Holding the hammer. Holding the hammer (answer A) is the only activity listed that requires gripping with the entire hand. Holding the stamping tools and needle (answers B and D) requires pinch patterns. Squeezing the sponge (answer C) offers less resistance than holding the hammer, and would, therefore, be less effective for strengthening. See reference: Breines: Folkcraft.

194. (B) The patients' written consents to take the photographs and use them for publicity. A photograph of a person who is being treated at a health care facility would release privileged information and would violate confidentiality just as much as releasing the individual's name or diagnosis (answers A and D). No information about a person may be released without a written consent. It is not necessary to obtain permission of the department head to use a photograph to promote a positive image for the facility (answer C). See reference: Bailey: Final preparation before implementing the research plan.

195. (A) Punctuality, accepting directions from a supervisor, and interacting with coworkers. Psychosocial components include time management, social conduct, interpersonal skills, and self-control. Punctuality and accepting feedback are examples of important prevocational skills within these psychosocial performance components. Memory, decision making, attention to tasks, and sequencing (answer B) are considered to be cognitive components. Standing tolerance, endurance, and eye–hand coordination (answer C) are categorized as sensorimotor components. Grooming and adhering to safety precautions (answer D) are work performance areas, not psychosocial performance components. See reference: AOTA: Uniform Terminology for Occupational Therapy, ed 3.

196. (C) recommend activities to develop fine coordination that teachers can incorporate into classroom programming. Recommending classroom activities that will develop the performance component of fine motor coordination would be the best population based intervention since it involves addressing the occupational performance needs of many students. Answers A, B, and D focus OT efforts on individual intervention approaches. See reference: AOTA: Guide To Occupational Therapy Practice:

197. (D) Family will demonstrate independence in current positioning and feeding techniques. Goals should be functional, measurable, and objective. In addition, short-term goals must relate to the long-term goal being addressed. Answer D meets those criteria. Answer A does not provide measurable criteria, nor does it directly relate to the long-term goal of family training. Answer B, while measurable, does not relate to the long-term goal. Answer C describes the long-term goal of family independence in the feeding program. See reference:

AOTA: Effective documentation for occupational therapy: Moorhead, P and Kannenberg, K: Writing functional goals.

198. (D) Electronic augmentative communication device. An augmentative communication keyboard is a high technology aid that can compensate for expressive deficits and assist a student with communication. Answer A is incorrect because an environmental control unit is a device that allows a person with severe disabilities to operate appliances or devices. It may be used to turn on a tape recorder for note taking, but it would not be used as the primary method for conversation and graphics in the classroom. Answers B and C are incorrect because both the Wanchik's writer and a head pointer are low technology aids for communication, rather than high-technology devices. See reference: Angelo and Lane (eds): Angelo, J: Written and spoken augmentative communication.

199. (A) make recommendations for ways of operating the technology. The OT practitioner on the assistive technology team usually determines which part of the body has sufficient motor control for operating the technology and then recommends the type of input access device (switch, keyword, software, etc.) that will best meet the client's needs. Answer B, recommending communication strategies, is most often the job of the speech and language pathologist. A social worker or other specialist in funding is usually responsible for seeking funding sources (answer C). Answer D, solving mechanical and software problems, is usually the role of the rehabilitation engineer. See reference: Angelo and Lane (eds): Angelo, J: A guide for assistive technology therapists.

200. (B) Performing a clerical task such as sorting papers. The most appropriate type of activities to begin treatment for a person with severe depression are repetitive, structured and simple enough to ensure success, such as "...housework, folding laundry, simple cooking, sanding, clerical tasks, and sewing." (p. 246). Engagement in leisure exploration (answer A), meditation (answer C), and stress management activities (answer D) would eventually be relevant intervention activities for a person with depression. However, in the early stages of depression, attention span, concentration and energy level may to be too impaired to benefit from these types of activities. See reference: Early: Responding to symptoms and behaviors.

BIBLIOGRAPHY

Allen, CK, Earhardt, CA, and Blue, T: Occupational Therapy Treatment Goals for the Physically and Cognitively Disabled. The American Occupational Therapy Association, Rockville, MD, 1992.

American Occupational Therapy Association, Inc.: Commission on Practice: Guide for supervision of occupational therapy personnel in the delivery of occupational therapy services. Am J Occup Ther 53:592-594, 1999.

American Occupational Therapy Association, Inc.: Effective Documentation for Occupational Therapy. American Occupational Therapy Association, Rockville, MD, 1991.

American Occupational Therapy Association, Inc.: Guidelines for the use of aides in occupational therapy practice. Am J Occup Ther 53:595-597, 1999.

American Occupational Therapy Association, Inc.: Intercommission Council: Occupational Therapy Roles. Am J Occup Ther 47:1087-1099, 1993.

American Occupational Therapy Association, Inc.: Occupational Therapy Code of Ethics. Am J Occup Ther 54:614-616, 2000.

American Occupational Therapy Association, Inc.: Policy: Registered Occupational therapists and certified occupational therapy assistants and modalities. Am J Occup Ther 45:1112-1113, 1991.

American Occupational Therapy Association, Inc.: Standards of practice for occupational therapy. Am J Occup Ther 52:866-869, 1998.

American Occupational Therapy Association, Inc.: Statement of occupational therapy referral. Am J Occup Ther 48:1034-1035, 1994.

American Occupational Therapy Association, Inc.: Statement: Purpose and value of occupational therapy fieldwork education. Am J Occup Ther 50:845, 1996.

American Occupational Therapy Association, Inc.: Statement: The role of occupational therapy in the independent living movement. Am J Occup Ther 47:1079-1080, 1993.

American Occupational Therapy Association, Inc.: Terminology task force: Uniform terminology for occupational therapy - third edition. Am J Occup Ther 48: 1047-1054, 1994.

American Occupational Therapy Association, Inc.: The Guide to Occupational Therapy Practice. Am J Occup Ther 53:247-322, 1999.

American Occupational Therapy Association, Inc.: The Occupational Therapy Manager, revised edition. American Occupational Therapy Association, Rockville, MD, 1996.

American Occupational Therapy Association Practice Department. (1999 revised). Guide to Role Performance: OT, OTA, Aide. Retrieved October 15, 2001 from the American Occupational Therapy Association website: http://www.aota.org/members/area2/links/link13.asp?PLACE.

Americans with Disabilities Act. Appendix to Part 1191 ADA - Accessibility Guidelines for Buildings and Facilities. Federal Register, Vol 56. No 134, 1991. US Architectural & Transportation Barriers Compliance Board.

Angelo, J and Lane, S (eds): Assistive Technology for Rehabilitation Therapists. FA Davis, Philadelphia, 1997.

Bailey, DM: Research and the Health Professional: A Practical Guide, ed 2. FA Davis, Philadelphia, 1997.

Bernstein, LC (ed): Aging: The Health Care Challenge, ed 2. FA Davis, Philadelphia, 1990.

Bonder, BR: Psychopathology and Function, ed 2. Slack, Thorofare, NJ, 1995.

Bonder, BR and Wagner, MB (eds): Functional Performance in Older Adults, ed 2. FA Davis, Philadelphia, 2001.

Borcherding, S: Documentation Manual for Writing SOAP Notes in Occupational Therapy. Slack, Thorofare, NJ, 2000.

Breines, EB: Occupational Therapy Activities from Clay to Computers: Theory and Practice. FA Davis, Philadelphia, 1995.

Bruce, MA and Borg, B: Psychosocial Occupational Therapy: Frames of Reference for Intervention, ed 2. Slack, Thorofare, NJ, 1993.

Cailliet, R: Soft Tissue Pain and Disability, ed 3. FA Davis, Philadelphia, 1996.

Case-Smith, J (ed): Occupational Therapy for Children, ed 4. CV Mosby, St. Louis, 2001.

Christiansen, C (ed): Ways of Living: Self-Care Strategies for Special Needs. American Occupational Therapy Association, Bethesda, MD, 1994.

Christiansen, C and Baum, C (eds): Occupational Therapy: Enabling Function and Well-Being, ed 2. Slack, Thorofare, NJ, 1997.

Cole, MB: Group Dynamics in Occupational Therapy, ed. 2. Slack, Thorofare, NJ, 1998.

Cottrell, RP (ed): Proactive Approaches in Psychosocial Occupational Therapy. Slack, Thorofare, NJ, 2000.

Denton, PL: Psychiatric Occupational Therapy: A Workbook of Practical Skills. Little Brown, Boston, 1987.

Dutton, R: Clinical Reasoning in Physical Disabilities. Williams & Wilkins, Baltimore, 1995.

Early, MB: Mental Health Concepts and Techniques for the Occupational Therapy Assistant. Lippincott Williams & Wilkins, Philadelphia, 2000.

Fazio, L: Developing Occupation-Centered Programs for the Community: A Workbook for Students and Professionals. Prentice Hall, Upper Saddle River, NJ, 2001.

Fisher, AG, Murray, EA, and Bundy, AC (eds): Sensory Integration: Theory and Practice. FA Davis, Philadelphia, 1991.

Gillen, G and Burkardt, A (eds): Stroke Rehabilitation: A Function-Based Approach. Mosby, St. Louis, 1998.

Glantz, C and Richman, N: OTR-COTA Collaboration in Home Health: Roles and Supervisory Issues. Am J Occup Ther 51:446-452, 1997.

Griffin, ER and Lember, S: Sexuality and the Person with Traumatic Brain Injury: A Guide for Families. FA Davis, Philadelphia, 1993.

Hellen, CR: Alzheimer's Disease: Activity-Focused Care, ed 2. Butterworth-Heinemann, Boston, 1998.

Hemphill, BJ (ed): Mental Health Assessment in Occupational Therapy. Slack, Thorofare, NJ, 1988.

Hunter, J, Schneider, M, Mackin, E, and Bell, J (eds): Rehabilitation of the Hand: Surgery and Treatment, ed 3. CV Mosby, Philadelphia, 1990.

Kettenbach, G: Writing SOAP Notes, ed 2. FA Davis, Philadelphia, 1995.

Kornblau, BL and Starling, SP: Ethics in Rehabilitation: A Clinical Perspective. Slack, Thorofare, NJ, 2000.

Kramer, P and Hinojosa, J (eds): Frames of Reference for Pediatric Occupational Therapy, ed 2. Lippincott Williams & Wilkins, Philadelphia, 1999.

Larson, O, Stevens-Ratchford, RG, Pedretti, LW, and Crabtree, J (eds): ROTE: The Role of Occupational Therapy with the Elderly. American Occupational Therapy Association Inc., Bethesda, MD, 1996.

Logigian, MK and Ward, JD, (eds): A Team Approach for Therapists: Pediatric Rehabilitation. Little Brown, Boston, 1989.

Mattingly, C and Fleming, MH: Clinical Reasoning: Forms of Inquiry in a Therapeutic Practice. FA Davis, Philadelphia, 1994.

Mosey, AC: Activities Therapy. Raven Press, NY, 1973.

Neistadt, ME and Crepeau, EB (eds): Williard & Spackman's Occupational Therapy, ed 9. Lippincott Williams & Wilkins, Philadelphia, 1998.

Occupational Safety and Health Administration: Standard #1910.1030,1 FR 5507, February, 1996.

Palmer, ML and Toms, JE: Manual for Functional Training, ed 3. FA Davis, Philadelphia, 1992.

Pedretti, LW and Early, ME (eds): Occupational Therapy: Practice Skills for Physical Dysfunction, ed 5. Mosby, St. Louis, 2001.

Piersol, CV and Ehrlich, PL (eds): Home Health Practice: A Guide for the Occupational Therapist. Imaginart, Bisbee, AZ, 2000.

Posthuma, BW: Small Groups in Counseling and Therapy: Process and Leadership, ed 3. Allyn & Bacon, Boston, 1999.

Reed, KL and Sanderson, SN (eds): Concepts of Occupational Therapy, ed 3. Williams and Wilkins, Baltimore, 1992.

Richard, RL and Staley, MJ (eds): Burn Care and Rehabilitation: Principles and Practice. FA Davis, Philadelphia, 1994.

Ross, M and Bachner, S (eds): Adults with Developmental Disabilities: Current Approaches in Occupational Therapy. American Occupational Therapy Association, Bethesda, MD, 1998.

Rothstein, JM, Roy, SH, and Wolf, SL: The Rehabilitation Specialist's Handbook. FA Davis, Philadelphia, 1991.

Sabonis-Chafee, B and Hussey, SM: Introduction to Occupational Therapy, ed 2. Mosby, St. Louis, 1998.

Scaffa, ME (ed): Occupational Therapy in Community-Based Practice Settings. FA Davis, Philadelphia, 2001.

Sladyk, K (ed): OT Student Primer: A Guide to College Success. Slack, 1997.

Sladyk, K and Ryan, SE (eds): Ryan's Occupational Therapy Assistant: Principles, Practice Issues and Techniques, ed 3. Slack, Thorofare, NJ, 2001.

Smith, LK, Weiss, EL, and Lehmkuhl, LD: Brunnstrom's Clinical Kinesiology, ed 5. FA Davis, Philadelphia, 1996.

Solomon, JW (ed): Pediatric Skills for Occupational Therapy Assistants. Mosby, St. Louis, 2000.

Stein, F and Cutler, SK: Psychosocial Occupational Therapy - A Holistic Approach, ed 2. Singular Publishing Group, Inc., Delmar, NY, 2001.

Trombly, CA (ed): Occupational Therapy for Physical Dysfunction, ed 4. Williams & Wilkins, Baltimore, 1995.

Unsworth, C (ed): Cognitive and Perceptual Dysfunction: A Clinical Reasoning Approach to Evaluation and Intervention. FA Davis, Philadelphia, 1999.

Zoltan, B: Vision, Perception and Cognition: A Manual for the Evaluation and Treatment of the Neurologically Impaired Adult, ed 3. Slack, Thorofare, NJ, 1996.